Stroke in Blacks

A Guide to Management and Prevention

Editors

R.F. Gillum, Hyattsville, Md.
P.B. Gorelick, Chicago, Ill.
E.S. Cooper, Philadelphia, Pa.

18 figures and 31 tables, 1999

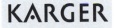

Basel · Freiburg · Paris · London · New York ·
New Delhi · Bangkok · Singapore · Tokyo · Sydney

••••••••••••••••••••••

Richard F. Gillum, MD, FACC

Centers for Disease Control and Prevention,
Hyattsville, Md., USA

Philip B. Gorelick, MD, MPH, FACP

Department of Neurological Sciences,
Rush Medical College and Program Director,
African-American Antiplatelet Stroke Prevention Study,
Chicago, Ill., USA

Edward S. Cooper, MD, MACP

University of Pennsylvania School of Medicine,
Philadelphia, Pa., USA

Library of Congress Cataloging-in-Publication Data
Stroke in blacks: a guide to management and prevention / editors, R.F. Gillum, P.B. Gorelick, E.S. Cooper.
Includes bibliographical references and indexes.
1.Cerebrovascular disease.   2. Blacks – Diseases.   3. Afro-Americans – Diseases.
I. Gillum, R.F. (Richard F.), 1944–   .   II. Gorelick, Philip B.   III. Cooper, Edward S.
[DNLM: 1. Cerebrovascular Disorders – ethnology.   2. Cerebrovascular Disorders – therapy.
3. Cerebrovascular Disorders – prevention & control.   4. Blacks.]
RC685.C6S773   1999   616.8′1–dc21
ISBN 3–8055–6713–8 (hardcover: alk. paper)

Drug Dosage. The authors and the publisher have exerted every effort to ensure that drug selection and dosage set forth in this text are in accord with current recommendations and practice at the time of publication. However, in view of ongoing research, changes in government regulations, and the constant flow of information relating to drug therapy and drug reactions, the reader is urged to check the package insert for each drug for any change in indications and dosage and for added warnings and precautions. This is particularly important when the recommended agent is a new and/or infrequently employed drug.

© Copyright 1999 by S. Karger AG, P.O. Box, CH–4009 Basel (Switzerland)
Printed in Switzerland on acid-free paper by Reinhardt Druck, Basel
ISBN 3–8055–6713–8

To Brenda S. Gillum, Faith M. Gillum, and to the memory of Roy E. Gillum and Margaret J. Gillum. *Richard F. Gillum*

To Leonidas Berry, MD, Richard Palmore and Edward Billingsley, African-Americans who made life's journey and inspired us, and all the patients of the African-American Antiplatelet Stroke Prevention Study and Studies of Dementia in the Black Aged Program, who have unselfishly participated to improve health care for all African-Americans. *Philip B. Gorelick*

To the memory of E. Sawyer Cooper, Jr. Proceeds from this book will be donated to the E. Sawyer Cooper, Jr. Scholarship Fund at the University of Pennsylvania for needy medical students from underserved populations. *Edward S. Cooper*

Contents

Contents

Foreword

'This time, like all times, is a very good one, if we but know what to do with it.'

Emerson

Stroke in Blacks is not only a guide to the management and prevention of strokes in the African-American population, but is an extraordinary compilation of recent research information and current management practices for patients who have suffered a stroke. Its encyclopedic approach provides under one cover some of the most useful information necessary for setting management guidelines and research agendas for the next millennium. Epidemiologic data has been drawn from population-based studies located, for example, in northern Manhattan, New York, Cincinnati, Ohio, and the Philadelphia, Pennsylvania areas, as well as larger multicentered studies such as ARIC and CHS. National data has been drawn from Medicare files and national databases such as the CDC, as well as from cluster states in the Stroke Belt. While focused upon the Black population within the United States, the presentation of comparative data from other countries with large Black populations enhances our understanding.

The mortality rate from cerebrovascular disease has decreased across the United States in all populations for the last four decades. Nevertheless, African-Americans of both genders have continuously had a higher death rate due to stroke compared to White Americans. In the last few years even the less impressive rate of decline in mortality appears to be leveling out and there is evidence that it may be on the increase. This alarming finding will require considerable effort to try to specifically identify the cause-and-effect relationships in what is obviously a continuously moving target as the American population continues to mix and move about the country on a regular basis. Information derived from as little as a decade ago is of interesting historic value and provides a basis for trend analysis, but in all probability such analysis will need to be repeated in the light of today's rapidly changing management of health care, increasingly complex risk factors associated with stroke, and the availability of new, safe and effective treatments. The aging population of African-Americans presents a particular challenge, and the continued need for current information and future projections is apparent.

This volume points out the subtle and not so subtle pathophysiologic and anatomic variations that lead to intracerebral hemorrhage, subarachnoid hemorrhage, lacunar strokes, cerebral embolism and infarct, and their impact in the Black population. While current diagnostic techniques, when available, can help differentiate the etiology of symptoms, the management of the underlying causal pathophysiology is clearly much less well understood in the Black population. There are numerous physical, psychological and cultural barriers that must be overcome, and only longitudinal data collected from a population likely to be more mobile and diverse will enable us to assess progress.

The variety of *risk factors* that have been identified and their greater or lesser incidence in the African-American population have been carefully reviewed. While some of the more traditional risk factors such as heart disease, prior stroke, diabetes and hypertension are more precisely evaluated, additional risk factors such as physical activity, lifestyle, socioeconomic status, obesity and urbanization are being identified and quantitated. From the field of molecular biology, for example, platelet glycoproteins IIb/IIIa, a specific membrane receptor, has been shown to be associated with hypertension in the Black population. However, the association of the glycoprotein IIIa polymorphism PIa2, a risk factor for stroke in young women in general, was not found to be associated with a higher incidence of stroke in Black women. How to interpret these findings and then apply them to improve health is not clear. Over the course of the next decade, some of the genetic as well as immunologic associations with stroke may help us more clearly define those at risk and focus our attention on those at higher risk.

There are few effective treatments either for the prevention or the acute management of stroke and this is as true for the Black American population as it is for all other ethnic groups. This volume outlines the importance of preventing stroke related to atrial fibrillation, the use of anticoagulation and antiplatelet agents, acute thrombolytic therapy and the value of carotid endarterectomy for the Black population. While most studies are designed to evaluate treatment in all Americans, particular attention has been paid to pharmacological differences in the ongoing African-American Antiplatelet Stroke Prevention Study (AAASPS), designed specifically to determine the efficacy of ticlopidine in this *at-risk* population. Both the value and difficulty of mounting such a study is instructive, and can serve as a model for future trials. Hypertension has long been identified as a risk factor for stroke; it is seen more frequently and with greater severity in the Black population than the White population. Valuable insights into the extraordinary importance of the identification, management and continuous maintenance of even mild hypertension control is reinforced in several chapters. There is no more critical message nor manageable risk factor than that associated with the management of blood pressure before, during and after a stroke. This is clearly something we can do right now, but it is relatively poorly managed by patients and physicians alike. Useful guidelines are clearly enunciated in this illuminating volume.

Much of *Stroke in Blacks* is devoted to providing specific epidemiologic and research data. One of its most valuable chapters relates to the practical guidelines for the diagnosis and management of stroke in Blacks today. However, as we look forward to new and better treatments for the management of stroke in the African-American patient, it is inevitable that we will see increased vascular dementia in an aging Black population. In addition, the hospitalization and management of acute stroke in a number of areas such as the Stroke Belt is suboptimal, while the rehabilitation after stroke, a cost-effective procedure, is under-utilized for a variety of sociologic factors.

While the search goes on for more effective treatment and management, we can certainly optimize the care of the Black stroke patient, and be sure that ethnic differences in such diverse areas as communication, physiology, pharmacology and expectations are taken into account. Furthermore, for the benefit of all Americans, particularly our minority populations, we must continue to engage in a strong and progressive research agenda so as to reduce the ravages of the third leading cause of death and the prime cause of disability in this country.

Michael D. Walker, MD
Director, Division of Stroke
Trauma and Neurodegenerative Disorders
National Institute of Neurological Disorders and Stroke
National Institutes of Health
Bethesda, Md.

Audrey S. Penn, MD
Deputy Director, National Institute of
Neurological Disorders and Stroke
National Institutes of Health
Bethesda, Md.

Preface

Since the early part of this century, data on mortality in the United States have shown a dramatic excess of stroke in Blacks. This devastating problem has been the subject of numerous articles in the *Journal of the National Medical Association* since its inception in 1902 but was generally ignored in other scientific writings over the first 70–80 years of this century. Only in the past two decades have we witnessed regular reports on stroke in Blacks in the medical literature. The epidemic risk of stroke and risk of dying from stroke that afflict African-Americans raise many important questions relating to why Blacks may be more prone to stroke. Is it an excess of cardiovascular disease risk factors? Is it severity of the risk factors or a greater susceptibility to them? Is it lack of access to medical care including medications or some other barrier? Is it stress? Is it racism, or gene-environmental interaction(s)? Presently, these and many other questions that relate to stroke in Blacks are the focus of scientific inquiry. Answers to these important questions promise to lead to improvements in prevention and treatment of stroke in Blacks and other minorities.

As researchers in the field, we have accepted the challenge of presenting in a single text, reviews of key topics on stroke in Blacks in an up-to-date, easy-to-access format. We have brought together experts in the areas of epidemiology, public health, clinical investigation, and clinical practice to provide in one volume state-of-the-art information on prevention, diagnosis, and treatment in persons of Black-African ancestry. Much of the information in this text emanates from studies of African-Americans as there has been recent and substantial interest in stroke in this high-risk group. One will also find information on native Africans and those of the African diaspora.

We emphasize the special features of the epidemiology, clinical presentation, prognosis, response to treatment, and access to health care that may be unique in Blacks. It is hoped that this book will aid practitioners in caring for patients with stroke and in preventing stroke in high-risk individuals. This book is also intended for public health workers, health planners and medical researchers as we provide information of interest that is not currently available in any other single text source.

The challenge to reduce the burden of stroke in Blacks is substantial. We hope that this text will not only provide important insights about prevention, diagnosis and treatment of stroke in Blacks, but will also provoke thought about reasons for excess stroke in Blacks and other high-risk groups. We hope this book will stimulate you to join us in meeting the challenge to better understand, prevent, diagnose, and treat stroke in Blacks.

Richard F. Gillum
Philip B. Gorelick
Edward S. Cooper

Gillum RF, Gorelick PB, Cooper ES (eds): Stroke in Blacks. Basel, Karger, 1999, pp 1–6

....

Introduction and Overview Commentary

Observations, Implications and Recommendations

Lewis H. Kuller

Department of Epidemiology, University of Pittsburgh, Graduate School of Public Health, Pittsburgh, Pa., USA

The decline in stroke mortality rates for both Blacks and Whites in the United States has been one of the most successful public health advances since the development of the polio vaccine [1]. Reduction in stroke mortality is a model of a successful basic and applied research program.

The stroke death rates were declining long before the introduction of effective antihypertensive therapy [2, 3]. The decline in stroke mortality appeared to be real and not an artifact of certification practices of the causes of death [2]. We reported in 1968 that the stroke death rates in Baltimore had declined 58% for Black men and 53% for Black women aged 45–54 between 1930 and 1961. This tremendous decline in stroke rates was also noted in Memphis, Tennessee, 1930–1961 [2]. It cannot be explained by drug treatment of hypertension. It must have been related to change in lifestyles.

Stroke mortality rates are only a crude reflection of the incidence of stroke, primarily reflecting the acute case-fatality and not long-term mortality after stroke. Most individuals who survive the initial acute event are more likely to die from cardiovascular disease.

After the widespread use of antihypertensive drug therapy, the slope of the decline in stroke mortality was accelerated. This experience is similar to trends for tuberculosis mortality; much of the decline in mortality began prior to the introduction of specific therapies, and was likely due to changes in environment and nutrition.

The initial phases of stroke research began with the observations in both experimental animals and human studies that elevated blood pressure was the most important determinant of the risk of stroke, both hemorrhagic and nonhemorrhagic. Epidemiological studies determined that there was a very great variation in stroke mortality among countries and within the United States. The stroke death rates in the United States were much higher in Blacks than Whites at least from the year 1915 and in the southeastern United States [2, 4]. The stroke belt in the southeastern United States was identified as early as the 1950s and persisted through the present time [5]. Studies in Baltimore in the 1960s and other communities showed that there was an important inverse association between socioeconomic status and stroke mortality [6]. This has been consistent across populations in most countries and has persisted to the present time. For example, recent follow-up from the Multiple Risk Factor Intervention Trial (MRFIT) showed that for Black men, aged 35–57, the all-cause, age-adjusted, death rates varied from 137/10,000 person-years in communities with average income < USD7,500 to 57.2/10,000 person-years for the living-in communities with incomes > USD27,500 (relative risk 2.5) (1.45–3.00) [5]. For stroke, it was estimated that the death rate increased 40% for each USD10,000 difference in family income in census tract.

The Nine-Area Stroke Study begun in the 1960s and early 1970s evaluated the geographic variations in stroke mortality in the United States [7–9]. The study verified that stroke death rates were much higher in the southeastern United States, especially in the eastern parts of Georgia, South Carolina, and North Carolina. In 1969–71 the death rate due to stroke for White men aged 45–54 was 21/100,000 in Colorado as compared to 379/100,000 for Black men in Savannah, Georgia, a remarkable 15-fold difference. The subsequent morbidity study verified that the stroke incidence rates [9], especially for men, were higher in the southeastern United States.

The Three-Area Risk Factor Study [10] demonstrated that blood pressure levels were much higher for Blacks than Whites, that obesity was strongly related to blood pressure levels, especially for Black women, that Black women in a high stroke rate area had much higher prevalence of obesity than White women in Savannah, and there was a higher prevalence of obesity in Black women in Savannah, Georgia, than Black women in Pueblo, Colorado, a low stroke rate area. The prevalence of obesity, however, was not different for Black and White men [11]. Blacks had a higher prevalence of diabetes that was related to their greater obesity and lower socioeconomic status [11].

The amount of sodium excreted in an overnight urine sample was much greater for Blacks than Whites, while potassium excretion was lower for Blacks, especially in Savannah [12]. The high sodium and low potassium urinary excretion in Blacks as compared to Whites was similar to previous studies by Dr. Herb Langford and others in Jackson, Mississippi [13, 14]. It was not possible, however, to determine an association of either sodium or potassium in overnight urine samples and blood pressure levels. The INTERSALT Study, with a larger sample size, and better collection of 24-hour urines, documented the association of salt intake and blood pressure levels [15]. Tobian [16] showed that increased potassium intake in rat models was associated with a decrease in the risk of cerebral vascular lesions, even independent of blood pressure changes. The Evans County Georgia studies [17, 18] were the model of efforts to understand the relationship between lifestyle, risk factors and stroke, and clearly documented the higher levels of blood pressure among Blacks, associated with socioeconomic factors and increased incidence of stroke among Blacks as compared to Whites. More recent studies have further documented the higher incidence of stroke among Blacks [19].

The high stroke rates in the southeast, and low socioeconomic status were all consistent with a dietary hypothesis. These observations suggest that either excess nutrients, such as salt or a deficiency of a nutrient such as potassium or specific amino acid or protein, or possibly an infectious etiology especially related to renal disease, might be the cause of the higher stroke rates in both the south and among Blacks and lower socioeconomic status groups.

Baker and Resch at the University of Minnesota developed unique pathology studies to evaluate the geographic epidemiology and pathology of cerebral vascular disease [20]. They determined that estimation of the premorbid blood pressure levels was strongly related to the extent of atherosclerosis in the circle of Willis at postmortem examination. They also determined that there were populations such as in Japan with a high prevalence of atherosclerosis in the circle of Willis, and yet relatively little atherosclerosis in the coronary arteries. The atherosclerosis in the coronary arteries was more closely related to higher blood cholesterol and high saturated fat and cholesterol in the diet, while the atherosclerosis in the circle appear to be more closely linked to elevated blood pressure. This led to the hypothesis that variations in blood cholesterol level, cigarette smoking, diabetes, and hypertension played a major role, not only in the extent, but also in the distribution of atherosclerotic disease, especially as related to cerebral vascular disease [21]. Baker and Resch initially found very little atherosclerosis in the circle of Willis in Black populations outside the United States, such as West Africa, i.e., Nigeria. The African population had a low prevalence of hypertension. However, subsequent studies in more urban Nigerian populations showed an increasing prevalence of disease in the circle of Willis associated with probable high blood pressure levels.

The MRFIT screenees provided the largest longitudinal study of risk of stroke mortality among Blacks and Whites [22]. The distribution of blood pressure in this study, and as well as in other studies, tended to be unimodel, Blacks having higher blood pressures than Whites, and perhaps a higher number of Blacks with very high blood pressure, i.e., at the tails of the higher levels of distribution. The risk of stroke death was 1.8 times higher for Black men aged 35–57 at entry than for White men, including 2.5 times as high for intracerebral hemorrhage (1.6 times for nonhemorrhagic stroke). The study clearly documented that the risk of stroke death, both hemorrhagic and non-hemorrhagic, was higher in Blacks than Whites, and was directly related to blood pressure levels especially the systolic blood pressure [22]. The lower the blood pressure, the lower the risk of stroke. The study also documented the positive association of smoking, cholesterol and diabetes, with risk of stroke.

Major clinical trials in the 1960s that have included both Blacks and Whites have shown unequivocally that reduction of blood pressure was associated with a substantial decrease in the risk of stroke, both hemorrhagic and nonhemorrhagic stroke [23, 24]. The reduction in risk occurs within a relatively short time after randomization into these trials.

A major result of these trials was that high blood pressure could be safely treated, that excellent control of blood pressure reduced risk of stroke and that nurses and other health professionals could play a primary role in hypertension treatment programs.

The results of the clinical trials led to the National High Blood Pressure Education Program and major efforts for identification, treatment, and control of hypertension among all age, race, and sex groups in the United States [25].

The majority of strokes occur among older individuals, 65+. Until the 1980s, there had been little interest among physicians that elevated systolic blood pressure, especially among older individuals, was an important risk factor, a normal component of aging. The pilot and subsequent full-scale trials of the Systolic Hypertension in the Elderly Program (SHEP) documented the benefits of treating systolic hypertension in the elderly [26].

One of the major outcomes of stroke is the development of dementia or decreased cognitive function. It has been estimated that 20% of stroke patients develop poststroke dementia [27, 28]. The risk of poststroke dementia may be related to prevalence of ApoE genotype, and to prior levels of cognitive function, before stroke. Blacks may be particularly vulnerable to poststroke dementia or cognitive decline, which may be associated with substantial morbidity and disability, especially in the older age group. A major effort therefore to prevent stroke disability, especially poststroke dementia, must be a high priority.

Conclusions

We have been extremely successful in reducing the incidence, mortality and disability associated with stroke among both Blacks and Whites. The incidence [29] and stroke death rates [30] are still too high among Blacks given our ability to identify the major determinants of stroke and the availability of very effective therapy. The high prevalence of hypertension among Blacks remains a major problem. The recent slowing of the decline in stroke mortality is of great concern. The slowing of the decline in stroke mortality is probably greater in Blacks than Whites. It may reflect a reduction in quality and quantity of antihypertensive programs as well as other possible factors. Traditional clinical approaches for the delivery of antihypertensive therapy have failed to reach the majority of Blacks in terms of controlling blood pressure levels. This is especially true in poorer and less educated populations in the community.

The goal of the next 10 years must be to reduce stroke incidence and mortality by at least 50%, especially for individuals < 75 or 80 years of age, and reduce the morbidity associated with stroke, especially dementia and major disability [31]. The difference in stroke morbidity and mortality between Blacks and Whites should be reduced or eliminated by successful primary and secondary prevention. There is absolutely no reason why we cannot reduce morbidity and mortality from stroke by at least 50% in the Black population at the present time. A decrease of about 5%/year is feasible and should be the minimum goal of our current public health and medical efforts.

References

1   Gillum RF, Sempos CT: The end of the long-term decline in stroke mortality in the United States? Stroke 1997;28:1527–1529.
2   Kuller L, Seltser R, Paffenbarger RS Jr, Krueger DE: Trends in cerebrovascular disease mortality based on multiple cause tabulation of death certificates 1930–1960. A comparison of trends in Memphis and Baltimore. Am J Epidemiol 1968;88:307–317.
3   Bonita R, Beaglehole R: Increased treatment of hypertension does not explain the decline in stroke mortality in the United States, 1970–1980. Hypertension 1989;13(suppl I):69–73.
4   Pickle LW, Mungiole M, Gillum RF: Geographic variation in stroke mortality in Blacks and Whites in the United States. Stroke 1997;28:1639–1647.
5   Nefzger MD, Kuller LH, Lilienfeld AM, Diamond EL, Miller GD, Stolley PD, Tonascia S: Three-Area Epidemiological Study of geographic differences in stroke mortality. I. Background and methods. Stroke 1977;8:546–550.
6   Kuller LH, Seltser R: Cerebrovascular disease mortality in Maryland. Am J Epidemiol 1967;86: 442–450.
7   Kuller LH, Bolker A, Saslaw MS, Paegel BL, Sisk C, Borhani N, Wray JA, Anderson H, Peterson D, Winkelstein W, Jr, Cassel J, Spiers P, Robinson AG, Curry H, Lilienfeld AM, Seltser R: Nationwide Cerebrovascular Disease Mortality Study. Accuracy of the clinical diagnoses of cerebrovascular disease. Am J Epidemiol 1969;90:556–566.
8   Kuller LH, Bolker A, Saslaw MS, Paegel BL, Sisk C, Borhani N, Wray JA, Anderson H, Peterson D, Winkelstein W, Jr, Cassel J, Spiers P, Robinson AG, Curry H, Lilienfeld AM, Seltser R: Nationwide cerebrovascular disease mortality study. I. Methods and analysis of death certificates. Am J Epidemiol 1969;90:536–544.
9   Kuller L, Anderson H, Peterson D, Cassel J, Spiers P, Curry H, Paegel B, Saslaw M, Sisk C, Wilber J, Millward D, Winkelstein W, Jr, Lilienfeld A, Seltser R: Nationwide cerebrovascular disease morbidity study. Stroke 1970;1:86–99.
10   Stolley PD, Kuller LH, Nefzger MD, Tonascia S, Lilienfeld AM, Miller GD, Diamond EL: Three-Area Epidemiological Study of geographic differences in stroke mortality. II. Results. Stroke 1977;8:551–557.

11   Brancati FL, Whelton PK, Kuller LH, Klag MJ: Diabetes mellitus, race, and socioeconomic status. A population-based study. Ann Epidemiol 1996;6:67–73.

12   Dai WS, Kuller LH, Miller G: Arterial blood pressure and urinary electrolytes. J Chron Dis 1984; 37:75–84.

13   Langford HG, Marino T, Watson RL: Electrolyte intake in the treated and untreated hypertensive patient; in Gross F, Strasser T (eds): Mild Hypertension: History and Management. Tunbridge Wells, Pitman, 1979.

14   Langford HG: Nonpharmacological therapy of hypertension. Commentary on diet and blood pressure. Hypertension 1989;13(Suppl I):98–102.

15   Stamler J: The INTERSALT Study: Background, methods, findings, and implications. Am J Clin Nutr 1997;65(suppl):626–642.

16   Tobian L: Dietary sodium chloride and potassium have effects on the pathophysiology of hypertension in humans and animals. Am J Clin Nutr 1997;65(suppl):606–611.

17   Grimm CE: Racial differences in blood pressure in Evans County, Georgia: Relationship to sodium and potassium intake and plasma renin activity. J Chron Dis 1980;33:87–94.

18   Heyman A, Karp HR, Heyden S, Bartel A, Cassel JC, Tyroler HA: Cerebrovascular disease in the biracial population of Evans County, GA. Arch Intern Med 1971;128:949–955.

19   Bunker CH, Ukoli FA, Nwankwo MU, Omene JA, Currier GW, Holifield-Kennedy L, Freeman DK, Vergis EN, Yeh LLL, Kuller LH: Factors associated with hypertension in Nigerian civil servants. Prev Med 1992;21:710–722.

20   Kuller LH: Epidemiology of stroke. Adv Neurol 1978;19:281–310.

21   Kuller L, Reisler DM: An explanation of variations in distribution of stroke and arteriosclerotic heart disease among populations and racial groups. Am J Epidemiol 1971;93:1–9.

22   Neaton JD, Wentworth DN, Cutler J, Stamler J, Kuller L, for the Multiple Risk Factor Intervention Trial Research Group: Risk factors for death from different types of stroke. Ann Epidemiol 1993; 3:493–499.

23   Veterans Administration Cooperative Study Group on Antihypertensive Agents: Effects of treatment on morbidity in hypertension. Results in patients with diastolic blood pressures averaging 115 through 129 mm Hg. JAMA 1967;202:116–122.

24   Veterans Administration Cooperative Study Group on Antihypertensive Agents: Effects of treatment on morbidity in hypertension. II. Results in patients with diastolic blood pressure averaging 90 through 114 mm Hg. JAMA 1970;213:1143–1152.

25   National High Blood Pressure Education Program, US Department of Health, Education and Welfare; in Borhani NO (ed): Medical Basis for Comprehensive Community Hypertension Control Programs. DHEW Publ No (NIH) 75–715, (formerly DHEW Publ No. (HRA) 74-3800).

26   SHEP Cooperative Research Group: Prevention of stroke by antihypertensive drug treatment in older persons with isolated systolic hypertension: Final results of the Systolic Hypertension in the Elderly Program (SHEP). JAMA 1991;265:3255–3264.

27   Kokmen E, Whisnant JP, O'Fallon WM, Chu CP, Beard CM: Dementia after ischemic stroke: A population-based study in Rochester, Minnesota (1960–1984). Neurology 1996;19:154–159.

28   Prencipe M, Ferretti C, Casini AR, Santini M, Giublei F, Culasso F: Stroke, disability, and dementia: Results of a population survey. Stroke 1997;28:531–536.

29   Sacco RL, Boden-Albala B, Gan R, Chen X, Kargman DE, Shea S, Paik MC, Hauser WA, and the Northern Manhattan Stroke Study Collaborators: Stroke incidence among White, Black, and Hispanic residents of an urban community. Am J Epidemiol 1998;147:259–268.

30   Gillum RF, Wilson JB: The burden of stroke and its sequelae; in Disease Manage Health Outcomes 1997, Feb 1 (2):84–94. Adis International Limited.

31   Gillum RF: Secular trends in stroke mortality in African Americans: The role of urbanization, diabetes and obesity. Neuroepidemiol 1997;16:180–184.

Dr. Lewis H. Kuller, Department of Epidemiology, University of Pittsburgh, 130 DeSoto Street, Pittsburgh, PA 15261 (USA)

Gillum RF, Gorelick PB, Cooper ES (eds): Stroke in Blacks. Basel, Karger, 1999, pp 7–18

....

Cerebral Ischemia and Infarction in Blacks

Clinical, Autopsy, and Angiographic Studies

Louis R. Caplan

Beth Israel Deaconess Medical Center, Harvard Medical School,
Boston, Mass., USA

Stroke, the third leading cause of death throughout the world, is an even more important cause of prolonged disability. Compared to White populations, African-Americans, and Blacks throughout the world, have a higher frequency of stroke, and have more severe strokes, and more fatal strokes [1–4]. Although stroke is a major public health problem among Blacks all over the world, the nature, location, and severity of the causative vascular diseases has not been as thoroughly studied as in White patients. Strokes are in some ways qualitatively different in Blacks and Whites although detailed information about stroke subtypes in racially mixed studies is sparse. Racial differences in the distribution of atherosclerotic-related stenosis and occlusion of extracranial and intra-cranial arteries have been described [5]. This chapter reviews available in-formation that compares the frequency of various stroke mechanisms and subtypes, the distribution of vascular occlusive lesions, and differences in clinical findings among Black and White patients with cerebrovascular disease. I close by commenting on the possible pathogenesis of the racial differences described.

Stroke Mechanisms and Subtypes

Some studies suggest that intracerebral hemorrhages are more common in Blacks compared to Whites. Table 1 shows comparative data from represen-tative studies and registries [6–14] concerning the frequency of brain hemor-rhages and infarcts. Among three racially mixed patient groups, hemorrhages

Table 1. Frequency of hemorrhage vs. ischemia in representative registries and studies

Study	Population	Race, sex	Hemorrhage %	Ischemia %
Kuhlemeier and Stiens [6]	Maryland, patients 46–106 years old	Black men	16	84
		Black women	11	89
		White men	10	90
		White women	9	91
Mohr et al. [7]	Harvard Stroke Registry	Whites	10	84
Bamford et al. [8]	Oxfordshire Stroke Project	Whites	10	81
Bogousslavsky et al. [9]	Lausanne Stroke Registry	Whites	11	89
Rosman [10]	Urban South African Blacks	Black men	32	68
		Black women	33	67
Quereshi et al. [11]	Blacks in Georgia 15–44 years old	Blacks	34	54
Friday et al. [12]	Lehigh Valley Stroke Registry	Blacks	13.3	86.7
		Whites	8.9	91.1
Kunitz et al. [13]	Pilot Stroke Data Bank	Black men	12.6	80.3
		Black women	11.4	73.5
		White men	5.9	88.5
		White women	6	78.7
Foulkes et al. [14]	Stroke Data Bank	Blacks	13	76
		Whites	13.5	69.5

represented significantly higher percentages of strokes among Blacks compared to Whites [6, 12, 13] but in the Stroke Data Bank [14] the proportion of hemorrhages was the same among Blacks and Whites. In two studies that included only Blacks [10, 11], there was at least 3 times the frequency of hemorrhages found in the three studies that involved exclusively White patients [7–9].

Table 2 shows the distribution of ischemic stroke subtypes in various studies and registries [7, 9, 10–16]. Blacks had more infarcts classified as lacunar and fewer embolic strokes compared to Whites. In a population-based study of stroke in South Alabama, Blacks had a higher frequency of brain hemorrhage and Black women had the highest frequency of lacunar infarction in the population [17].

The increased frequency of intracerebral hemorrhages and lacunar strokes is mostly attributable to the relatively greater burden of hypertension among

Table 2. Ischemic stroke subtypes in various studies and registries

Study	Atherothrombosis %	Embolism %	Lacunae %	Others %
Lehigh Valley [12]				
Blacks	57.8	6.7	20	2.2
Whites	60.7	19.9	9.2	1.3
Quereshi et al. [11], Blacks	9	20	21	50
Rossman [10], Blacks	32	14	20	1
Wityk et al. [15]				
Blacks	19	13	27	40
Whites	17	31	24	30
Harvard Stroke Registry [7]	34	31	19	–
Northern Manhattan Stroke Study [16]				
Blacks	14	17	30	36
Whites	12	38	16	31
Pilot Stroke Data Bank [13]				
Blacks	15.4	15.6	11.8	23.4
Whites	14.5	18.7	6.3	18.7
Lausanne Stroke Registry [9]	43	20	13	8
Stroke Data Bank [14]				
Blacks	5	13	20	38
Whites	7	14	17	31

Blacks in the various studies. These two stroke subtypes are caused predominantly by hypertension. The reason for the reduced frequency of cardiac embolic mechanisms of stroke is less clear. Blacks in past studies have had less coronary artery disease and fewer myocardial infarcts than Whites and ischemic heart disease is one of the most important cardiac sources for brain embolism. Either Blacks had fewer cardiac potential sources of emboli or the heart was less intensively studied in Blacks.

Racial Differences in the Distribution and Severity of Atherosclerosis Derived from Autopsy Studies

Necropsy studies during the years 1950 to 1970 established the usual pattern of cervicocranial atherosclerosis in predominantly and often exclusively

White individuals [18–25]. The greatest burden of occlusive disease in White men was in the proximal portions of the internal carotid and vertebral arteries in the neck. When cervical atherosclerosis was severe, the intracranial internal carotid and middle cerebral arteries and the intracranial vertebral and basilar arteries often also showed atherostenotic lesions. Predominant disease in the large intracranial arteries of the circle of Willis was less common. White men with extracranial carotid and vertebral arterial stenosis often had coexistent coronary and peripheral vascular occlusive disease, hypertension, and elevated serum cholesterol levels.

All of the autopsy studies available that studied the comparative frequency, location, and severity of cervicocerebral atherosclerosis in mixed racial populations [26–31] (except data from South Africa [32]) share three major flaws: (1) Nearly all were performed in the 1960s before knowledge gained from close study of the morphology of atherosclerotic lesions removed from the carotid arteries during endarterectomies [33]. The presence of ulcerations, complex atherosclerotic lesions, and mural thrombi were not commented upon in the early studies of atherosclerosis. (2) The early morphological studies analyzed the extent of the surface area of arteries that showed atherosclerosis but did not study severity of stenosis or occlusions. (3) The studies concentrated on intimal lesions and did not analyze qualitative or quantitative changes in the connective tissue in the arterial media.

The International Atherosclerosis Project was a very industrious study of atherosclerosis in various White and Black individuals that came to autopsy [26–30]. The aorta, coronary, carotid, and large intracranial arteries (middle cerebral and basilar arteries) were analyzed for the presence and extent of surface arterial areas that had fatty streaks, fibrous plaques, calcified lesions, and raised lesions. Solberg and colleagues reported the results of analysis of 1,547 sets of cervicocerebral arteries among New Orleans Whites and Blacks, Jamaican Blacks, and Whites from Oslo, Norway, Santiago, Chile, and Gautemala [27, 28]. Coronary artery and aortic atherosclerotic lesions were more prevalent among Whites. The frequency of raised lesions in the extracranial carotid arteries was about equal in Whites and Blacks. New Orleans Blacks had more intracranial raised lesions than New Orleans Whites. New Orleans Blacks had more intracranial atherosclerosis than Jamaican Blacks and each group of Blacks had more intracranial disease than Whites from Oslo, Santiago, and Guatemala [17, 18].

Resch, Williams and colleagues studied the intracranial arteries of the circles of Willis from 5033 autopsies among Maryland and Alabaman Whites and Blacks, Minnesota Whites, and Nigerian and Senagalese Blacks [29, 30]. Similar to the International Atherosclerosis Project, the grading system used included mostly calcification and surface area and did not study severity of stenosis. American Blacks had more intracranial disease than Whites, and Blacks from Nigeria and Senegal had less extensive disease than American individuals [27, 28]. Reef and Isaacson [31] studied systemic and cerebral arteries among Bantus and found a very low frequency of coronary, carotid, and cerebral atherosclerotic disease. Joubert et al. [32] showed that carotid artery disease was rare among 30 autopsied South African Black patients but lacunar infarcts were present in 43% of individuals studied.

Racial Differences Derived from Arterial Investigations Performed during Life

The introduction of cerebral angiography into medicine during the last half of the twentieth century made it possible to study the presence of cervicocranial occlusive disease during life. Angiography, in contrast to necropsy, showed the extent of luminal stenosis and occlusion but did not give qualitative or quantitative information about the arterial walls.

Bauer et al. [34] in 1962 reported the results of cervicocranial angiography in a racially mixed group of patients in Detroit and found that occlusive lesions causing more than 25% stenosis or complete occlusion of cervical arteries were more common in White patients compared to Blacks. Heyden et al. [35] in 1970 reported the racial differences among patients with angiographically documented severe carotid and middle cerebral artery (MCA) occlusive disease studied at Duke University Hospital. Among the 85 patients with internal carotid artery (ICA) occlusion, 57 were White men, 27 White women, and only 1 patient was Black. Intracranial disease of the MCAs and combined ICA/MCA disease was, in contrast, more common in Blacks. Coronary artery disease, claudication, and high serum cholesterol correlated with the presence of ICA disease but not intracranial disease. Hypertension was about equally present in those with ICA and MCA disease [35].

Russo [36] analyzed the angiographc findings among 50 patients (25 Whites and 25 Blacks) who had anterior circulation transient ischemic attacks. Twice as many Whites (14 vs. 7) had ICA occlusive disease [36]. In the large Joint Study of Extracranial Arterial Occlusion, severe occlusive disease of extracranial arteries was much more common in Whites compared to Blacks [37]. Unilateral ICA occlusions were found in 956 patients and 88 patients had bilateral ICA occlusions [38]. Ninety-one percent of the patients with ICA occlusions were White and only 9% were Black [38]. Ninety-eight percent of patients with subclavian artery occlusive disease and subclavian steal were White [39]. In contrast, intracranial occlusive disease was more prevalent in Blacks [40].

During the mid-1980s, Gorelick, Hier, myself and others reported the results of angiographic studies among a racially mixed patient population studied predominantly at the Michael Reese Hospital in Chicago [5, 41–43]. Among 71 angiogrammed patients with anterior circulation ischemia, Whites had more important disease of the ICA in the neck (more angiographic lesions, more high-grade stenotic lesions, and greater mean degree of stenosis) while Blacks had more frequent and severe occlusive disease of the intracranial supraclinoid ICA and the MCA (more angiographic lesions and higher mean stenosis at these two intracranial sites) [41]. Coronary artery disease, claudication, and high serum cholesterol were more common in Whites and correlated with the presence of extracranial ICA disease, but race was the only significant factor that predicted the location of vascular disease [41]. Among 51 patients who had angiography because of posterior circulation ischemia, Whites had more frequent and severe disease of the vertebral artery in the neck while Blacks had more lesions of the distal basilar artery and intracranial arterial branches [42]. Blacks had significantly higher mean diastolic blood pressures and more diabetes mellitus but race was the only factor that increased the risk of having intracranial posterior circulation occlusive lesions [42]. In another study that compared patients with angiographically documented severe ICA disease in the neck with those that had MCA occlusive disease, ICA lesions correlated with male sex, White race, high cholesterol levels, and coronary artery disease [43]. MCA occlusive disease patients were more often Black, female, and younger than ICA disease patients. As in the other two Chicago studies [41, 42], hypertension was common in both ICA and MCA disease patients [43].

The Pilot Stroke Data Bank [13] and the Stroke Data Bank [14] were large multi-institutional studies that included racially mixed patients. The Pilot Stroke Data Bank contained 1,144 patients among whom 43% were Black, and one-third of patients had cerebral angiography [5, 13]. Among the 44 patients with angiographically documented > 50% stenosis of the extracranial ICA, only 6 (13.6%) were Black. In this study few patients had intracranial arterial stenosis [5, 13]. In the Stroke Data Bank, among 816 patients (60.8% Black), angiography was performed in 275 [5, 14]. Only 40% of patients with severe ICA stenosis in the neck (> 50% luminal narrowing) were Black but Blacks made up 82.6% of the patients with severe intracranial stenosis of the intracranial ICA and MCAs [5, 14].

Umerah [44] in 1980 studied 113 Zambian Black patients during a period of 3.5 years with cerebral angiography. Thirty-two patients had occlusion of a cerebral vessel. Severe stenosis or occlusion of the intracranial carotid artery was found in 19 patients. Fifteen had occlusion of the internal carotid artery, bilateral in 7 while all 4 patients with intracranial ICA stenosis had bilateral disease. Extracranial atherosclerosis was extremely rare [44]. Joubert et al. [32] studied 304 South-African stroke patients. Very few had TIAs (1.9%) or carotid bruits (0.6%). Arch and carotid angiography were performed on a random sample of 30 Black stroke patients and extracranial lesions were found in only 5 patients [32]. Quereshi et al. [11] studied the nature and etiology of stroke among young (15–44 years old) Black stroke patients admitted to the Grady Memorial Hospital in Atlanta Georgia during a 3.5-year period. Angiography was performed in 100 of the 248 stroke patients. Atherosclerotic vasculopathy was rare, occurring in only 10 patients, 3 extracranial and 7 intracranial [11].

Some more recent studies have used extracranial and intracranial ultrasound and magnetic resonance angiography (MRA), as well as contrast cerebral angiography, to evaluate the presence and severity of occlusive vascular lesions. Wityk et al. [15] studied the etiology and vascular lesions found among a racially mixed (50% Black) group of stroke patients studied in Baltimore, Md. during a 2-year period using ultrasound, MRA, and contrast angiography. White patients were more than twice as likely to have extracranial carotid artery disease than Blacks (33% of White patients vs. 15% of Blacks); intracranial lesions were equally distributed among Blacks and Whites but Whites had significantly more tandem lesions, i.e. both extracranial and intracranial stenotic lesions (17 vs. 2%) [15].

In one study, among 99 Black and 106 White patients evaluated by Duplex ultrasound of the carotid arteries, White vs. Black race was found to be an independent risk factor for predicting carotid artery stenosis [45]. Tell et al. [46] analyzed carotid plaque disease among 1,578 individuals referred for extracranial ultrasound evaluations. White patients had significantly more plaque than Blacks in the internal and external carotid arteries in the neck but not in the common carotid artery. The Northern Manhattan Stroke Study [47] examined the maximum internal carotid artery plaque thickness (MICPT) among 526 racially mixed stroke-free individuals that lived in Northern Manhattan. The mean MICPT was equal (1.7 ± 1.3 mm) in Black and White patients but was less in Hispanics (1.2 ± 1.5 mm). The mean MICPT was higher in patients with hypertension, hypercholesterolemia, smoking, and elevated fasting blood glucose levels. The Northern Manhattan Stroke Study [16] also analyzed the presence of atherosclerotic disease among 438 hospitalized acute stroke patients. Extracranial atherosclerotic occlusive disease accounted for stroke in 11% of Whites and 8% of Blacks while 6% of Blacks and 1% of Whites had intracranial occlusive lesions. The ratio of extracranial/intracranial occlusive disease was 9.0 in Whites and 1.2 in Blacks. Ryu et al. [48] compared the extracranial ultrasound findings among 50 White and 25 Black patients with transient ischemic attacks. The extent of atherosclerosis as measured by B-mode ultrasound was similar in Blacks and Whites. However, when the 32 patients with the most severe extracranial carotid artery disease ipsilateral to the ischemic hemisphere were analyzed, this group included 66% (23 of 35) of Whites and 43% (9 of 21) Blacks [48].

In summary, studies of arterial lesions among racially mixed individuals indicate that severe extracranial internal carotid artery and vertebral artery atherosclerotic occlusive disease occurs more commonly among Whites while intracranial disease is more common among Blacks. Early studies seem to show more impressive racial differences than more recent analyses. Among all racial groups, men have more extracranial disease while women seem to have proportionally more severe intracranial occlusive disease.

Clinical Differences among Stroke Patients

A few studies suggest the possibility that there may be racial differences in the clinical course and response to treatment among Black and White patients with cerebrovascular disease. Three small studies analyzed the clinical findings and outcomes in predominantly or exclusively White patients with MCA disease [49–51]. Corston et al. [49] reported 21 patients with MCA occlusive disease studied at the National Hospital, Queens Square, London. Among 21 patients, 15 (71%) had TIAs, 8 occurring prior to strokes. After treatment (11 with anticoagulants, 4 antiplatelet drugs) only 2 patients had further TIAs. Hinton et al. [50] studied 16 patients with MCA occlusive disease at the Massachusetts General Hospital in Boston, among whom 15 (94%) had TIAs. Twelve of the patients were treated with anticoagulants and did quite well. Among 13 patients with MCA occlusive disease studied in Lausanne, 9 had TIAs [51]. Among these 50 patients, 39 (78%) had TIAs, and the outcome was usually favorable especially when patients were treated with anticoagulants.

My colleagues and I compared the clinical findings among patients selected because they had MCA (20 patients) or ICA (25 patients) occlusive disease [43]. 85% of patients with intracranial disease were Black. Only 4 of the patients with MCA disease had TIAs and all developed strokes and brain infarcts visible on CT scans. Anticoagulants were not effective usually in preventing strokes in patients with MCA stenosis. Progressive and fluctuating deficits often developed during a period of 1 week, suggesting a hemodynamic, low-flow, mechanism of their MCA territory brain infarcts.

Although the data are sparse, they suggest that MCA, and possibly other intracranial vascular occlusive disease, may be different in Blacks and Whites. The presence of TIAs responsive to anticoagulants and platelet antiaggregants in White patients is most consistent with a mechanism of intimal irregularities with distal intra-arterial embolism as the most likely stroke mechanism. In contrast, progressive ischemia unresponsive to substances that modify platelet function and coagulation, suggest a low-flow mechanism of ischemia perhaps caused by fibromuscular thickening of the media rather than intimal disease. Carotid artery disease in the neck, a condition most often found in White men, is known to be mostly associated with intimal irregularities and the formation of white platelet-fibrin and red erythrocyte-fibrin thromboemboli that cause TIAs and strokes. Strokes in patients with carotid artery disease in the neck are mostly related to intra-arterial embolism to the MCA and its branches. The posited racial differences in intracranial arterial morphology is purely hypothetical since there are no modern studies that compare the morphological changes within the large intracranial arteries in symptomatic White and Black patients.

Possible Pathogenesis of the Racial Differences in the Distribution of Vascular Lesions

Many physicians and researchers have tried to explain the predominance of severe extracranial occlusive disease in Whites, especially White men, and the predominance of intracranial occlusive disease in Black men and women. The commonest explanation proferred is that the racial differences are caused by the higher frequency of hypertension, especially severe uncontrolled hypertension in Blacks. The data available argue strongly against this simple explanation. Hypertension in Whites is more associated with extracranial disease than intracranial and the presence of hypertension or even severe hypertension does not predict the occurrence of intracranial occlusive disease.

Hypertensive disease is somewhat different in Whites and Blacks. Blacks, as well as Asians, retain more of a sodium load and hypertension responds better to diuretics in Blacks compared to Whites [52, 53]. Hypertension can be related to high-resistance or high volume states. Blacks, and Asians, as well as menstruating women and women who are pregnant or who take female sex hormones often have higher blood volumes compared to White normotensive and hypertensive men. Diabetes is also a disorder often associated with high blood volume. All the conditions associated with high blood volume – female sex, diabetes, hypertension in Blacks and Asians – are associated with intracranial disease. In contrast, hypertension in Whites, often of the high-resistance type, is associated with extracranial carotid and vertebral artery disease in the neck. The morphology of the extracranial and intracranial arteries is different. The media is more important in intracranial arteries. Perhaps high-resistance hypertension affects more the extracranial arteries while high-volume states tend to cause more stress and disease in intracranial arteries.

Clearly more data are needed about the morphology of occlusive vascular disease in different locations in different racial groups and in men and women. Modern technology especially ultrasound now provides an opportunity to study the arterial wall during life. The hypothetical difference herein posited between high-resistance and high-volume hypertension and other high volume states is testable. Clearly more research is necessary.

Conclusions

Cerebrovascular disease and strokes are a particularly serious problem among Blacks. Blacks have disproportionately more strokes, more fatal strokes, and more disabling strokes than Whites. Necropsy and data bank and registry studies show that Blacks have more intracerebral hemorrhages and lacunar infarcts than Whites.

The distribution of occlusive cervicocranial disease differs between Whites and Blacks. White men have a predominance of extracranial occlusive disease involving the internal carotid and vertebral arteries in the neck while Blacks and women have more intracranial artery occlusive disease especially involving the middle cerebral arteries.

Although hypertension is more prevalent, more severe, and less well controlled among Blacks, hypertension alone cannot account for the racial and sex differences in the distribution of atherosclerotic occlusive disease. High volume states that are associated with hypertension are posited to predispose to intracranial disease.

References

1   Gillum R: Stroke in Blacks. Stroke 1988;19:1–9.
2   Caplan LR: Strokes in African-Americans. Circulation 1991;83:1469–1471.
3   Howard G, Anderson R, Sorlie P, Andrews V, Backlund E, Burke GL: Ethnic differences in stroke mortality between non-Hispanic Whites, Hispanic Whites, and Blacks: The National Longitudinal Mortality Study. Stroke 1994;25:2120–2125.
4   Otten MW, Teutsh SM, Williamson DF, Marks JJ: The effect of known risk factors on the excess mortality of black adults in the United States. JAMA 1990;263:845–850.
5   Caplan LR, Gorelick PB, Hier DB: Race, sex, and occlusive cerebrovascular disease: A review. Stroke 1986;17:648–655.
6   Kuhlemeir KV, Stiens SA: Racial disparities in severity of cerebrovascular events. Stroke 1994;25: 2126–2131.
7   Mohr JP, Caplan LR, Melski J, Duncan G, Goldstein R, Kistler JP, Pessin MS, Bleich H: The Harvard Cooperative Stroke Registry: A prospective registry. Neurology 1978;28:754–762.
8   Bamford J, Sandercock P, Dennis M, Burn J, Warlow C: A prospective study of acute cerebrovascular disease in the community: The Oxfordshire Community Stroke Project – 1981–1986. J Neural Neurosurg Psychiatry 1990;53:16–22.

9   Bogousslavsky J, Van Melle G, Regli F: The Lausanne Stroke Registry: Analysis of 1,000 consecutive patients with first stroke. Stroke 1988;19:1083–1092.

10   Rosman K: The epidemiology of stroke in an urban population. Stroke 1986;17:667–669.

11   Quereshi AI, Safdar K, Patel M, Janssen RS, Frankel MR: Stroke in young Black patients: Risk factors, subtypes, and prognosis. Stroke 1995;26:1995–1998.

12   Friday G, Lai SM, Alter M, Sobel E, LaRue L, Gil-Peralta A, McCoy RL, Levitt LP, Isack T: Stroke in the Lehigh Valley: Racial/ethnic differences. Neurology 1989;39:1165–1168.

13   Kunitz SC, Gross CR, Heyman A, Kase C, Mohr JP, Price T, Wolf P: The Pilot Stroke Data bank: Definition, design, and data. Stroke 1984;15:740–746.

14   Foulkes MA, Wolf PA, Price TR, Mohr JP, Hier DB: The Stroke Data Bank: Design, methods, and baseline characteristics. Stroke 1988;19:547–554.

15   Wityk RJ, Lehman D, Klag M, Coresh J, Ahn H, Litt B: Race and sex differences in the distribution of cerebral atherosclerosis. Stroke 1996;27:1974–1980.

16   Sacco RL, Kargman DE, Gu Q, Zamanillo MC: Race-ethnicity and determinants of intracranial atherosclerotic cerebral infarction: The Northern Manhattan Stroke Study. Stroke 1995;26: 14–20.

17   Gross CR, Kase CS, Mohr JP, Cunningham SC, Baker WE: Stroke in South Alabama: Incidence and diagnostic features – A population based study. Stroke 1984;15:249–255.

18   Fisher CM: Occlusion of the internal carotid artery. Arch Neurol Psychiatry 1951;65:346–377.

19   Hutchinson EC, Yates PO: The cervical portion of the vertebral artery: A clinicopathological study. Brain 1956;79:319–331.

20   Whisnant JP, Martin MJ, Sayre GP: Atherosclerotic stenosis of cervical arteries. Arch Neurol 1961; 5:429–432.

21   Schwartz CJ, Mitchell JRA: Atheroma of the carotid and vertebral arterial systems. Br Med J 1961; 2:1057–1063.

22   Torvik A, Jorgenson L: Thrombotic and embolic occlusions of the carotid arteries in an autopsy material. 1. Prevalence, location, and associated diseases. J Neurol Sci 1964;1:24–39.

23   Fisher CM, Gore I, Okabe N, White PD: Atherosclerosis of the carotid and vertebral arteries – Extracranial and intracranial. J Neuropathol Exp Neurol 1965;24:455–476.

24   Blackwood W, Hallpike JF, Kocen RS, Mair WGP: Atheromatous disease of the carotid arterial system and embolism from the heart in cerebral infarction: A morbid anatomical study. Brain 1969; 92:897–910.

25   Castaigne P, Lhermitte F, Gautier JC, Escourolle R, Derouesne C: Internal carotid artery occlusion: A study of 61 instances in 50 patients with post-mortem data. Brain 1970;93:231–258.

26   McGill HC, Arias-Stella J, Carbonell L, Correa P, deVeyra E, Donoso S, Eggen DA, Galindo L, Guzman M, Lichtenberger E, Loken AC, McGarry PA, McMahan CA, Montenegro M, Moosy J, Perez-Tamayo R, Resrepo C, Robertson WB, Salas J, Solberg LA, Strong JP, Tejada S, Wainwright J: General findings in the International Atherosclerosis Project. Lab Invest 1968;18:38–42.

27   Solberg LA, McGarry PA, Moosy J, Tejada C, Loken AC, Robertson WB, Donoso S: Distribution of cerebal atherosclerosis by geographic location, race, and sex. Lab Invest 1968;18:144–152.

28   Solberg LA, McGarry PA: Cerebral atherosclerosis in Negroes and Caucasians. Atherosclerosis 1972;16:141–154.

29   Williams AO, Resch JA, Loewenson RB: Cerebral atherosclerosis: A comparative autopsy study between Nigerian Negroes and American negroes and Caucasians. Neurology 1969;19:205–210.

30   Resch JA, Williams AO, Lemercier G, Loewenson RB: Comparative autopsy studies on cerebral atherosclerosis in Nigerian and Senegal negroes, American negroes and Caucasians. Atherosclerosis 1970;12:401–407.

31   Reef H, Isaacson C: Atherosclerosis in the Bantu: The distribution of atheromatous lesions in Africans over 50 years of age. Circulation 1962;25:66–72.

32   Joubert J, Lemmer LB, Fourie PA, van Gelder AL: Are clinical differences between Black and White stroke patients caused by variations in the atherosclerotic involvement of the arterial tree? S Afr Med J 1990;77:248–251.

33   Fisher CM, Ojemann RG: A clinico-pathological study of carotid endarterectomy plaques. Rev Neurol 1986;142:573–589.

34   Bauer RB, Sheehan S, Wechsler N, Meyer JS: Arteriographic study of the sites, incidence, and treatment of arteriosclerotic cerebrovascular lesions. Neurology1962;12:698–711.

35   Heyden S, Heyman A, Goree JA: Nonembolic occlusion of the middle cerebral and carotid arteries: A comparison of predisposing factors. Stroke 1970;1:363–369.

36   Russo LS: Carotid system transient ischemic attacks: Clinical, racial, and angiographic correlations. Stroke 1981;12:470–473.

37   Hass WK, Fields WS, North RR, Kricheff II, Chase NE, Bauer RB: Joint Study of Extracranial Arterial Occlusion. II. Arteriography, techniques, sites, and complications. JAMA 1968;203:961–968.

38   Fields WS, Lemak N: Joint Study of Extracranial Arterial Occlusion. X. Internal carotid artery occlusion. JAMA 1976;235:2734–2738.

39   Fields WS, Lemark N: Joint Study of Extracranial Arterial Occlusion. VII. Subclavian steal. JAMA 1972;222:1139–1143.

40   Heyman A, Fields WS, Keating RD: Joint Study of Extracranial Arterial Occlusion. VI. Racial differences in hospitalized patients with ischemic stroke. JAMA 1972;222:285–289.

41   Gorelick PB, Caplan LR, Hier DB, Parker SL, Patel D: Racial differences in the distribution of anterior circulation occlusive disease. Neurology 1984;34:54–59.

42   Gorelick PB, Caplan LR, Hier DB, Patel D, Langenberg P, Pessin MS, Biller J, Kornack D: Racial differences in the distribution of posterior circulation occlusive disease. Stroke 1985;16:785–790.

43   Caplan L, Babikian V, Helgason C, Hier D, DeWitt LD, Patel D, Stein R: Occlusive disease of the middle cerebral artery. Neurology 1985;35:975–982.

44   Umerah BC: Angiography of stroke in central africa. AJR 1980;134:963–965.

45   Gil-Peralta A, Alter M, Lai SM, Friday G, Otero A, Katz M, Comerota AJ: Duplex Doppler and spectral flow analysis of racial differences in cerebrovascular atherosclerosis. Stroke 1990;21:740–744.

46   Tell GS, Howard G, McKinney WM: Risk factors for site specific extracranial carotid artery plaque distribution as measured by B-mode ultrasound. J Clin Epidemiol 1989;42:551–559.

47   Sacco RL, Roberts JK, Boden-Albala B, Gu Q, Lin I-F, Kargman DE, Berglund L, Hauser WA, Shea S, Paik MC: Race-ethnicity and determinants of carotid atherosclerosis in a multiethnic population: The Northern Manhattan Stroke Study. Stroke 1997;28:929–935.

48   Ryu JE, Murros K, Espeland MA: Extracranial carotid atherosclerosis in Black and White patients with transient ischemic attacks. Stroke 1989;20:1133–1137.

49   Corston R, Kendall B, Marshall J: Prognosis in middle cerebral artery stenosis. Stroke 1984;15: 237–241.

50   Hinton R, Mohr JP, Ackerman R, Adair L, Fisher CM: Symptomatic middle cerebral artery stenosis. Ann Neurol 1979;5:152–157.

51   Feldmeyer J, Merendaz C, Regli F: Stenoses symptomatiques de l'arter cerebral moyenne. Rev Neurol 1983;139:725–736.

52   Veterans Administration Cooperative Study Group on Antihypertensive Agents: Comparison of propanolol and hydrochlorothiazide for the initial treatment of hypertension. 1. Results of short-term titration with emphasis on racial differences in response. JAMA 1982;248:1996–2003.

53   Veterans Administration Cooperative Study Group on Antihypertensive Agents: Comparison of propanolol and hydrochlorothiazide for the initial treatment of hypertension. 2. Results of long-term therapy. JAMA 1982;248:2004–2011.

Louis R. Caplan, MD, Beth Israel Deaconess Medical Center,
Harvard Medical School, Boston, MA 02163 (USA)

Gillum RF, Gorelick PB, Cooper ES (eds): Stroke in Blacks. Basel, Karger, 1999, pp 19–28

....

Lacunar Stroke in Black Patients

Clinical Presentation and Detection

Gwendolyn F. Ford Lynch[a]*, Jaqueline Washington*[b]*, Philip B. Gorelick*[a]

[a] Department of Neurology, Rush Medical College, Chicago, Ill., and
[b] Department of Neurology, Emory University, Atlanta, Ga., USA

Lacunes, as the name suggests, are small 'lakes' or cavities that occur deep in the brain. The underlying vascular pathology is lipohyalinosis, a degenerative vessel-wall disease that is unique to smaller cerebral arteries. Lacunar infarction, however, may also be caused by microatheroma, microemboli, or other arteriopathies. Lacunar infarcts are common among African-Americans. In this chapter, we review the history, epidemiology, clinical presentation and diagnosis, and prognosis of lacunar strokes.

Brief History

Lacunar infarctions, as described by Fisher, are 'small infarcts that lie in the deeper non-cortical parts of the cerebrum and brainstem and result from occlusion of penetrating branches of the large cerebral arteries – middle cerebral, posterior cerebral, basilar, and less commonly, anterior cerebral and vertebral arteries' [1, 2]. These small infarcts (up to 1.5–2.0 cm in size) are thought to be largely due to occlusion of subcortical cerebral arteries that may be 100–500 μm in diameter.

The first written description of lacunes was provided by Pierre Marie who described these lesions as 'a cavity as a result of a healed infarct resulting from obstruction or rupture of a small perforating artery, most commonly in the lenticular nucleus' [3, 4]. Much of our current understanding of lacunar pathology, clinical presentation and epidemiology stems from the work of Fisher, Mohr, Caplan, and others [2, 5, 6].

The introduction of brain computed tomography (CT) and magnetic resonance imaging (MRI) was a major advance in our understanding of this stroke subtype. These imaging modalities provided pre-mortem visualization of the location, size, and number of lacunar strokes. Such information may be especially useful in the study of hyperacute stroke therapies or vascular dementia. In the former case, acute lacunar infarction may be excluded from the administration of neuroprotective therapies.

Epidemiology

Lacunar infarction occurs more commonly in African Americans when compared to European-Americans [7]. Data from the Lehigh Valley Study showed that the percentage of lacunar infarction was nearly two times higher in Blacks (20%) than Whites (9.2%). The Northern Manhattan Stroke Study included 225 patients with incident stroke between 1975 and 1984 [8]. The study population was 20% Black, 63% Hispanic, and 15% White. 31% of Blacks with first ever stroke had lacunar syndromes, compared to 17% of Whites.

Lacunar infarction may be common among young African-American stroke patients. In a hospital-based study of stroke in 219 Black patients between the ages of 15 and 44 years, lacunar infarction was the most common ischemic stroke subtype, accounting for 21% of cerebral infarcts in this group [9]. These results differ from other studies of stroke in the young adult that emphasize cardioembolic strokes or strokes due to nonatherosclerotic mechanisms. The reason for these differences is not clear, but it may be related to the higher prevalence of hypertension in young African-Americans.

In the South Alabama Study the incidence of lacunar infarction was highest in Black women [10]. As this was the first large-scale study to demonstrate a predilection by sex for lacunar stroke in a population, further study is needed to confirm this association.

Risk Factors

Hypertension

Hypertension is thought to be a major risk factor for lacunar infarction. This is supported by pathologic studies that show blood vessel changes that may be associated with chronic hypertension, including lipohyalinosis, microatheroma, fibrinoid necrosis, and Charcot-Bouchard aneurysms.

The association of stroke and hypertension has been demonstrated in numerous stroke studies involving both large and small vessel disease. There appears to be a preponderance of hypertension, however, in patients who have

Table 1. Risk factors for lacunar stroke in Blacks (mean age 65.3 years)

Risk factor	Percentage
Hypertension	70.6
Diabetes	42.3
History of smoking	65.4
Family history of stroke	49.0
Preceding TIA	24.0
Prior stroke	23.5

Nonpublished data from the Henry Ford Stroke Data Bank [with permission].

suffered lacunar infarctions. In a study of 121 stroke patients, 93% of patients with lacunar infarction (23% of the study population) had either a history of hypertension or echocardiographic evidence of left-ventricular hypertrophy [11]. In a Mayo Clinic population study lacunar infarcts accounted for 12% of annual stroke incidence and the prevalence of hypertension in lacunar and nonlacunar stroke patients was 81 and 70%, respectively [12].

African-Americans have a higher incidence and prevalence rate of hypertension [13]. In studies of Blacks with lacunar infarction, hypertension appears to play an important role. In the study of young Black stroke patients mentioned above, there was a higher frequency of hypertension in young Black stroke sufferers, most of whom had lacunar infarcts, when compared to non-Blacks (55 vs. 24%, p=0.003) [9]. The Henry Ford Stroke Data Base rated hypertension as the number one risk factor in Black lacunar stroke patients (table 1). In the South Alabama Study, for every stroke subtype (including lacunar strokes), a history of hypertension was more prevalent in Blacks when compared to Whites [10].

Diabetes and Smoking

The causal relationship between diabetes mellitus (DM) and lacunar strokes is less well defined than that for hypertension. There are data, however, which support the relationship between DM and lacunar infarction [14]. In a population-based study from Rochester Minnesota no significant difference, in percentage of diabetics, was found between patients with lacunar stroke (14%) and non-lacunar stroke (16%) [12]. In a study of 203 consecutive patients with first-ever stroke due to lacunar infarction, diabetes was observed as the third most common risk factor (odds ratio 2.3 [95% confidence interval 1.0–5.5]) after hypertension (8.9 [4.2, 18.8]) and smoking (6.6 [2.9,14.8]) [15]. In a study of 637 lacunar stroke patients from the Stroke Data Bank, Mast et al. [16] showed that diabetes was an independent risk factor for multiple but not single lacunes (odds ratio 2.3, 95% confidence interval 1.1–4.5). No studies to date have specifically addressed the relationship between DM and lacunar strokes in Blacks. Data from the Henry Ford Stroke Data Bank show that diabetes is the third most common risk factor, after hypertension and smoking, for lacunar stroke in Black patients (table 1).

Thus, DM and smoking [17] may be risk factors for lacunar infarction (table 1). Both DM and smoking are prevalent in African-Americans. Lacunar infarction might also be associated with large artery intracranial disease [18] or family history of stroke (table 1).

Presentation and Diagnosis

The presentation and diagnosis of lacunar syndrome in Blacks does not differ from that of other racial/ethnic groups. As the penetrating arteries perfuse only a limited area of the brain, the spectrum of neurologic deficits is less diverse than with large artery occlusive disease. Furthermore, since pathologic correlation is rare in lacunar stroke, the diagnosis is based on clinical signs and symptoms consistent with the recognized lacunar syndromes and supporting lab tests. It is presumed that there is corresponding disease of small penetrating arteries, and, thus, the designation lacunar 'hypothesis' has been used to refer to this phenomenon [19].

Clinical Syndromes

The most commonly occurring lacunar syndromes are pure motor hemiparesis, pure sensory stroke, ataxic hemiparesis, sensorimotor syndrome and the dysarthria clumsy hand syndrome [20]. Others including hemiballismus, acute hemidystonia, and the hemiathetosis occur rarely. Data on the clinical presentation of lacunar stroke in Blacks are sparse. Though the diagnosis is made on clinical grounds, one must keep in mind that it is a syndrome and in one study 25% of patients who presented with lacunar syndromes had alternate etiologies [8].

Pure motor hemiparesis was defined by Fisher and Curry [21] as unilateral paralysis without other neurologic findings. Motor weakness presenting in isolation, without signs of sensory loss, visual defect, or neuropsychological dysfunction is consistent with the diagnosis. In the first reports lesions were in the centrum semiovale. Lesions may also be found in the internal capsule, basis pontis and the cerebral peduncle.

The Northern Manhattan Stroke Study showed that 45% of all lacunar strokes were in the category of pure motor hemiparesis [8]. Three percent

(25 patients) of 850 stroke registry patients presenting to Harlem hospital had pure motor hemiparesis [22].

Pure sensory lacunar syndrome is characterized by a persistent or transient 'numbness' with or without sensory loss involving the face, arm, and leg. The numbness and sensory loss are seen in isolation and are not accompanied by neuropsychological disturbance, motor weakness, abnormalities of extraocular movements, dysarthria, vertigo, or visual field defect [23]. The pure sensory syndrome was seen in 7% of patients presenting with lacunar syndrome in the Northern Manhattan Stroke Study [8]. Lesions resulting in this syndrome are most often located in the thalamus.

The syndrome of ataxic hemiparesis was first described in 1965 [24]. The syndrome is apparent when upper motor neuron pattern weakness and cerebellar dysfunction are present unilaterally. The motor weakness is associated with cerebellar signs of dysmetria, adiadokokinesis, and rarely hypotonia. Cerebellar signs are out of proportion to the degree of weakness. Hyperesthesia has been reported as an associated symptom. Ataxic hemiparesis is associated with lesions of the upper basis pontis and internal capsule. Frequency data for this syndrome in the Black population are generally lacking. Overall, the syndrome accounted for 21% of patients with lacunar strokes in one series [17] and 18% in another [8].

The sensorimotor lacunar syndrome consists of isolated sensorimotor deficit. The syndrome was first described by Mohr et al. [25] in 1977. The clinical findings are associated with thalamocapsular lacunar lesions. Sensory loss and motor weakness can occur disproportionately. This syndrome occurred in 20% of patients presenting with a first-time lacunar syndrome. Finally, dysarthria clumsy hand syndrome occurs with basis pontis lesions and those of the genu of the internal capsule. There is dysarthria, dysphagia, facial weakness and clumsiness of the hand.

Diagnostic Studies

A screening brain computerized tomography scan is usually performed on all patients who present with a lacunar stroke syndrome. The purpose of this scan is to identify hemorrhage, infarctions, or edema. Typical small, deep lacunar type infarctions are the most common finding in those patients with a positive scan [26]. However, a significant percentage of patients with positive CT scans will have larger infarctions, or small hemorrhages that account for their 'lacunar' stroke syndrome [27, 28]. These findings indicate that a medium to large vessel occlusion or hypertensive intracerebral hemorrhage, respectively, may be the primary cause of the stroke, and not small vessel lipohyalinosis.

The sensitivity of CT and MRI in documenting lacunar syndromes varies. This may be related to differences in the radiologic definition of lacunar infarction. In one study a lacune was defined as a sharply marginated, hypo-dense, round, ovoid, or linear lesion without mass effect that measured less than 2 cm in its longest dimension. In another study this definition was expanded to clarify its location to be limited to the basal ganglia, internal capsule, deep hemispheric white matter, thalamus, or pons [8]. The radiologic definition of lacune has been alternatively defined as a small deep lesion on CT or MRI with signal intensity consistent with infarction that is usually less than or equal to 1 cm in diameter. This radiologic diagnosis is also dependent on the consistency of the location of the lesion and the clinical syndrome [8]. Using the latter criteria, CT or MRI demonstrates appropriately located deep infarcts in 84% of cases of lacunar syndromes. MRI, however, is superior to CT in evaluating lesions especially in the posterior fossa. Some lacunes are probably too small to be seen on CT or MRI.

As mentioned above, the etiology of lacunar infarction is often small vessel occlusive disease. Some individuals with lacunar syndrome have evidence of other potential causes for infarction, such as intracranial large artery athero-sclerosis, cardiac source embolism (i.e. atrial fibrillation, cardiomyopathy, or valvular abnormality), or extracranial cerebrovascular atherosclerosis [12, 29, 30] causing some to question the use of the term lacunar infarction in specifying stroke etiology [31]. Other etiologies such as cardiac embolism and large artery occlusive disease should be ruled out.

It has been shown that African-Americans may have a greater predilection for intracranial large artery occlusive disease [18, 32]. These observations suggest that African-American patients presenting with a lacunar syndrome may have other causes for their stroke and investigations for these causes should be considered. Transcranial doppler ultrasound and magnetic reson-ance angiography have been shown to be useful screening tools for large vessel intracranial disease [33–36]. The use of these safe, noninvasive diagnostic tools may help to identify individuals at risk for future ischemic events associated with intracranial arterial stenosis (e.g., sickle cell patients).

It has become apparent that a significant percentage of individuals with lacunar infarction have significant extracranial carotid stenosis. It has been postulated that the presence of internal carotid artery stenosis is not necessarily a cause of the lacunar infarction in all cases, but simply a general marker of atherosclerosis [37]. Studies that specifically address this issue in African-Americans are lacking. However, in a study of 55 patients with lacunar infarc-tion, 13% had ≥50% carotid stenosis (by doppler criteria) ipsilateral to the clinical event, and 4% had high grades of stenosis on the contralateral side [38]. Salgado et al. [39] found that 37% of patients with lacunar infarction had some degree of carotid stenosis but only 3% had stenosis greater than 50%. 31% (14 of 45 patients) of lacunar stroke patients who underwent selective angiography demonstrated carotid stenosis in a prospective study conducted by Kappelle et al. [37]. These findings support the notion that a subgroup of lacunar stroke patients will have other markers of cerebrovascular disease. While the presence of carotid stenosis may not be directly associated with the lacunar infarction, identification of such a lesion may be particularly important in light of the results of the Asymptomatic Carotid Artery Surgery Trial [40]. This clinical trial demonstrated a statistically significant reduction in the risk of stroke with carotid endarterectomy combined with medical management, compared to medical management alone, in individuals with asymptomatic carotid stenosis. Given these facts, a noninvasive screening for carotid stenosis with carotid ultrasound should be considered for all lacunar stroke patients.

Cardiac abnormalities are not a rare finding in patients with lacunar infarction. As with carotid stenosis, the presence of a cardiac abnormality does not necessarily indicate a cardioembolic cause for the infarction, but may simply be a marker of a concomitant condition [41]. Salgado et al. [41] found that 10% of 145, first-ever lacunar stroke patients had a potential cardiac source of embolism. In another study, atrial-septal aneurysm was noted in 46% of lacunar stroke patients by transesphageal echocardiogram [42]. Other studies have suggested that cardiac embolism is the most likely stroke etiology in 10% of lacunar stroke cases [43–48]. These data strongly support the argument for performing an echocardiogram for any patient who presents with lacunar infarction.

Conventional cerebral angiography is, of course, the gold standard to which the screening studies, carotid doppler, transcranial doppler, and MR angiography, have been compared [33, 35, 46–54]. The unacceptable rates of false-positives or false-negatives associated with these screening studies, and the potential complicating factor of an intracranial vascular abnormality (i.e. tandem stenosis, arteriovenous malformation, intracranial aneurysm) warrants a conventional cerebral angiogram to confirm significant findings from screening studies. This is particularly important when a change in treatment (e.g. oral anticoagulation), which might be associated with greater risk, is being considered.

Prognosis

There is little prognostic data regarding lacunar infarction specific to race. In the South Alabama Study case fatality rates among different stroke subtypes were compared. This study reported on 160 incident strokes. 107 of the reported strokes occurred in Blacks. 13 of 20 lacunar strokes occurred in Blacks. The case fatality rates among all patients was lowest (10%) among lacunar stroke cases [10]. Overall, lacunar stroke is associated with lower case fatality rates, frequency of recurrent stroke [55] and death at 1 year and 5 years [12].

Specific data regarding the rate of recurrent stroke in Blacks is generally lacking. Unpublished data from the Henry Ford Hospital Stroke Data Bank report a history of previous stroke in 23.5% of patients with lacunar stroke between the years 1987 and 1993. Sacco et al. [12] reported a 4% cumulative probability of recurrent stroke at 1 month and 10% at 12 months. A 26% rate of recurrence at 5 years in the same group was similar to the Henry Ford Hospital experience. Cerebral infarcts accounted for 85% of recurrent strokes. A second lacunar stroke was reported in 17% of patients with lacunar stroke.

References

1   Fisher CM: Lacunar strokes and infarcts: A review. Neurology 1982;32:871–876.
2   Fisher CM: Lacunes: Small deep infarcts. Neurology 1965;15:774–784.
3   Marie P: Des foyers lacunaires de desintigration et de differents antres états carrtaires du cerveau. Rev Méd (Paris) 1901;21:281.
4   Millikan C, Futtrell N: The fallacy of the lacune hypothesis. Stroke 1990;21:1251–1257.
5   Mohr JP: Lacunes. Neurol Clin 1983;1:201–221.
6   Caplan LR: Penetrating branch artery disease; in Caplan LR (ed): Stroke: A Clinical Approach, ed 2. Boston, Butterworth-Heinemann, 1993, pp 273–297.
7   Friday G, Lai SM, Alter MD, Sobel E, LaRue L, McCoy RL, Levitt LP, Isack T: Stroke in the Lehigh Valley: Racial/ethnic differences. Neurology 1989;39:1165–1168.
8   Gan R, Sacco RL, Kargman DE, Roberts JK, Boden-Albala B, Gan Q: Testing the validity of the lacunar hypothesis: The Northern Manhattan Stroke Study experience. Neurology 1997;48: 1204–1210.
9   Qureshi AI, Safdar K, Patel M, Jannsen RS, Frankel MR: Stroke in young Black patients: Risk factors, subtypes, and prognosis. Stroke 1995;26:1995–1998.
10 Gross CR, Kase CS, Mohr JP, Cunningham SC, Baker WE: Stroke in South Alabama: Incidence and diagnostic features – A population based study. Stroke 1984;15:249–255.
11 Reimers J, deWytt C, Senevirantne B: Lacunar infarctions: A twelve month study. Clin Exp Neurol 1987;24:27–28.
12 Sacco SE, Whisnant JP, Broderick JP, Phillips SJ, O'Fallon WM: Epidemiologic characteristics of lacunar infarcts in a population. Stroke 1991;22:1236–1241.
13 Flack JM, Wiist WH: Epidemiology of hypertension and hypertensive target-organ damage in the United States. J Assoc Acad Minority Phys 1991;2:143–150.
14 Bell DS: Stroke in the diabetic patient. Diabetes Care 1994;17:213–219.
15 You R, Mcneil JJ, O'Malley HM, Davis SM, Donnan GA: Risk factors for lacunar infarction syndromes. Neurology 1996;47:1109–1110.
16 Mast H, Thompson JL, Lee S, Mohr JP, Sacco RL: Hypertension and diabetes mellitus as determinants of multiple lacunar infarcts. Stroke 1995;26:30–33.
17 You R, McNeil JJ, O'Malley HM, Davis SM, Donnan GA: Risk factors for lacunar infarction. Neurology 1995;45:1483–1487.
18 Caplan LR, Gorelick PB, Hier DB: Race, sex, and occlusive cerebrovascular disease: A review. Stroke 1986;17:648–655.
19 Bamford JM, Warlow CP: Evolution and testing of the lacunar hypothesis. Stroke 1988;19:1074–1082.

20   Besson G, Hommel M: Lacunar syndromes. Adv Neurol 1993;62:187–192.

21   Fisher CM, Curry HB: Pure motor hemiplegia of vascular origin. Arch Neurol 1965;13:130–140.

22   Richter RW, Brust JCM, Bruun B, Shafer SQ: Frequency and course of pure motor hemiparesis: A clinical study. Stroke 1977;8:58–70.

23   Fisher CM: Lacunar infarcts: A review. Cerebrovasc Dis 1991;4:311–320.

24   Fisher CM, Cole M: Homolateral ataxia and crural paresis: A vascular syndrome. J Neurol Neurosurg Psychiatry 1965;28:48–55.

25   Mohr JP, Kase CS, Meckler MD, Fisher CM: Sensorimotor stroke due to thalamocapsular ischemia. Arch Neurol 1977;34:739–741.

26   Nelson FR, Pullicino P, Kendall BE, Marshall J: Computed tomography in patients with lacunar syndromes. Stroke 1980;11:256–261.

27   Scharf J, Brauherr E, Forsting M, Sartor K: Significance of haemorrhagic lacunes on MRI in patients with hypertensive cerebrovascular disease and intracerebral haemorrhage. Neuroradiology 1994;36:504–508.

28   Iwasaki Y, Kinoshita M: Lacunar syndrome and intracerebral hemorrhage: Clinico-computed tomographic correlations. Comput Med Imaging Graph 1988;12:359–363.

29   Cacciatore A, Russo LS: Lacunar infarction as an embolic complication of cardiac and arch angiography. Stroke 1991;22:1603–1605.

30   Bogousslavsky MD, Barnett HJM, Fox AJ, Hachinski VC, Taylor W: Atherosclerotic disease of the middle cerebral artery. Stroke 1986;17:1112–1120.

31   Millikan C, Futrell N: The fallacy of the lacune hypothesis. Stroke 1990;21:1251–1257.

32   Heyman A, Fields WS, Keating RD: Joint study of extracranial arterial occlusion in hospitalized patients with ischemic stroke. JAMA 1972;222:285–289.

33   Rorick MB, Nichols FT, Adams RJ: Transcranial Doppler correlation with angiography in detection of intracranial stenosis. Stroke 1994;25:1931–1934.

34   Ley-Pozzo J, Ringelstein EB: Noninvasive detection of occlusive disease of the carotid siphon and middle cerebral artery. Ann Neurol 1990;28:640–647.

35   Zannette EM, Fieschi C, Bozzao L, Roberti C, Toni D, Angentino C, Lenzi GL: Comparison of cerebral angiography and transcranial doppler sonography in acute stroke. Stroke 1989;20:899–903.

36   D'Aprile P, Federico F, Medicamento N, Conte C, Carella A: Cerebral Ischemia: Magnetic resonance angiography and transcranial doppler evaluation. Ital J Neurol Sci 1994;15:39–47.

37   Kappelle LJ, Koudstall PJ, van Gijn J, Ramos LMP, Keunen JEE: Carotid angiography in patients with lacunar infarction: A prospective study. Stroke 1988;19:1093–1096.

38   Tegeler CH, Fenglin S, Terumi M: Carotid stenosis in lacunar stroke. Stroke 1991;22:1124–1128.

39   Salgado AV, Ferro JM, Gouveia-Oliveira A: Long-term prognosis of first ever lacunar strokes: A hospital-based study. Stroke 1996;27:661–666.

40   Anonymous: Carotid Endarterectomy for patients with symptomatic internal carotid artery stenosis. National Institute of Neurologic Disorders and Stroke. J Neurol Sci 1995;129:76–77.

41   Salgado AV, Ferro JM, Gouveia-Oliveira A: Long-term prognosis of first-ever lacunar strokes: A hospital-based study. Stroke 1996;27:661–666.

42   Albers GW, Comess KA, DeRook FA, Bracci P, Atwood JE, Bolger A, Holson J: Transesophageal echocardiographic findings in stroke subtypes. Stroke 1994;25:23–28.

43   Bogousslavsky J, Cahin C, Regli F, Despland PA, van Melle G, Kappenberger L: Cardiac sources of embolism and cerebral infarction-clinical consequences and vascular concomitants: The Laussanne Stroke registry. Neurology 1991;41:855–859.

44   Lodder J, Bamford JM, Sandercock PA, Jones LN, Warlow CP: Are hypertension or cardiac embolism likely causes of lacunar infarction? Stroke 1990;21:375–381.

45   Timsit SG, Sacco MS, Mohr JP, Foulkes MA, Tatemichi TK, Wolf PA, Price TR, Hier DB: Early clinical differentiation of cerebral infarction from severe atherosclerotic stenosis and cardioembolism. Stroke 1992;23:486–491.

46   Horowitz DR, Tuhrim S, Weinberger JM, Rudolf SW: Mechanisms in lacunar infarction. Stroke 1992;23:325–327.

47   Cerebral Embolism Task Force: Cardiogenic brain embolism. Arch Neurol 1989;46:727–734.

48 Tuszinsky MH, Petito CK, Levy DE: Risk factors and clinical manifestations of pathologically verified lacunar infarctions. Stroke 1989;20:990–999.

49 Bowen BC, Quencer RM, Margosian P, Pattany PM: Magnetic Resonance Angiography of occlusive disease of the arteries in the head and neck: Current concepts. Am J Roentgenol 1994;162:9–18.

50 Yin D, Takeuchi J: Comparison of MR angiography with x-ray angiography in patients with ischemic cerebrovascular diseases. Nippon Geka Hokan – Arch Jpn Chir 1993;62:241–248.

51 Wilterdink JL, Feldman E: Carotid stenosis: A neurologist's perspective. Neuroimag Clin N Am 1996;6:831–841.

52 Johnson BA, Heiserman JE, Drayer BP, Keller PJ: Intracranial MR angiography: Its role in the integrated approach to brain infarction. Am J Neuroradiol 1994;15:901–908.

53 Bridgers SL: Clinical correlates of Doppler/ultrasound errors in the detection of internal carotid artery occlusion. Stroke 1989;20:612–615.

54 Bornstein NM, Beloev ZG, Norris JW: The limitations of diagnosis of carotid occlusion by Doppler ultrasound. Ann Surg 1988;207:315–317.

55 Bramford J, Sandercock P, Dennis M, Burn J, Warlow C: Classification and natural history of clinically identifiable subtypes of cerebral infarction. Lancet 1991;337:1521–1525.

Gwendolyn F. Ford Lynch, MD, Department of Neurology,
Rush Medical College, Chicago, IL 60612 (USA)

Gillum RF, Gorelick PB, Cooper ES (eds): Stroke in Blacks. Basel, Karger, 1999, pp 29–35

....

Primary Intracerebral Hemorrhage and Subarachnoid Hemorrhage in Black Patients: Risk Factors, Diagnosis, and Prognosis

Jim Gebel, Joseph Broderick

Stroke Research Center, University of Cincinnati, Department of Neurology, Cincinnati, Ohio, USA

Primary or spontaneous intracerebral hemorrhage (ICH) and subarachnoid hemorrhage (SAH) comprise a disproportionate fraction of stroke-related morbidity and mortality in the Black population. This chapter begins with a brief review of the clinical presentation and diagnosis of ICH and SAH, and concludes with a brief review of their treatment. Its principal focus, however, is to summarize the available information on the known risk factors for these entities in Blacks. In so doing, we provide a frame of reference from which to consider future clinical and epidemiologic investigation.

Clinical Presentation and Diagnosis

The typical presentation of ICH and SAH in Blacks does not appreciably differ from that of other persons. The clinical triad of ICH includes abrupt onset of progressive focal neurologic deficits, headache, and diminished level of consciousness. ICH is clinically distinguished from thromboembolic ischemic stroke by a smooth progression of symptoms crossing vascular territories rather than abrupt and maximal symptoms at onset or a stepwise symptom progression more characteristic of cerebral infarction. The presence of headache and depressed level of consciousness, while possible in ischemic stroke, are more frequent and severe in ICH, and more often out of proportion to the anticipated size of the stroke as defined by its clinical signs and symptoms.

Despite these characteristic clinical features, our ability to properly diagnose ICH, particularly of small size, based on clinical grounds alone is poor. Computerized tomography (CT) scanning of the brain has dramatically improved our ability to diagnose ICH and to differentiate ICH from acute ischemic stroke. CT scanning is part of the standard diagnostic work-up for patients presenting with signs or symptoms of acute stroke.

The one nearly constant clinical symptom of SAH in those patients that retain consciousness is abrupt onset of severe headache, typically described as the worst headache of the patient's life. Immediate or subsequent loss of consciousness is frequent in severe SAH, and particularly in instances when there is intraventricular blood. Focal neurologic deficits, when present, may range from isolated cranial nerve palsies in cases where no parenchymal blood is present, to severe deficits where parenchymal blood is extensive. Although the clinical features of SAH are somewhat distinctive, our ability to clinically differentiate SAH from ICH, migraine, and ischemic stroke is at best fair. Again, CT of the brain has greatly improved our ability to detect acute SAH, being up to 92% sensitive within 24 h of SAH [1]. Lumbar puncture to detect red blood cells and/or xanthochromia in the cerebrospinal fluid is useful in instances where clinical suspicion is high but radiologic evidence is lacking. The most frequent reasons for failure of CT to detect SAH include delay in imaging after symptom onset, a very small amount of SAH, or rare instances where bleeding is confined to the spinal subarachnoid space. The most frequent underlying etiology of nontraumatic SAH is rupture of a berry aneurysm. Less frequent causes include rupture of an arteriovenous malformation, rupture of a mycotic aneurysm, and spontaneous SAH with no identified cause (often confined to the perimesencephalic cisterns). Four-vessel cerebral angiography is indicated to differentiate between these underlying causes, and is particularly important when the suspected cause is a berry aneurysm, since up to 20% of aneurysmal SAHs prove to have more than one aneurysm.

Incidence and Risk Factors

Although the overall incidence of stroke fell significantly during the 1960s and 1970s, the incidence rate of all strokes plateaued in the 1980s [2–4]. The incidence rate estimates reported for ICH during this same time period have varied widely from 9/100,000 to 80/100,000 [5], largely due to the lack of consistent verification of ICH by CT or autopsy in many of the earlier studies. These earlier studies were ethnically homogeneous (usually all White) and did not include Blacks or Hispanics in any significant number.

Table 1. Incidence of SAH and ICH among Blacks and Whites by age in 1988[1]

Age group	ICH		SAH	
	Blacks	Whites	Blacks	Whites
0–34	2	0.5	4	1
35–54	27	7	21	10
55–74	58	33	21	12
75+	36	156	19	21

[1] Crude (unadjusted) rate per 100,000 population. Data reproduced with permission.

The first reliable estimates of ICH incidence in Blacks became available during the CT era. In Greater Cincinnati in 1982, the annual incidence rate of ICH was found to be 17.5/100,000 per year [6] in Blacks as compared to 13.5/100,000 per year in Whites. In this study, a history of hypertension was more prevalent in Blacks (74%) versus Whites (40%, p=0.003). In a later study from Greater Cincinnati during 1988, the overall incidence rate of ICH in Blacks, age- and sex-adjusted to the 1980 US population, was 19/100,000 per year (95% CI of 12–26) [7, 8]. While this overall rate was not significantly different from the overall rate of ICH in Whites (15/100,000 per year, 95% CI of 12–17) during this same time period, the rate of ICH by age categories differed substantially between Blacks and Whites. Rates of ICH in Blacks peaked in the sixth and seventh decades of life and were significantly higher than in Whites of similar age up to the age of 75. The odds ratio of ICH for Blacks up to age 55, as compared to Whites of similar age, was 3.7, and 1.8 for Blacks ages 55–74. Above age 75, the incidence of ICH decreased in the Black population while exponentially increasing in Whites. This resulted in an odds ratio of ICH in Blacks age 75 and older of 0.23 as compared to Whites. However, the very small number of Blacks in this oldest age category in this study makes this estimate of ICH incidence in Blacks ages 75 and older less reliable (table 1). Rates of CT imaging of all stroke patients were similar (85% for Blacks and 84% for Whites), suggesting that a difference in detection rate does not explain the differences observed. This relationship of higher ICH incidence rates in young Blacks as compared to Whites has also been observed in a population-based study of stroke in the young in Baltimore County, Maryland, during 1988 [9].

More recent data from Greater Cincinnati during the first 6 months of 1993 [10] demonstrated an increase in the incidence rate of ICH in Blacks to 38/100,000 per year (95% CI of 25–52), which is over twice the rate of ICH observed in Greater Cincinnati during 1982 and 1988. Additional analysis is proceeding to determine whether this difference reflects a true change in the incidence of ICH among Blacks, is due to the smaller (6-month) sampling period, or represents an unrecognized detection bias. It is noteworthy that 98% of patients in this study had brain CT.

The reasons why young and middle-aged Blacks are at greater risk for ICH than other Americans are not clear. Although an increased prevalence of hypertension among Blacks may explain some of the increased incidence, it is unlikely to be the sole underlying cause. Additional factors may include increased rates of smoking or alcohol abuse, or additional unrecognized genetic or environmental risk factors. To better understand what factors may underlie the differences in the incidence rates of ICH between Blacks and Whites, we are conducting a systematic study of potential environmental and genetic risk factors among Blacks and Whites in the Greater Cincinnati region. We also plan to study the anatomic and radiologic patterns of ICH for Blacks and Whites.

Similar to ICH, the lack of consistent autopsy or CT confirmation of diagnosis and lack of demographic generalizability have plagued the early epidemiologic studies of SAH. Again, information regarding SAH incidence and pathogenesis in Blacks is limited. The age- and sex-adjusted annual incidence rate of SAH in Blacks from June 1987 to June 1989 in King County, Washington (10/100,000 per year) and in 1988 in Greater Cincinnati (12/100,000 per year) was twice that of Whites in these two communities [7, 11, 12]. Recent data from the Greater Cincinnati population indicate that the rate of SAH did not change during the first 6 months of 1993. This contrasts to the increase observed in ICH incidence rates in Blacks during this same time period as compared to 1988 [10]. In Greater Cincinnati during 1988, SAH incidence rates in Blacks and Whites increased with age, and the relative risk of SAH in Blacks in any given age group from 35 years on up remained approximately twice that of Whites [7]. The 30-day mortality rate of 44% in Blacks was identical to that observed in Whites. Rates of hypertension, a weaker risk factor for SAH than for ICH, were again comparable in Blacks (56%) with SAH as compared to Whites (50%). However, smoking, the strongest risk factor for SAH, was more prevalent among Blacks [8]. As for ICH, there is a clear need for systematic large-scale clinical and genetic studies of SAH in Blacks (tables 2, 3).

Treatment

The first and foremost treatment for ICH or SAH is prevention. The high prevalence of hypertension and smoking in the Black community make these

Table 2. Median (25th, 75th percentile) volumes (cm^3) of ICH in Blacks and Whites in Greater Cincinnati in 1988[1]

	Blacks (n=27)	Whites (n=161)
ICH	9 (6, 28)	24 (8, 59)
IVH	1 (0, 16)	0.7 (0, 17)
ICH, IVH	16 (8, 48)	36 (11, 78)

[1] Includes isolated intraventricular hemorrhage.

Table 3. Anatomic locations of ICH in Blacks and Whites in Greater Cincinnati in 1988[1]

Anatomic location	Blacks (n=27)	Whites (n=161)
Lobar	10 (37%)	64 (40%)
Deep hemisphere[1]	10 (37%)	79 (49%)
Pons	4 (15%)	6 (4%)
Cerebellum	2 (7%)	12 (7%)
Unknown	1 (4%)	0 (0%)

[1] Includes isolated intraventricular hemorrhage.

two risk factors ideal targets for primary prevention. Although the prevalence of untreated hypertension and hypertension-related morbidity and mortality have declined in Blacks since the introduction of antihypertensive therapy, the rate of this decline has lagged behind that of the general population [2, 3]. Unless these two treatable risk factors are more successfully controlled, it will be difficult to make a major impact on the morbidity and mortality of ICH and SAH in the Black community. Improved detection of persons at higher risk based upon genetic risk factors offers another primary prevention strategy insofar as that identification of relevant genes and testing thereof would offer the opportunity to periodically screen high-risk persons and to counsel them regarding smoking cessation and hypertension control.

The treatment of ICH once it has occurred has limited scientific basis and disappointingly, no treatment has been proven to favorably alter long-term outcome. Potential interventions include surgical evacuation of the hematoma mass by craniotomy or stereotactic aspiration; mannitol and other osmotic diuretics for treatment of perihematoma edema; blood pressure control in cases of severe hypertension; and corticosteroids for delayed edema formation.

Whether any or all of these modalities are used and in what circumstances varies greatly among treating physicians [13]. Randomized trials of ultra-early surgical intervention versus best medical therapy are needed to provide data for more rational therapeutic decision-making for clinicians who treat patients with ICH.

The treatment of acute SAH involves eliminating the underlying cause of SAH by clipping or coiling the responsible aneurysm(s) whenever feasible, and secondly, preventing and treating the delayed complications of SAH: hydrocephalus, salt wasting, and vasospasm. Acute hydrocephalus (typically within 24–48 h) is usually due to obstruction of the ventricular system by intraventricular blood whereas delayed (typically 2 weeks or later post-SAH) hydrocephalus is usually due to blockage of Pachonian (arachnoid) granulation from large amounts of subarachnoid blood, preventing absorption of cerebrospinal fluid. Both may respond to ventriculostomy and shunting. Cerebral arterial vasospasm is a delayed sequela of SAH, typically appearing between 4 and 14 days posthemorrhage. Treatment of vasospasm should consist of nimodipine administered orally every 4 h for all nonhypotensive patients with SAH. This has been shown to improve outcome in two major trials [14, 15]. Hypervolemic and hypertensive therapy are additional medical options for the treatment of symptomatic vasospasm. Intra-arterial papaverine infusion and/or angioplasty are more aggressive, invasive approaches to the treatment of arterial vasospasm. The cerebral salt wasting syndrome often observed after SAH can be a difficult problem, since it may trigger a precipitous diuresis of intravascular volume, resulting in acute hypotension and reflex plateau waves of increased intracranial pressure. Because Black patients with SAH are often chronically hypertensive, the associated shrinkage and lability of intravascular volume may make them susceptible to the adverse effects of salt wasting. Thus, an aggressive, proactive approach to maintain intravascular volume repletion and cerebral perfusion pressure is warranted. Treatment should consist of cm^3 for cm^3 replacement of fluid losses with isotonic crystalloid with or without colloid solution(s), in addition to appropriate maintenance fluids.

Conclusion

ICH and SAH are an important cause of an increased burden of disability and death in Blacks as compared to the general population, and comprise a larger proportion of the total (increased) stroke morbidity in this population. Because both types of hemorrhage occur at younger ages in Blacks as compared to Whites, the impact of this mortality as measured by person years of lost life is even greater than the differences in incidence rates. Increased prevalence of hypertension and smoking may explain some of the observed differences between Blacks and Whites and represent important targets of primary prevention for both SAH and ICH. However, other potentially important environmental factors and predisposing genetic factors should be a focus of future investigations.

References

1   Ho HW, Batjer HH: Aneurysmal subarachnoid hemorrhage: Pathophysiology and Sequelae; in Batjer H (ed): Cerebrovascular Disease. Philadelphia, Lippincott-Raven, 1997.
2   Brown RD, Whisnant JP, Sicks JD, O'Fallon WM, Wiebers DO: Stroke incidence, prevalence, and survival: Secular trends in Rochester, Minnesota, through 1989. Stroke 1996;27:373–380.
3   Broderick JP, Phillips SJ, Whisnant JP, O'Fallon WM, Bergstrahl MS: Incidence rates of stroke in the eighties: The end of the decline in stroke? Stroke 1989;20:577–582.
4   Gillum RF: The epidemiology of cardiovascular disease in Black Americans. N Engl J Med 1996; 335:1597–1599.
5   Broderick JP: Natural history of primary intracerebral hemorrhage; in Whisnant JP (ed): Population-Based Clinical Epidemiology of Stroke. Oxford, Butterworth-Heinemann, 1993.
6   Brott TG, Thalinger K, Hertzberg V: Hypertension as a risk factor for spontaneous intracerebral hemorrhage. Stroke 1986;17:1078–1083.
7   Broderick JP, Brott TG, Tomsick T, Miller R, Huster G: Intracerebral hemorrhage is more than twice as common as subarachnoid hemorrhage. J Neurosurg 1993;78:188–191.
8   Broderick JP, Brott TG, Tomsick T, Huster G, Miller R: The risk of subarachnoid and intracerebral hemorrhages in Blacks as compared with Whites. N Engl J Med 1992;326:733–736.
9   Kittner SJ, McCarter RJ, Sherwin RW, Sloan MA, Stern BJ, Johnson CJ, Buchholz D, Seipp MJ, Price TR: Black-White differences in stroke risk among young adults. Stroke 1993;24(suppl I):13–15.
10 Broderick JP, Brott TG, Kothari R, Miller R, Khoury J, Pancioli A, Gebel J, Mills D, Minneci L, Shukla R: The Greater Cincinnati/Northern Kentucky Stroke Study: Preliminary first-ever and total incidence rates of stroke among Blacks. Stroke 1998;29:415–421.
11 Longstreth WT, Nelson LM, Koepsell TD, van Belle G: Clinical course of spontaneous subarachnoid hemorrhage: A population-based study in King County, Washington. Neurology 1993;43:712–718.
12 Longstreth WT: Nontraumatic subarachnoid hemorrhage; in Gorelick P (ed): Handbook of Neuro-epidemiology. New York, Dekker, 1994.
13 Broderick J, Brott T, Zuccarello M: Management of Intracerebral Hemorrhage; in Batjer H (ed): Cerebrovascular Disease. Philadelphia, Lippincott-Raven, 1997.
14 Allen GS, Ahn HS, Preziosi TJ, Battye A, Boone SC, Chou SN, Kelly DL, Weir BK, Crabbe RA, Lavik PJ, Rosenbloom SB, Dorsey FC, Ingram CA, Mellits DE, Bertsch LA, Boisvert DP, Hundley MB, Johnson RE, Strom JA, Transon LA: Cerebral arterial spasm – A controlled trial of nimodipine in patients with subarachnoid hemorrhage. N Engl J Med 1983;308:619–624.
15 Pickard JD, Murray GD, Illingworth R, Shaw MDM, Teasdale GM, Foy PM, Humphrey PR, Lang DA, Nelson R, Richards P, et al: Effect of oral nimodipine on cerebral infarction and outcome after subarachnoid hemorrhage: British aneurysm nimodipine trial. Br Med J 1989;298:636–642.

Dr. Joseph Broderick, Stroke Research Center, University of Cincinnati, Department of Neurology, 4010 Medical Science Building, 231 Bethesda Avenue, Cincinnati, OH 45267-0525 (USA)

Gillum RF, Gorelick PB, Cooper ES (eds): Stroke in Blacks. Basel, Karger, 1999, pp 36–48

....
Cerebral Embolism and Procoagulant States

Bradley S. Jacobs [a] *, Ralph L. Sacco* [a] *, Milton Alter* [b]

[a] Neurological Institute, New York Presbyterian Hospital, New York, N.Y., and
[b] Division of Neurology, Lankenau Hospital, Wynnewood, Pa., USA

Cerebral embolism and procoagulant states are frequent causes of ischemic stroke. Many embolic sources and procoagulant states have only recently been established as risk factors for ischemic stroke and several are in the process of being evaluated. Some of these newly discovered stroke risk factors may help to explain a portion of strokes previously thought to have a cryptogenic etiology. The recognition of a cardiac etiology of stroke is critical, since specific treatments, such as anticoagulation, may significantly decrease the risk for stroke recurrence. The prevalence of some of these sources has been shown to differ in Blacks when compared to other race-ethnic populations; however, differences in treatment efficacy in Blacks when compared to other populations have not been well studied. In this chapter, we will discuss the most common sources of cerebral embolism, approaches to diagnosis and management, differences between African-American and Caucasian populations, less common cardioembolic sources, and some of the causes of hypercoagulable states.

Cerebral Embolic Stroke

Cardiogenic brain embolism, which accounts for the majority of cerebral emboli, is found to be the cause of ischemic stroke in approximately 15–20% of all such cases [1]. Three general categories of cardiac emboli are cardiac dysrhythmias, cardiac valve disorders, and cardiac wall disorders (table 1). The most common dysrhythmia associated with stroke is nonvalvular atrial fibrillation. The more common valvular diseases associated with stroke include

Table 1. Potential cardiac sources of emboli

Dysrhythmias
Definite
Atrial fibrillation
Possible
Sick sinus syndrome
Valvular disorders
Definite
Rheumatic heart disease
Infective endocarditis
Noninfective endocarditis
Prosthetic valves
Possible
Mitral annular calcification
Calcific aortic stenosis
Mitral valve prolapse
Bicuspid aortic valve
Wall disorders
Definite
Recent myocardial infarction
Left ventricular aneurysm
Cardiomyopathy
Cardiac tumors
Possible
Patent foramen ovale
Atrial septal defect
Atrial septal aneurysm

rheumatic heart disease, infective endocarditis, and noninfective ('marantic') endocarditis. The most common disorder of the cardiac wall associated with stroke is acute myocardial infarction with an associated left ventricular thrombus. In addition to the cardiac sources, aortic atherosclerosis has recently been found to be a source of emboli in persons with stroke.

Few stroke studies have included sufficient numbers of Blacks to make race-ethnic comparisons by stroke subtypes. Those studies that have evaluated the frequency of cerebral embolism in Blacks have yielded differences in the importance of cerebral embolism as a stroke subtype. Structural cardiac lesions were found to give rise to embolic stroke in 46% of South African Blacks admitted with stroke [2]. Only 20% of ischemic strokes in African-American patients less than 45 years old in Atlanta were found to have a cardioembolic etiology [3]. In Northern Manhattan, the proportion of cardioembolic stroke was less frequent in Blacks compared to Whites [4] (fig. 1) and the types of cardiac disease in stroke

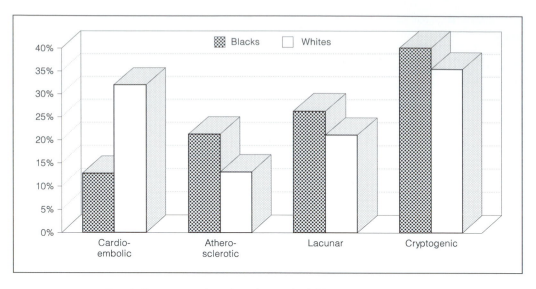

Fig. 1. Frequency of stroke subtypes in African-Americans and Whites in Northern Manhattan, 1993–1997.

patients varied as well (fig. 2) [5]. Moreover, the etiologic fraction of first ischemic strokes attributable to atrial fibrillation and other cardiac disease was lower in Blacks when compared to Whites and Hispanics [6].

Diagnosis of Cerebral Embolism

Past medical history, clinical presentation, neurologic exam, and brain imaging can assist in the diagnosis of cerebral embolism. Reports from the NINDS Stroke Data Bank have helped clarify some of the findings associated with cardiac embolism. When compared to large-vessel atherosclerotic stenosis, the more common clinical picture associated with cardioembolic infarct included a history of cardiac disease, decreased consciousness at onset of infarct, and language or visual field deficit. For atherosclerotic infarcts, the more common clinical findings included male gender, history of hypertension, diabetes, previous transient ischemic attack, previous stroke, and fractional arm weakness [7]. When classifying patients with a high, medium, or low risk of cardioembolic source, features consistent with a higher risk were history, or presence of, systemic embolism; abrupt onset of stroke; and decreased level of consciousness at onset [8]. Neurologic exam features suggestive of cardioembolism included diminished level of consciousness, visual field abnormalities, neglect, or aphasia. Pure motor hemiparesis was inversely associated with cardioembolic stroke [9]. Findings on computed tomography associated with

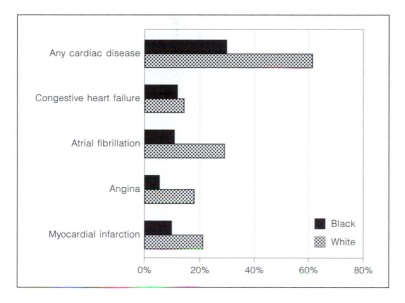

Fig. 2. Black-White differences in frequency of cardiac disease in patients with ischemic stroke in the Northern Manhattan Stroke Study [5].

a cardioembolic source include infarcts involving one half lobe or larger, or infarcts involving both superficial and deep structures. Small deep infarcts were inversely associated with cardioembolic stroke [10].

Diagnostic evaluation for these embolic sources includes electrocardiography and ambulatory EKG, chest X-ray, transthoracic echocardiography (TTE), and transesophageal echocardiography (TEE). The electrocardiogram can help determine any evidence of myocardial ischemia or dysrhythmia. If suspicion for arrhythmia is present from the clinical history but the electrocardiogram is normal, an ambulatory EKG should be obtained. Chest X-ray can be helpful in the diagnosis of heart failure.

TTE is helpful in determining the presence of valvular dysfunction and vegetations, wall motion abnormalities, thrombus, or masses. If a bubble study is performed with aerated saline, the presence of patent foramen ovale can be determined. TTE allows good visualization of left ventricular thrombus, large aortic and mitral valve vegetations, aortic and mitral stenosis, mitral valve prolapse, left ventricular wall motion abnormalities, left ventricular hypertrophy, and dilated cardiomyopathy [11]. The main disadvantage of TTE is that visualization of the left atrium and atrial appendage, interatrial septum, small valvular abnormalities, and the aortic arch may be inadequate. Moreover, poor chest acoustical penetration may limit the interpretation of some images.

While some abnormalities can be detected using TTE, assessment of the heart using TEE is a more sensitive test for certain types of cardiac dysfunction. TEE is performed by having the patient swallow a small ultrasound transducer and obtaining an image of the heart via the esophagus. Although this is a semi-invasive procedure with disadvantages of patient discomfort and cost, it is safe with very rare complications including arrhythmia, angina, bronchospasm, hypoxia, and pharyngeal or esophageal bleeding [12]. TEE is helpful in visualizing pathology including left atrial appendage thrombus, spontaneous echo contrast in the left atrium, patent foramen ovale or atrial septal defect, atrial septal aneurysm, atrial myxoma, small valvular vegetations, prosthetic valve vegetations, and aortic arch atherosclerosis [11].

Sources of Cerebral Embolism

Atrial Fibrillation (AF). In nonvalvular AF, stroke is most likely due to thrombus formation in the left atrium or left atrial appendage and subsequent embolism. AF is the etiology of 6–24% of all ischemic strokes. It is associated with an incidence of transient ischemic attack (TIA) or stroke of 8% per year in patients over 60 years old [1]. The risk of ischemic stroke associated with AF has been shown to increase with the presence of other risk factors including history of hypertension, prior stroke or TIA, diabetes, and age greater than 65 years. The absence of all of these high-risk variables reduces the risk of ischemic stroke to 1.0% per year. The presence of these high-risk variables can increase the risk of stroke to 4–8% per year [13]. Excess stroke risk associated with AF may be reduced through the use of warfarin. The risk of infarct with AF and treatment of AF have not been specifically studied in Black populations.

In Northern Manhattan, among hospitalized patients with cerebral infarction, fewer African-Americans (11%) and Hispanics (11%) than Whites (29%) had AF [5]. The attributable risk of AF for first ischemic stroke was 20% in Whites, while only 2% in Hispanics and 3% in Blacks [6] (fig. 3). Of consecutive patients hospitalized in Detroit, Michigan, 50% of patients without AF were African-American, whereas only 33% of patients with AF were African-American [14]. AF was present in only 0.74% of 267 South African Black patients admitted with stroke including infarct (71%), parenchymal hemorrhage (26%), and subarachnoid hemorrhage (3%) [2]. In summary, few studies have specifically addressed the frequency of AF and its association with stroke in Blacks. From the studies available, AF is possibly less common among African-Americans and is less often associated with stroke in African-Americans than in Whites.

Cardiac Valve Disorders. The cardiac valve disorders most clearly and commonly associated with stroke are rheumatic heart disease with mitral

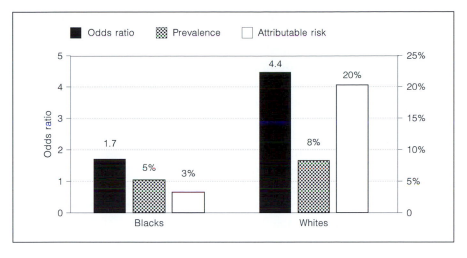

Fig. 3. Odds ratio, prevalence, and attributable risk of AF for ischemic stroke in African-Americans and Whites in the Northern Manhattan Stroke Study [6].

stenosis, infective and noninfective endocarditis, and prosthetic valves. Patients with rheumatic heart disease have approximately a 20% chance of systemic emboli with untreated disease and yearly rates of embolism of 4% per year. Thrombus, which forms in the left atrium, is often the source of embolism. Risk of embolization with rheumatic heart disease and AF is increased 17-fold compared to persons with no valvular disease or atrial fibrillation. After an initial embolic event, 30–75% of people not treated with anticoagulation have recurrence, usually within 6–12 months [15]. Overall rates of rheumatic heart disease have declined, but no studies address this specifically in African-Americans.

Infective endocarditis carries a risk of stroke of 15–20%. Diagnosis is based on blood cultures and echocardiography. Treatment consists of antibiotics, which usually prevents stroke occurrence. Noninfective ('marantic') endocarditis is seen in association with cancer and also with the antiphospholipid antibody syndrome and systemic lupus erythematosus (Libman-Sacks endocarditis). Treatment with anticoagulation is often recommended to prevent stroke recurrence. Mechanical prosthetic valves have a risk of embolism of about 2–4% per year when anticoagulated, which is similar to the embolic risk of a bioprosthetic valve without anticoagulation.

Cardiac Wall Disorders. Common cardiac wall disorders include myocardial infarction (MI), ventricular aneurysm, and patent foramen ovale (PFO). Approximately 3% of patients with acute MI have an ischemic stroke within the first 4 weeks of the event. Most of these strokes occur within the first 2 weeks and most are associated with anterior wall infarction and left ventricular mural thrombus. In Northern Manhattan, Whites with ischemic stroke have a greater frequency of history of MI (21%) than Blacks (10%) [5]. Among 116 South African Blacks over the age of 20 with stroke (67% ischemic and 33% hemorrhagic), none had evidence of cardiac disease by history or electrocardiography [16]. While it is likely that acute MI in blacks carries the same stroke risk as in Whites, MI may account for fewer strokes relative to the other stroke etiologies in Blacks. The treatment for prevention of stroke in acute MI is usually short-term anticoagulation.

PFO is commonly found in the general population (22–35%). Several studies have shown PFO to be more common among patients with cryptogenic stroke than in the general population [17]. Most studies of PFO as a risk factor have been conducted in predominantly White populations. In a preliminary report from Northern Manhattan, PFO was determined to be a more potent risk factor for ischemic stroke in Hispanics and Whites (with odds ratios of 2.7 and 1.8), than in African-Americans (odds ratio of 0.9) [18]. The mechanism of stroke with PFO is likely thrombus either in the lower extremity, pelvic venous circulation or heart. The optimal treatment has not been determined and ranges from antiplatelet agents to anticoagulants and depends on the stroke clinical syndrome, size of the PFO, and other associated features. The efficacy of mechanical closure of a PFO is currently being investigated.

Aortic Atheroma. Aortic atheroma has recently been found to be associated with ischemic stroke. The odds ratio of ischemic stroke was 9.1 (95% confidence interval of 3.3–25.2) in patients with atherosclerotic plaques ≥4 mm. In addition, patients without an obvious cause of infarct were more likely to have an atherosclerotic aortic arch than patients with a possible or known cause of stroke [19]. In Northern Manhattan, aortic atheroma was again found to be a significant independent stroke risk factor. No significant differences existed among different race-ethnic groups, but Hispanics had fewer small atheromas (2–4 mm) than Blacks or Whites [20]. Complex aortic lesions that are thought to be the cause of embolic stroke include highly mobile and pedunculated plaque protruding more than 7.5–10 mm, ulcerated plaque with a cavity of more than 5 mm in depth, and plaque with a mobile thrombus [21]. It is unclear whether antiplatelet agents or anticoagulation is the best treatment to prevent recurrence. The clinical stroke syndrome and complexity of the aortic lesion, among other factors, may help to determine the best treatment strategy.

Procoagulant States

Procoagulant states are a less common etiology of stroke, accounting for up to 8% of all ischemic strokes [22]. There is likely to be a greater incidence in young persons with stroke or older persons with a stroke but no clear etiology. As we gain a better understanding of the coagulation system and its disorders, the importance of procoagulant states as a risk factor for stroke is being clarified. Procoagulant states may uncommonly be a primary cause of stroke, but when combined with other stroke risk factors, it may significantly contribute to the development of stroke. The treatment of many of these disorders is anticoagulation.

Procoagulant states can be divided into subtypes of hematological abnormalities (table 2). Among the disorders of natural anticoagulants, activated protein C resistance is most common, followed by protein S, protein C, and antithrombin III deficiencies. These disorders are associated with thrombophilia, but their association with ischemic stroke is not as clear. Immune-mediated disorders associated with a hypercoagulable state and ischemic stroke are antiphospholipid antibody syndrome and, less commonly, thrombotic thrombocytopenic purpura. Disorders involving excess, deficient, and dysfunctional erythrocytes are associated with stroke. Most notable is sickle cell anemia in Blacks. Platelet disorders, most commonly essential thrombocythemia, and white blood cell disorders are also associated with procoagulant states and stroke. Our discussion will focus on defects of the natural anticoagulants and the antiphospholipid antibody syndrome.

Antithrombin III (ATIII) is a plasma glycoprotein synthesized in endothelial cells and hepatocytes. It inhibits thrombin and other factors in the coagulation cascade. Both hereditary and acquired deficiencies may predispose to thrombophilia. Venous thrombosis is more common than arterial thrombosis and stroke [22]. When evaluated in the acute phase of stroke, ATIII deficiency was found in 3.6% of Whites compared to 7.0% of Blacks. This was a nonsignificant difference in a prospective study of 128 ischemic stroke patients [23].

Protein S is a vitamin K-dependent glycoprotein synthesized in the liver and is a cofactor for activated protein C which inactivates factor V and factor VIII in the coagulation cascade (fig. 4). Protein S deficiency may be hereditary or acquired and results in a hypercoagulable state. Approximately 60% of protein S is bound in plasma, while 40% is free and active. Protein S deficiency may be responsible for about 5% of venous thromboses, but its association with ischemic stroke is less clear [22]. Of consecutive patients with ischemic stroke, 1.2% of Whites and 7.0% of Blacks had a free protein S deficiency. African-Americans also had a significantly lower mean level of free protein S than Whites [23]. In a case-control study which showed that free protein

Table 2. Procoagulant states potentially associated with
ischemic strokes

Anticoagulant disorders
    Antithrombin III
    Protein S
    Protein C
    Activated protein C resistance – factor V Leiden
    Plasminogen
    Plasminogen activator

Procoagulant excess
    Factor V
    Factor VIII
    Factor X
    Fibrinogen

Antiphospholipid antibody syndrome

Cellular hematological disorders
Erythrocyte disorders
    Disorders of hemoglobin
        Sickle cell disease
        Thalassemia
    Polycythemia
    Anemia
Leukocyte disorders
    Leukemia
    Lymphoma
    Plasma cell disorders
        Waldenström's macroglobulinemia
        Myeloma
        Cryoglobulinemia
Platelet disorders
    Thrombocytosis
    Thrombocytopenia

S deficiency was not more common in stroke patients when compared to
hospitalized controls, the frequency of deficiency was significantly greater in
Blacks (34%) compared to non-Blacks (13%) [24]. In a series of young Blacks
with stroke in Atlanta, 6% of 112 ischemic strokes were diagnosed with protein
S deficiency [3]. It is not clear from the above studies, whether lower protein
S levels are associated with an increased risk of stroke, but the prevalence of
this deficiency may be greater among African-Americans.

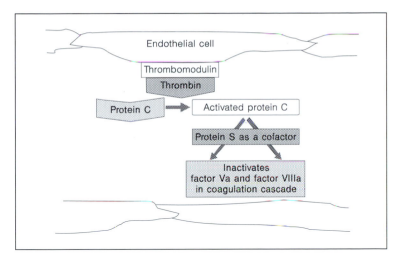

Fig. 4. Coagulation cascade involving protein C, protein S, and factors V and VIII.

Protein C is also vitamin K-dependent and synthesized in the liver. It is activated by thrombin and then inactivates factors V and VIII using protein S as a cofactor. Protein C deficiency may be acquired or hereditary and result in a hypercoagulable state. Congenital deficiency may result in approximately 6–10% of venous thromboses. Numerous case reports have shown stroke to be associated with protein C deficiency [22]. In Tennessee, low protein C levels were found more frequently among Blacks than Whites and the mean level of functional protein C was significantly lower in Blacks [23]. Again, it has yet to be shown whether protein C deficiency is a greater risk factor for stroke in Blacks than in Whites.

Activated protein C resistance has been found with a mutation in the factor V gene, namely factor V Leiden. This is the most common known etiology of venous thrombosis, resulting in about 20% of such cases. It is less clearly associated with ischemic stroke [22]. In New Haven, approximately equal percentages of Blacks (1.4%) and Whites (1.6%) were found to have factor V Leiden [25]. In the Physicians' Health Study and Women's Health Study, the carrier frequency of factor V Leiden was 5.27% in Whites compared to 1.23% in African-Americans [26]. In Virginia, healthy Whites had a prevalence of factor V Leiden of 3.3% compared to healthy Blacks with a prevalence of 1.25% [27]. The prevalence of factor V Leiden was 0.6% in a Black population with sickle cell trait or disease. It was not, however, more frequent in those patients with sickle cell disease who had stroke [28]. Factor V Leiden is likely a less important cause of stroke among African-Americans.

Antiphospholipid antibodies are polyclonal immunoglobulins that bind negatively charged or neutral phospholipids. Anticardiolipin antibodies and lupus anticoagulants are the major antiphospholipid antibodies and have been associated with venous and arterial thrombosis, including ischemic stroke. Anticardiolipin antibodies are found in approximately 10% of stroke patients [29] and are more common than lupus anticoagulant. The odds ratio for stroke given the presence of anticardiolipin antibodies is 2.31 after adjusting for other traditional stroke risk factors [29]. The stroke recurrence rate in patients with anticardiolipin antibodies is about 10% and is higher in young persons with stroke [22]. Lupus anticoagulant associated with stroke was found more frequently in Blacks (56%) compared to Whites (35%) [23]. The prevalence of antiphospholipid antibodies and their associated stroke risk has not been well studied in African-Americans. In one series of stroke in young Blacks in Atlanta, 4% of ischemic strokes were thought to have antiphospholipid antibody as an etiology [3].

Diagnosis of Procoagulant States

All patients with ischemic stroke do not require a complete hypercoagulable work-up. Every stroke patient should have a screening complete blood count, activated partial thromboplastin time, and prothrombin time. If the patient has a history of spontaneous abortions, previous thrombotic events, collagen vascular disease, or thrombocytopenia, an evaluation for antiphospholipid antibodies is required. If there is a family history of thrombophilia, then a search for a natural anticoagulant deficiency is warranted.

If the patient is relatively young (less than 50 years old) and without well-recognized stroke risk factors, then work-up for a hypercoagulable state should be pursued. The basic battery of tests would include measures of ATIII, protein C, protein S, lupus anticoagulant, anticardiolipin antibodies, and activated protein C resistance. If activated protein C resistance is present, then the patient should be tested for factor V Leiden. Most of these tests should not be ordered in the early phase of an acute stroke. Ideally, testing should be done several weeks after an acute stroke [22]. Some of these tests may have their results altered by anticoagulation or specific clinical circumstances. ATIII activity may be falsely lowered by heparin therapy, liver disease, nephrotic syndrome, disseminated intravascular coagulation, and possibly with oral contraceptives. Protein C and protein S activity may be falsely lowered with warfarin, vitamin K deficiency, liver disease, and DIC. In addition, protein S may be falsely lowered during pregnancy, with the use of oral contraceptives, and possibly with nephrotic syndrome. Activated protein C resistance and lupus anticoagulant testing may be affected by heparin.

Conclusion

Cerebral embolism and procoagulant states are frequently associated with ischemic stroke. Although not thoroughly studied within Black populations, it appears that certain types of stroke associated with embolism or procoagulant states may have different frequencies in the Black population. Cardiac disease, in particular MI, AF, and PFO, may be less frequently associated with ischemic stroke in Blacks than in Whites. Some procoagulant states, specifically protein S and protein C deficiencies, may be more common in Blacks, but it is not clear whether they increase the risk of ischemic stroke in Blacks. Further studies will be required to determine if the differences mentioned above contribute significantly to differences in stroke etiology within Black populations. These etiologic differences may be important in determining a more appropriate stroke work-up and choosing the best stroke therapy in Blacks.

References

1   Cerebral Embolism Task Force: Cardiogenic brain embolism: The second report of the cerebral embolism task force. Arch Neurol 1989;46:727–743.
2   Joubert J: The MEDUNSA Stroke Data Bank. South Afr Med J 1991;80:567–570.
3   Qureshi AI, Safdar K, Patel M, Janssen RS, Frankel MR: Stroke in young Black patients: Risk factors, subtypes, and prognosis. Stroke 1995;26:1995–1998.
4   Sacco RL, Kargman DE, Gu Q, Zamanillo MC: Race-ethnicity and determinants of intracranial atherosclerotic cerebral infarction: The Northern Manhattan Stroke Study. Stroke 1995;26:14–20.
5   Sacco RL, Kargman DE, Zamanillo MC: Race-ethnic differences in stroke risk factors among hospitalized patients with cerebral infarction: The Northern Manhattan Stroke Study. Neurology 1995;45:659–663.
6   Abel GA, Sacco RL, Lin IF, Boden-Albala B, Kargman DE, Paik MC: Race-ethnic variability in etiologic fraction for stroke risk factors: The Northern Manhattan Stroke Study (abstract). Stroke 1998;29:277.
7   Timsit SG, Sacco RL, Mohr JP, Foulkes MA, Tatemichi TK, Wolf PA, Price TR, Hier DB: Early clinical differentiation of cerebral infarction from severe atherosclerotic stenosis and cardioembolism. Stroke 1992;23:486–491.
8   Kittner SJ, Sharkness CM, Price TR, Plotnick GD, Dambrosia JM, Wolf PA, Mohr JP, Hier DB, Kase CS, Tuhrim S: Infarcts with a cardiac source of embolism in the NINCDS Stroke Data Bank: Historical features. Neurology 1990;40:281–284.
9   Kittner SJ, Sharkness CM, Sloan MA, Price TR, Dambrosia JM, Tuhrim S, Wolf PA, Mohr JP, Hier DB, Caplan LR: Infarcts with a cardiac source of embolism in the NINDS Stroke Data Bank: Neurologic examination. Neurology 1992;42:299–302.
10 Kittner SJ, Sharkness CM, Sloan MA, Price TR, Dambrosia JM, Tuhrim S, Wolf PA, Mohr JP, Hier DB: Features on initial computed tomography scan of infarcts with a cardiac source of embolism in the NINDS Stroke Data Bank. Stroke 1992;23:1748–1751.
11 Hart RG: Cardiogenic embolism to the brain. Lancet 1992;339:589–593.
12 Daniel WG, Erbel R, Kasper W, Visser CA, Engberding R, Sutherland GR, Grube E, Hanrath P, Maisch B, Dennig K, Schartl M, Kremer P, Angermann C, Iliceto S, Curtius JM, Mugge A: Safety of transesophageal echocardiography: A multicenter survey of 10,419 examinations. Circulation 1991;83:817–821.

13   Atrial Fibrillation Investigators: Risk factors for stroke and efficacy of antithrombotic therapy in atrial fibrillation. Arch Intern Med 1994;154:1449–1457.

14   Ali AS, Fenn NM, Zarowitz BJ, Niemyski P, Vitarelli A, Gheorghiade M: Epidemiology of atrial fibrillation in patients hospitalized in a large hospital. Panminerva Med 1993;35:209–213.

15   Streifler JY, Furlan AJ, Barnett HJM: Cardiogenic brain embolism: Incidence, varieties, treatment; in Barnett HJM, Mohr JP, Stein BM, Yatsu FM (eds): Stroke: Pathophysiology, Diagnosis, and Management. New York, Churchill Livingstone, 1992, pp 977–978.

16   Rosman KD: The epidemiology of stroke in an urban Black population. Stroke 1986;17:667–669.

17   Sacco RL, Homma S, DiTullio MR: Patent foramen ovale: A new risk factor for ischemic stroke. Heart Dis Stroke 1993;2:235–241.

18   Di Tulio MR, Sacco RL, Sciacca R, Savoia MT, Nahar T, Boden-Albala B, Mendoza L, Thompson E, Homma S: Patent foramen ovale as a risk factor for ischemic stroke in a multiethnic population (abstract). Stroke 1998;29:277.

19   Amarenco P, Cohen A, Tzourio C, Bertrand B, Hommel M, Besson G, Chauvel C, Touboul P, Bousser M: Atherosclerotic disease of the aortic arch and the risk of ischemic stroke. N Engl J Med 1994;331:1474–1479.

20   Di Tullio MR, Sacco RL, Gersony D, Nayak H, Weslow RG, Kargman DE, Homma S: Aortic atheromas and acute ischemic stroke: A transesophageal echocardiographic study in an ethnically mixed population. Neurology 1996;46:1560–1566.

21   Liebson PR, Soble JS, Neumann AL: Echocardiography in the assessment of cerebrovascular events; in Gorelick PB (ed): Atlas of Cerebrovascular Disease. Philadelphia, Current Medicine, 1996, pp 11.14–11.15.

22   Tatlisumak R, Fisher M: Hematologic disorders associated with ischemic stroke. J Neurol Sci 1996; 140:1–11.

23   Gaines KJ, Chesney C, Van der Zwaag R, Cape C: Racial differences in coagulation studies in stroke. Neurol Res 1992;14(suppl):103–108.

24   Mayer SA, Sacco RL, Hurlet-Jensen A, Shi T, Mohr JP: Free protein S deficiency in acute ischemic stroke: A case-control study. Stroke 1993;24:224–227.

25   Pottinger P, Sigurdsson F, Berliner N: Detection of the factor V Leiden mutation in a nonselected black population. Blood 1996;87:2091.

26   Ridker PM, Miletich JP, Hennekens CH, Buring JE: Ethnic distribution of factor V Leiden in 4,047 men and women. JAMA 1997;277:1305–1307.

27   Ferreira-Gonzalez A, Fisher LM, Lehman CM, Langley MH, Lofland DH, Xia Q, Nguyen NX, Modesto D, Willoughby JB, Wilkinson DS, Garrett CT: Detection of a common mutation in factor V gene responsible for resistance to activated protein C causing predisposition to thrombosis. J Clin Lab Anal 1997;11:328–335.

28   Kahn MJ, Scher C, Rozans M, Michaels RK, Leissinger C, Krause J: Factor V Leiden is not responsible for stroke in patients with sickling disorders and is uncommon in African-Americans with sickle cell disease. Am J Hematol 1997;54:12–15.

29   The Antiphospholipid Antibodies in Stroke Study (APASS) Group: Anticardiolipin antibodies are an independent risk factor for first ischemic stroke. Neurology 1993;43:2069–2073.

Ralph L. Sacco, MD, MS, Neurological Institute, Room 547,
710 West 168th Street, New York, NY 10032 (USA)

Gillum RF, Gorelick PB, Cooper ES (eds): Stroke in Blacks. Basel, Karger, 1999, pp 49–61

....

Clinical Assessment of Cerebrovascular Disease in African-Americans

Ultrasound, Neuroradiology, and Other Modalities

Kenneth Gaines[a], *Richard Levy*[a], *Mark DeLano*[b]

[a] Field Neuroscience Institute, St. Mary's Medical Center, Michigan State University, College of Human Medicine, Saginaw, Mich., and
[b] Department of Radiology, Michigan State University, College of Human Medicine, East Lansing, Mich., USA

Stroke affects African-Americans more frequently and at younger ages than most other Americans [1–12]. Neuroimaging and related diagnostic studies are useful in delineating the distribution and extent of occlusive cerebrovascular disease and, thus, may be useful in explaining racial differences in stroke. Although stroke mortality has been declining for the last 30 years, the stroke mortality in African-Americans remains almost twice as high as that in Whites [1]. Reasons for the mortality differential have been the topic of several reviews and much speculation, but an adequate explanation for this differential remains elusive [2]. Further information on the epidemiology of Black-White differences in stroke can be found in other chapters in this monograph.

This chapter will review the anatomic differences in stroke subtype and vessel pathology in Blacks that are relevant to radiological evaluation. We will discuss the role of standard imaging techniques, such as computerized tomography (CT), magnetic resonance imaging (MRI), and ultrasound, as well as newer imaging techniques such as magnetic resonance angiography (MRA), computerized tomographic angiography (CTA), transcranial Doppler (TCD) and functional MRI. This chapter will discuss the radiological evaluation of the acute stroke patient. This is important as many new therapies for stroke are being designed to salvage brain tissue in the acute stroke period. We will also discuss the economic aspects of the radiological evaluation as they might impact the African-American stroke patient. Finally, we will present an algorithm for clinicoradiologic evaluation of the acute stroke patient, discuss how this evaluation can be done in a cost-effective manner, and review the circumstances where such an evaluation might be tailored to the African-American stroke patient.

Neuroimaging in Stroke

Imaging tests used in the evaluation of the stroke patient provide both structural and functional information about the brain. CT and MRI define anatomic areas of stroke involvement. Angiography, MRA, CTA, and ultrasound define blood vessel lesion extent, type, and location. Single photon emission computed tomography (SPECT) and positron emission tomography (PET) have been, until recently, the only functional imaging techniques available. Functional MRI imaging, a newer technique, is becoming established as its usefulness in stroke diagnosis is being defined. Functional MRI imaging techniques include diffusion and perfusion imaging and magnetic resonance spectroscopy. In the sections that follow we will outline the relative merits of the various types of imaging modalities for defining the underlying pathophysiology of stroke.

CT Imaging in Stroke

The primary modality used in the evaluation of acute stroke is noncontrast CT. CT has wide availability and has a high sensitivity for detection of acute hemorrhage. Unfortunately, CT is relatively insensitive to the early changes of acute stroke. Detection of infarction is dependent on the development of edema with an associated decrease in CT density and swelling of the affected brain tissue. This results in a delay in the CT diagnosis of ischemic stroke, with changes developing in approximately 60% of patients at 24 h, and at least 90% of patients by 48 h. Some changes have been reported in large acute infarcts as early as 6 h post-ictus. The pathologic changes are mostly irreversible by this time, and the time window for effective acute therapeutic intervention to impact the natural history of cerebral ischemia has largely passed.

The CT findings of acute ischemic stroke are subtle mass effect with gyral swelling and sulcal effacement, loss of distinction between gray and white matter structures, and decreased density of edematous tissues. Other early signs of stroke include: (1) the loss of the insular cortical ribbon due to insular edema (insular ribbon sign), and (2) a thrombus in the middle cerebral artery (MCA) (dense MCA sign), which is an uncommon finding that can be seen in isolation of the other manifestations of stroke when imaging is obtained early. CT detection of infarcts in the posterior fossa is limited by artifact caused by the dense skull base and may not be seen until late or not at all depending on the size of the lesion. Likewise, lacunar infarction is difficult to detect acutely and is usually found late as a focal, round hypodense lesion less than 15 mm in diameter. Lacunar infarction may be difficult to differentiate from a dilated perivascular or Virchow-Robin space. Recognition of the typical location of these entities may resolve the dilemma. Identification of hemorrhagic infarction is much less problematic. The high contrast that is found between acute hematoma and surrounding normal brain parenchyma and the associated mass effect assure early detection of hemorrhagic infarction.

The added value of CT in acute stroke management has been to exclude those patients with acute hemorrhage, large completed infarction, and non-stroke diseases from treatment with thrombolysis. The presence of hemorrhage precludes thrombolysis as there is unacceptable morbidity and mortality associated with such treatment. Patients with large completed infarction are unlikely to realize benefit from delayed thrombolysis and may be at heightened risk of hemorrhagic conversion.

MR Imaging in Stroke

MRI affords greater sensitivity to anatomic changes, but is insensitive to acute hemorrhage when compared with CT. Tissue characterization in MRI is dependent on multiple parameters, primarily tissue proton density and the T1 and T2. Images are optimized or 'weighted' to emphasize signal from tissues with high proton density, short T1 times, or long T2 times. Conventional MR images reflect the variation in these parameters in normal and pathological tissue. Patient motion is an additional parameter that becomes important in the consideration of the MRA and the functional MRI techniques (see below).

MRI findings in brain ischemia include mass effect arising from edema, parenchymal signal alterations, and vascular flow abnormalities. The MRI features of acute cortical stroke result from gray matter edema with gyral swelling. This manifests as increased proton density and T2 prolongation and hyperintensity on proton density and T2-weighted images. Fluid attenuated inversion recovery (FLAIR) techniques nullify signal from cerebrospinal fluid (CSF) often making subtle cortical infarcts more conspicuous than seen on routine T2 or proton-density-weighted images. Although T1-weighted scans effectively demonstrate gyral swelling, decreased signal intensity due to edema is a late finding. Acute infarcts are more frequently detected with MRI than with CT. T2-weighted MRI imaging may be normal up to 8 h after the vascular insult [13], although in animal studies T2 changes have been detected as early as one hour after infarction [14]. Vascular flow abnormalities on MRI images during acute ischemia can be detected immediately as the loss of the normal vascular flow void in the affected vessel. This is indicative of either slow or absent flow in the involved vessel. The use of gadolinium-based contrast media can improve detection of acute infarction by the demonstration of intra-arterial enhancement. Vascular enhancement has been reported as early as 2 h after a complete occlusion and clinical onset of symptoms, and significantly before the onset of T2-weighted signal abnormality [15]. Others have found this sign within 3 days of the vascular insult in 75% of patients with supratentorial cortical infarction [16]. The sign is quite uncommon in brainstem and deep cerebral infarctions, and is transient and usually absent after the first postinfarct week [17].

Detection of white matter and lacunar infarcts is more difficult than detection of cortical infarction as changes are not typically seen until after 24 h. The MRI features of lacunar infarction are small, focal regions of hypointensity on T1 and hyperintensity on T2-weighted images with progressive change toward CSF signal characteristics. Lacunes typically remain slightly hyperintense relative to CSF on proton-density-weighted and FLAIR techniques into the chronic stage, but often become isointense to CSF making differentiation from a dilated perivascular space more difficult.

The subacute stage of infarction begins between 24 and 48 h after stroke onset. Infarcts achieve a chronic appearance by 4 weeks postinsult. The appearance of a subacute infarct on CT or MRI is dependent on the degree of edema, the state of reperfusion or collateral flow, and the presence or absence of hemorrhage. As the edema begins to resolve, an infarct begins to organize or develop petechial hemorrhage, and an infarcted region may become isodense with normal brain parenchyma on noncontrast CT. This phenomenon is known as 'fogging', alluding to the clouding or opacification of a previously hypodense region during the subacute stage. As the infarct evolves into a chronic lesion there is encephalomalacia and volume loss reflecting brain tissue necrosis.

Parenchymal enhancement with either CT or MRI contrast agents depends on the agent arriving at the site of insult. No contrast enhancement will be seen in complete occlusion unless collateral vascular channels deliver the agent to the injured brain tissue. Partial or transient occlusion with resultant brain injury may demonstrate enhancement independent of collateral circulation. Signs of contrast enhancement are also dependent on the disruption of the blood-brain barrier, which allows for abnormal local accumulation of contrast. CT scans demonstrate enhancement in the second week and maximal enhancement in the third week. Enhancement generally persists until the seventh week although it may persist for more than 6 months in large infarctions [18]. The development of contrast enhancement on MR is earlier than that seen with CT, although peak enhancement develops according to a similar time frame (7–30 days after cortical infarction).

Functional Neuroimaging

The primary utility of MRI in the management of acute stroke has, until recently, been limited to demonstrating the extent of irreversible change or infarction and vascular narrowing or occlusion. The introduction of diffusion-weighted techniques allows the detection of acute ischemic change within minutes of the vaso-occlusive event. Diffusion-weighted imaging is sensitive to the motion of water through the intracellular and interstitial spaces, making the scan exquisitely sensitive to the pathologic alterations induced by acute infarction. Early detection of these changes provides the opportunity to intervene with thrombolytic or neuroprotective agents prior to irreversible ischemic changes. Perfusion-weighted or so-called dynamic susceptibility contrast (DSC) imaging detects the arrival of an intravenous bolus of gadolinium contrast agent for the detection of regions with absent or diminished perfusion. The added value of DSC scans when used in conjunction with diffusion-weighted imaging is related to the identification of tissues at risk for infarction – the ischemic penumbra.

Radiological Evaluation in African-American Stroke Patients

Given differences between Blacks and Whites in the frequency of various stroke subtypes and in the location of atherosclerosis, clinicians should consider utilizing these differences to tailor the imaging evaluation. While extracranial occlusive disease and cardiac embolism may be more common among Whites, it is intracranial occlusive disease, lacunar infarct, and hypertensive intracranial hemorrhage that may be more common among Blacks; yet, these differences are only relative and not absolute. This was demonstrated in the South Alabama stroke incidence study where stroke subtypes were defined for Blacks and Whites [3]. In particular, where atherothrombotic vascular lesions are amenable to treatment (i.e. by endarterectomy or angioplasty), such lesions should be appropriately and aggressively sought to reduce recurrence rates following initial stroke.

Stroke is not a single disease but multiple syndromes that are the manifestation of different pathophysiologic mechanisms. Correctly defining the stroke pathophysiology – cardioembolic, hemodynamic, artery-to-artery embolus, coagulopathy, arteritis, and large or small vessel disease – is critical in the clinical decision regarding appropriate acute stroke intervention and secondary stroke prevention.

Distinguishing between intracranial atherosclerotic disease and other intracranial vascular lesions, i.e. arteritis, can occasionally be difficult. Figure 1a–e shows MRI and angiographic studies from a 60-year-old African-American

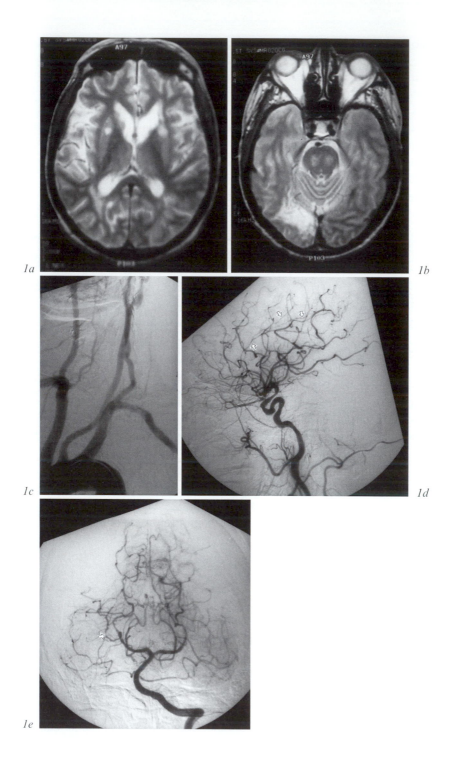

1a
1b
1c
1d
1e

male patient that presented with acute onset of progressive multifocal neurologic deficits. The MRI shows multiple lacunar infarcts and the angiographic study shows multiple areas of intracranial vessel stenosis. The radiological differential diagnosis is between atherosclerosis and arteritis. As there was clinical uncertainty, a biopsy of brain and overlying meningeal tissue was obtained which confirmed atherosclerotic disease. This case is an example of common cerebrovascular lesions in the African-American patient (i.e. intracranial atherosclerosis and lacunar infarction).

Our clinical imaging approach to evaluate the stroke patient is geared toward elucidation of the underlying pathophysiologic stroke mechanism and the extent and location of the vessel lesion. There are several areas, however, where the imaging approach might be tailored to the African-American stroke patient:

(1) As there may be a relatively high frequency of intracranial occlusive disease in African-Americans, an imaging approach should not only include images of the carotid bifurcation, but must also include the intracranial circulation. Although there are no currently established therapies for managing patients with acute intracranial occlusive disease, such patients could be appropriate for trials of angioplasty or intraarterial thrombolysis.

(2) As there are possible dangers of hyperosmolar contrast agents in the African-American population, low osmolar nonionic contrast agents should be used where indicated. Imaging modalities such as TCD and MRA may provide a better risk benefit profile than conventional catheter angiography.

Social and Economic Issues

Social and economic level issues in relation to delivery of neuroradiologic services to African-American stroke patients may be important. African-Amer-

Fig. 1. a Proton density, 5600/18/1 (TR/TE/NEX), fast spin echo MRI of the brain shows bilateral lenticulostriate arterial distribution lacunar infarcts and bilateral deep parieto-occipital white matter ischemic changes. *b* Proton density MRI, same patient as in figure 1a, shows bilateral pontomesencephalic ischemic change with a right occipital posterior cerebral arterial distribution infarct. Brain biopsy was negative for cerebral vasculitis. *c* Digital subtraction catheter angiogram (DSA) of the aortic arch vessels reveals no evidence of large vessel stenosis or atherosclerotic plaque. *d* Selective right common carotid DSA, lateral projection, reveals irregularity of the carotid siphon with pronounced narrowing of the supraclinoid internal carotid artery. There is diffuse narrowing of the pericallosal and internal parietal branches of the anterior cerebral artery (arrows) relative to the more proximal (A_2 segment) anterior cerebral artery. *e* Digital subtraction angiogram, frontal projection, of the right vertebral artery shows diffuse luminal irregularity with multiple segmental narrowing (arrows) in the right posterior cerebral artery distribution.

Table 1. Cost (USD) for radiologic procedures at two locations plus Medicare reimbursement

Radiologic procedure	Location I	Location II	Medicare reimbursement
Magnetic resonance imaging brain	1,550	1,300	1,042
Magnetic resonance angiogram	970	710	502
Computerized tomographic scan of brain without contrast	1,203	631	220
Carotid artery doppler ultrasound	440	388	55
Cerebral angiogram 3 vessel	9,373	–	2,233

Rates given are technical plus professional components. MRI of brain cost includes administration of gadolinium. Data are provided by two university-affiliated institutions in Michigan and by state Medicare agencies in Michigan. Location I is outpatient and location II is inpatient.

ican patients more frequently are uninsured or underinsured [1] and, therefore, potentially have more limited access to medical care. African-American patients have fewer high-cost, high-discretion procedures performed such as coronary angiography [19] and carotid endarectomy [20]. Reasons proposed to explain this disparity in utilization pattern include different rates of procedure refusals, levels of trust in the medical care system, and incidence of various disease types. There is limited additional data in stroke patients to suggest differential utilization of rehabilitative medical resources [21].

Cost data for various radiological procedures and combinations of procedures used in the stroke patient are given in table 1. A common clinical problem is deciding which non-invasive radiological procedures to utilize in screening patients for more invasive studies such as catheter angiography. One common approach would be to utilize MR angiography as the screening modality [22]. This has the advantage of an accurate visualization of both extracranial and large caliber intracranial vessels noninvasively with little risk. However, disadvantages include limited patient tolerability (claustrophobic and uncooperative patient), cost, overestimation of degree of stenosis, and lack of availability. An alternative approach would be to utilize carotid Doppler to image the extracranial carotid artery and TCD to image the intracranial circulation. This has the advantage of increased patient tolerability and lower cost. However, disadvantages include incomplete visualization at times of the vessels of interest and technical problems with acoustic windows in some patients. It is apparent that MRI of the brain and related cerebral vessels is more expensive when compared to the ultrasound approach. Most studies show the two imaging approaches to be of comparable although not identical accuracy in defining intracranial vessel stenosis greater than 60% [23, 24]. One recent trend has been to combine ultrasound with MRA to study the carotid artery in the neck and reserve conventional angiography for cases where there is disagreement between these modalities. This has resulted in a 100% sensitivity and 91–97% specificity in detecting surgically significant carotid stenotic disease in the neck [25], but with added cost. Detailed evaluation of the distal branches of the intracranial circulation with MRA remains problematic, and conventional angiography may be required in some cases.

Stroke Clinical Imaging Evaluation

An acute stroke treatment pathway is outlined in figure 2. This pathway contains key neuroradiologic branch points and treatment options. As the pathway is complex, it is advantageous to have a physician skilled in acute stroke treatment involved from the time of first medical contact.

Intracerebral hemorrhage (ICH) is more frequently seen in African-Americans than among Whites. An example of a CT scan showing an ICH in the common deep hemispheral location is given in figure 3. Some specific radiological features of ICH have important clinical correlation. CT evidence of enlargement of the hemorrhage over the ensuing 4 hours after onset may occur [26] and this change in hemorrhage size is often accompanied by clinical neurological deterioration. Therefore, if the hemorrhage patient begins to show clinical deterioration, evidence of hemorrhage enlargement should be sought with a repeat CT scan as medical and/or surgical intervention may be needed.

Since approval of acute cerebral infarct treatment with t-PA [27], the paradigm for appropriate imaging in the stroke patient has also shifted. If a patient arrives within the 3-hour t-PA treatment window and t-PA administration is being considered, then an immediate CT scan is appropriate. Given the relatively high frequency of ICH in the African-Americans, the difficulty distinguishing infarct from hemorrhage on clinical grounds, and the heightened risk of bleeding noted among African-American patients receiving t-PA for cardiac disease [28], early CT evaluation is important for the African-American stroke patient. If available, use of SPECT and diffusion-weighted MRI to help identify those patients who might benefit from acute treatment is reasonable in a research setting. For patients presenting beyond the 3-hour t-PA treatment window, there is no currently approved intervention to alter the degree of cerebral tissue damage. However, such cases may be appropriate for clinical

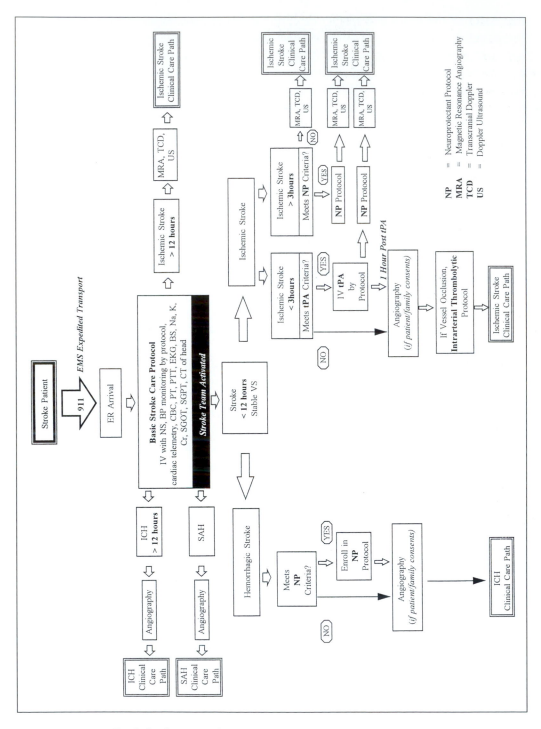

Fig. 2. Stroke protocol.

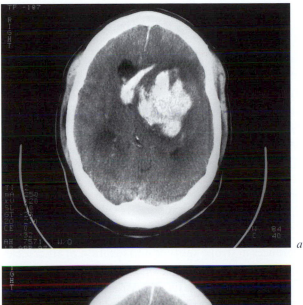

a

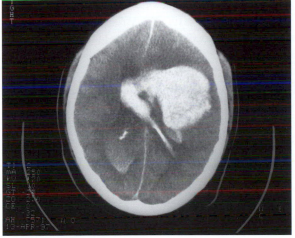

b

Fig. 3. a Noncontrasted CT scan of an African-American patient that presented with right hemiparesis and rapid progression to a comatose state. This slice shows a large irregular mass in the basal ganglia on the left that results from a hypertensive intracerebral hemorrhage. There is shift of midline structures and obliteration of the lateral ventricle on the left. *b* Noncontrasted CT of the same patient in (*a*) at a higher level showing extension of the hemorrhage into the deep frontal and parietal lobe on the left. Blood has extended into the right lateral ventricle.

research trials of intraarterial thrombolysis or neuroprotective agents (see fig. 2). Referral of selected patients to centers with expertise in acute stroke management should be considered.

The number of brain and cerebrovascular imaging modalities for stroke has increased in recent years offering more options for clinicoradiologic evaluation. In the evaluation of acute stroke patients for thrombolytic therapy, CT and conventional cerebral angiography are the more useful techniques. Uniform application of these procedures by race, gender, and ethnic group is important. There is no indication that African-Americans nor any other racial or ethnic groups benefit less from acute stroke treatments such as thrombolysis [28].

Conclusion

Since there may be differences in stroke subtype and location of atherosclerosis by race, application of this information to the radiological evaluation of an individual stroke patient could prove useful. As African-Americans may be more prone to large artery intracranial occlusive disease, lacunar infarction, and hypertensive intraparenchymal hemorrhage, the neurodiagnostic approach must include studies that define the brain areas and blood vessels involved with these lesions. Acute stroke interventions should be offered to appropriate African-American stroke patients, but only after a careful neuroradiologic evaluation to assess risk and benefit. Community education should be undertaken to heighten awareness of acute stroke treatment options among African-Americans. The health care system must continue to evaluate and eliminate differentials in access to health care.

References

1 Gaines K, Burke G: Ethnic differences in stroke: Black-White differences in the United States population. Neuroepidemiology 1995;14:209–239.
2 Gorelick P: Distribution of athrosclerotic cerebrovascular lesions: Effects of age, race, and sex. Stroke 1993;24(suppl 1):I-16–19.
3 Gross C, Kase C, Mohr J, Cunningham S, Baker W: Stroke in South Alabama: Incidence and diagnostic features in a population-based study. Stroke 1984;15:249–254.
4 Friday G, Lai S, Alter M, LaRue J, Gil-Peralta A, McCoy R, Levitt L, Isack T: Stroke in Lehigh Valley: Racial and ethnic differences. Neurology 1989;39:1165–1168.
5 Broderick J, Brott T, Tomsick T, Huster G, Miller R: The risk of subarachnoid hemorrhage in Blacks as compared to Whites. NEJM 1992;326:733–736.
6 Klastky A, Armstrong M, Friedman G: Racial differences in cerebrovascular disease hospitalizations. Stroke 1991;22:299–304.
7 Baum H, Goldstein M: Cerebrovascular disease type specific mortality: 1968–77. Stroke 1982;13: 810–817.

8   Kittner S, White L, Losonczy K, Wolf P, Hebel R: Black-White differences in stroke incidence in a national sample: The contribution of hypertension and diabetes mellitus. JAMA 1990;264: 1267–1270.

9   Taylor G, Barber J, Jackson M, Resch J, Loufemi W: Lipid composition of cerebral vessels in American Negroes, Caucasians, and Nigerian Africans: A comparative study. Stroke 1975;6:298–300.

10 Linn S, Fulwood R, Carroll M, Brook J, Johnson C, Kalesbeek W: Serum total cholesterol/HDL cholesterol ratios in U.S. White and Black adults by selected demographic and socioeconomic variables. Am J Publ Health 1991;81:1038–1043.

11 Schreiner P, Chambless L, Brown S, Watson R, Toole J, Heiss G: Lipoprotein (a) as a correlate of stroke and transient ischemic attack prevalence in a biracial cohort: The ARIC Study. Ann Epidemiol 1994;4:351–359.

12 Kane W, Aronson S: Cerebrovascular disease in the Negro male: A retrospective study. Trans Am Neurol Assoc 1968;93:225–226.

13 Yuh WT, Crain MR, Loes DJ, Greene GM, Ryals TJ, Sato Y: MR imaging of cerebral ischemia: Findings in the first 24 hours. Am J Neuroradiol 1991;12:621–629.

14 Brandt-Zawadzki M, Pereira B, Weinstein P, Moore S, Kucharczyk W, Berry I, McNamara M, Derugin N: MR imaging of acute experimental ischemia in cats. Am J Neuroradiol 1986;7:7–11.

15 Crain MR, Yuh WTC, Greene GM, Loes DJ, Ryals TJ, Sato Y, Hart MN: Cerebral ischemia: Evaluation with contrast enhanced MR imaging. Am J Neuroradiol 1991;12:631–639.

16 Elster AD, Moody DM: Early cerebral infarction: Gadopentetate dimeglumine enhancement. Radiology 1990;177:627–632.

17 Elster AD: MR contrast enhancement in brainstem and deep cerebral infarction. Am J Neuroradiol 1991;12:1127–1132.

18 Norton GA, Kishore PRS, Lin J: CT contrast in cerebral infarction. Am J Roentgenol 1978;131: 881–885.

19 Wenneker M, Epstein A: Racial inequalities in the use of procedures for patients with ischemic heart disease in Massachusetts. JAMA 1989;261:253–257.

20 Maxwell JG, Rutherford EJ, Covington C, Clancy T, Tackett D, Robinson N, Johnson G: Infrequency of Blacks among patients having carotid endarectomy. Stroke 1989;20:22–26.

21 Horner R, Hoenig H, Sloane R, Rubenstein L, Kahn K: Racial differences in the utilization of inpatient rehabilitation services among elderly stroke patients. Stroke 1997;28:19–25.

22 Hoeffner E: MRA in cerebrovascular disease. Clin Neuroscience 1997;4:117–122.

23 Baumgartner R, Mattle H, Aaslid R: Transcranial color-coded duplex sonography, magnetic resonance angiography, and computed tomography angiography: Methods, applications, advantages, and limitations. J Clin Ultrasound 1995;23:89–111.

24 Bowen B, Quencer R, Margosian P, Pattany P: MR angiography of occlusive disease of the arteries in the head and neck: Current concepts. Am J Radiol 1994;162:9–18.

25 DeMarco J, Schonfeld S, Wesbey G: Can noninvasive studies replace conventional angiography in the preoperative evaluation of carotid stenosis? Neuroimaging Clin N Am 1996;6:911–929.

26 Brott T, Broderick J, Kothari R, Barsan W, Tomsick T, Sauerbeck L, Spilker J, Duldner J, Khoury J: Early hemorrhage growth in patients with intracerebral hemorrhage. Stroke 1997;28:1–5.

27 NINDS, National Institute of Neurologic Disorders and Stroke Study Group: Tissue plasminogen activator for acute ischemic stroke. N Engl J Med 1995;333:1581–1587.

28 The NINDS t-PA Stroke Study Group: Intracerebral hemorrhage after intravenous t-PA therapy for ischemic stroke. Stroke 1997;28:2109–2118.

29 NASCET Collaborators, North American Symptomatic Carotid Endarectomy Trial Collaborators: Beneficial effect of carotid endarectomy in symptomatic patients with high-grade carotid stenosis. N Engl J Med 1991;325:445–453.

Kenneth Gaines, MD, Field Neuroscience Institute,
4677 Towne Centre Rd., Suite 103, Saginaw, MI 48604 (USA)

Gillum RF, Gorelick PB, Cooper ES (eds): Stroke in Blacks. Basel, Karger, 1999, pp 62–69

....
Sickle Cell Disorders and Cerebrovascular Disease

Adeeb Ahmed, Robert J. Adams

Department of Neurology, Medical College of Georgia, Augusta, Ga., USA

Sickle cell disorders include all states where a sickle gene is inherited. The term sickle cell anemia is usually reserved for the homozygous state of hemoglobin S (SSD).

Epidemiology

About 1 in every 400 births in African-Americans is identified with newborn screening to have SSD. SSD also occurs among Hispanics but rarely Caucasians. Stroke is relatively common in SSD. A population study from Jamaica indicated an incidence of 7.4% by age 14 years [Balkaran et al., 1992]. The best estimates are from the Cooperative Study of Sickle Cell Disease (CSSCD) [Frempong et al., 1998]. In that study the risk of having a stroke by 20, 30 and 45 years of age was 11, 15 and 24% respectively for SSD patients. Hemoglobin (Hb) SC is a condition where the sickle gene is combined with a Hb C gene. The resulting anemia is less severe. Stroke rates for Hb SC patients at 20, 30 and 40 years were 2, 4 and 10% respectively.

In the CSSCD, data were collected from 4,082 sickle cell disease patients enrolled from 1978 to 1988. This long-term observational study demonstrated the incidence of first-time stroke, either cerebral infarction or hemorrhage, to be highest in early childhood, age 2–5 years (1.02/100 patient-years), followed by 6–9 years (0.79) and falling to 0.41 between 10 and 19 years [Frempong et al., 1998]. Cerebral infarction accounts for most strokes (75%) and is the most common manifestation of stroke in SSD children [Powars et al., 1978].

In the CSSCD, hemorrhage accounted for 33% of first strokes in adults. The risk of hemorrhage was fairly low in children less than age 20 and was highest in young adults [Frempong et al., 1998].

Pathogenesis

Hb in the red cells in adults exists as a tetramer of two α- and two β-chains. Alterations in the amino acid sequence of one of the globin chains gives rise to hemoglobinopathies while decrease in quantity of globin chains causes the thalassemias. Hemoglobinopathies are categorized as sickle cell trait (one normal β-globin and other sickle β-globin), sickle cell disease (both β-globin are sickle β-globins), and hemoglobin SC (one sickle β-globin and the other C β-globin).

How SSD causes stroke is not clear. The fundamental pathology of SSD is the formation of Hb polymer strands within the erythrocyte causing profound distortions of shape and deformability. Sickled cells do not pass well through the microcirculation but occlusion from microcirculatory obstruction is not sufficient to explain the large territorial infarcts often seen in these children. While the cause of stroke is probably multi-factorial, it is clear that the large basal arteries are often occluded or stenotic in symptomatic patients. This vasculopathy, which can be severe, may be initiated by endothelial injury. Recently, a possible coagulopathic state with decreased levels of both protein C and S activities [Tam, 1997] has been reported in some patients, and elevated homocysteinemia [Houston et al., 1997] may increase stroke risk in some cases. Endothelial dysfunction and stimulation of growth factors causing fibrosis may also add to the vessel stenosis associated with SSD [Touhy et al., 1997]. Anemia is associated with high flow rates [Adams and Nichols, 1989; Brass et al., 1988] which may predispose to vessel damage. Finally, abnormal adherence of red blood cells to vascular endothelium may be involved [Hebbel, 1997].

Risk Factors

Clearly established risk factors for cerebral infarction in SSD are homozygous state (Hb SS), young age, prior stroke [Powars et al., 1978], and elevated blood flow velocities in basal brain arteries by transcranial Doppler (TCD) [Adams et al., 1992, 1997, 1998]. Large-vessel arterial lesions [Adams and Nichols, 1989], older age [Frempong et al., 1998], prior ischemic stroke and arterial aneurysms predispose to hemorrhage.

Clinical Manifestations

As in patients without SCD, brain infarction typically presents with the sudden onset of symptoms of acute hemispheric dysfunction including hemiparesis, altered speech or aphasia, hemisensory and visual deficits without alteration of consciousness [Powars et al., 1978; Pavlakis et al., 1989; Adams and Nichols, 1989]. Seizures, especially partial in onset, accompany about 20% of cases and should alert the clinician to the possibility of cerebrovascular disease. Transient ischemic attacks are not commonly reported. Children presenting with cerebral infarction often show CT evidence of prior undetected brain lesions ('silent infarcts'). Neurological examination usually shows some degree of hemiparesis. Typically motor symptoms improve but patients, especially children, are left with significant cognitive deficits [Hariman et al., 1991; Cohen et al., 1994; Armstrong et al., 1996]. Bilateral infarctions may be devastating leaving patients with pseudobulbar palsy. Posterior circulation syndromes are unusual but have been reported. Death after cerebral infarction is rare. Silent or hyposymptomatic brain infarction has been detected in 10–20% of SSD patients studied with magnetic resonance imaging (MRI) and other techniques [Pavlakis et al., 1988; El Gammal et al., 1986].

The CSSCD performed MRI screening on 312 patients and found that 17% of patients without a history of stroke had MRI lesions consistent with ischemia [Moser et al., 1996]. In addition, the CSSCD performed neuropsychological testing on 135 children aged 6–12 years along with MRI of the brain [Armstrong et al., 1996]. Nine (6.6%) had a history of stroke and these had abnormal MRI and neuropsychological testing. Twenty-one others (15.6%) had no stroke history but MRI lesions indicative of infarction and 105 (77.8%) had normal MRI. Abnormal MRI was associated with abnormalities on one or more cognitive tests. 'Silent' MRI lesions are not uncommon and are associated with cognitive deficits. However, it is not clear whether these lesions predispose to subsequent clinical stroke.

Intracranial hemorrhage is less common than infarction and tends to occur in older SSD patients. It is manifested by sudden severe headache usually with alteration of consciousness with or without focal findings [Powars et al., 1978]. Hemorrhage is more likely to be fatal than infarction. In the CSSCD, 9 of the 11 fatal strokes were hemorrhages and the other 2 were undetermined for a 26% risk of death from hemorrhage [Frempong et al., 1998]. Symptoms and findings depend on whether bleeding is subarachnoid, intraparenchymal or intraventricular. Convulsions and coma suggest massive subarachnoid or intraventricular bleeding. Parenchymal bleeding is usually subcortical and presents with depressed alertness or stupor and focal findings [Adams, 1994].

Prevention

Because of the ability of TCD to predict stroke, primary prevention has now been shown to be feasible. TCD studies have shown a strong association with stroke, approximately 40%, if the time-averaged mean blood flow velocity was 200 cm/s or greater [Adams et al., 1992, 1997, 1998]. This was the basis for the Stroke Prevention Trial in Sickle Cell Anemia (STOP) [Adams et al., 1998] which demonstrated the feasibility of primary prevention of stroke in patients with sickle cell disease.

In the STOP trial, children with sickle cell anemia aged 2–16 years with no history of stroke were screened with TCD. Time-averaged mean velocity (as opposed to peak systolic velocity) in the intracranial internal carotid artery or the middle cerebral artery ≥200 cm/s were required for randomization to either standard care or regular blood transfusions. Exchange or simple transfusion were allowed.

The incidence of stroke (cerebral infarction or intracranial hemorrhage) was over 90% lower in the transfusion group when the study was halted. There were 11 strokes in the standard care arm and 1 in the transfusion arm. TCD proved to be an effective predictor of stroke with a risk of 10% per year in those receiving standard care. It is unclear how long the prophylactic transfusion should be continued. There have been reports which have documented a high risk of stroke recurrence after stopping transfusion [Wang et al., 1991; Rana et al., 1997] when it was used for secondary prevention. The results of the STOP study led to recommendations for screening children with SSD. The decision to initiate transfusion should be made after careful consideration of the risks and benefits and treatment given in a setting experienced with transfusion and its complications.

Transfusion has been the standard of care for secondary prevention. It is associated with reduction in recurrence from as high as 47–90% to about 10% [Russell et al., 1984; Balkaran et al., 1992]. The maintenance of Hb S at a level less than 30% appears to be effective in reducing the rate of recurrent infarction but does not prevent transient neurological events [Pegelow et al., 1995]. Hydroxyurea can increase fetal Hb and improve the clinical course of sickle cell disease patients [Charache et al., 1991], but as yet there is no evidence that this drug will be an effective alternative to transfusion for stroke prevention and at least one intracranial hemorrhage has been reported in a child on hydroxyurea [Vichinsky and Lubin, 1994].

Few have used antiplatelet agents or anticoagulants for either primary or secondary prevention of SSD-related stroke. Anticoagulation may be especially hazardous if moyamoya vessels are present. The use of aspirin cannot be casually recommended because those at highest risk are children in whom aspirin use has been curtailed due to an association with Reye's syndrome. Similarly, experience with ticlopidine in children or adults with SSD is limited. Warfarin has been tried in adults with stroke, but there is no systematic experience and the bleeding risk of moyamoya would dictate caution in patients with this finding.

Patients with intracranial hemorrhage due to aneurysm probably should be put on chronic transfusion after surgical clipping of accessible lesions to prevent rebleeding. Whether incidentally discovered aneurysms should be operated to prevent expansion or rupture is unknown. Although there is little support in the literature, transfusion for intracranial hemorrhage not associated with aneurysm seems reasonable. In some cases the angiogram may show no aneurysm or obstructive vasculopathy. In such cases we recommend short-term transfusion (for 1–2 years) only.

Diagnostic Work-Up

Although there is a strong association between SSD and stroke, it is crucial to consider non-SSD-related causes as well. Upon presentation it is important to rule out intracranial hemorrhage with a noncontrast CT. CT contrast agents may be used but preferably after hydration of the patient with intravenous fluids. An EKG and basic labs should also be obtained. Special tests for coagulopathies or cardiac sources of stroke are not performed routinely in most centers but may be appropriate in some patients, especially those with recurrent stroke despite transfusion. If the CT does not show stroke or another lesion responsible for the patient's symptoms, MRI should be performed. The CT or MRI typically show cortical and subcortical areas of ischemic damage in either territorial or 'borderzone' patterns and often old lesions in asymptomatic areas [Zimmerman et al., 1987]. Once the patient is stabilized, TCD can be used to examine the intracranial vessels. Unlike patients at risk before onset of stroke, TCD in patients who already have had stroke and advanced disease leading to symptoms may not show high velocity [Adams, 1996]. In addition, the indication for chronic transfusion, at least in children, is ischemic stroke as documented by clinical and radiographic methods. Even if the patient has no demonstrable vasculopathy, most would recommend transfusion at least for a few years.

Cerebral angiography is indicated in all cases of intracranial hemorrhage (except epidural and subdural) to detect surgically correctable aneurysm or AVMs. Angiography is also useful in patients presenting with transient symptoms with negative confirmation of ischemia on parenchymal imaging. In this situation angiography is used to determine the extent of large vessel disease which, if present, strengthens the case for placing that patient on chronic transfusion [Frempong, 1991]. Angiography can be safely used if patients are prepared by reduction of Hb S to less than 30% of the total Hb and with vigorous hydration.

In all neurologically asymptomatic children with sickle cell disease, we recommend screening with transcranial Doppler because it can predict risk and could lead to prophylactic transfusion to prevent stroke [Adams et al., 1998]. The role of TCD in adults with SSD has not been established.

Management

In children, acute cerebral infarction is treated with blood transfusion using concentrated erythrocytes on an emergent basis [Adams, 1994]. The optimal method (simple vs. exchange), extent and efficacy of acute transfusion have not been established. It is reasonable in all patients to provide aggressive hydration (unless there is concern for massive cerebral edema) which may decrease blood viscosity and to administer aspirin to adults. Our practice is to manage younger patients with exchange transfusion avoiding hypotension during phlebotomy and attempting to reduce the Hb S to less than 30% within 48–96 h. Patients with altered sensorium, massive stroke or requiring central venous access are treated initially in an intensive care setting. In most cases these patients go on to chronic transfusion programs in which they receive 10–15 cm^3/kg packed erythrocyte transfusions every 3 - 4 weeks for an indefinite period [Charache et al., 1991].

Adults with SSD should be considered for TPA treatment of acute ischemic stroke if they present within 3 h of onset of symptoms and have an appropriate CT scan.

For those patients with intracranial hemorrhage: (1) treat increased intracranial pressure and prevent brain herniation in parenchymal bleeds; (2) prevent deterioration from acute hydrocephalus using ventriculostomy drainage in cases with intraventricular blood and/or (3) give nimodipine in patients with subarachnoid hemorrhage 60 mg every 4 h; (4) reduce Hb S by exchange transfusion and hydration in an intensive care setting, and (5) perform cerebral angiography as soon as feasible. For aneurysm or arteriovenous malformation, surgery should be considered. Surgery should be followed by chronic transfusion in younger patients to decrease hemodynamic stress on vessels. If extensive occlusive disease and moyamoya is revealed, patients should be treated with chronic transfusion until age 21 or offered the option to continue indefinitely after considering the risks of prolonged transfusion.

References

Adams RJ: Neurological complications; in Embury SH, Hebbel RP, Mohandas N, Steinberg MH (eds): Sickle Cell Disease: Scientific Principles and Clinical Practice. New York, Raven Press, 1994, pp 599–621.

Adams RJ, McKie VC, Carl EM, Nichols FT, Perry R, Brock K, McKie K, Figueroa R, Litaker M, Weiner S, Brambilla D: Long-term stroke risk in children with sickle cell disease screened with transcranial doppler. Ann Neurol 1997;42:699–704.

Adams RJ, McKie VC, Hsu L, Files B, Vichinsky E, Pegelow C, Abboud M, Gallagher D, Kutlar A, Nichols FT, Bonds D, Brambilla D, Woods G, Olivieri N, Driscoll C, Miller S, Wang W, Hurlett A, Scher C, Berman B, Carl E, Jones A, Roach S, Wright E, Zimmerman R, Waclawiw M: Prevention of a first stroke by transfusions in children with sickle cell anemia and abnormal results on transcranial Doppler ultrasonography. N Engl J Med 1998;339:5–11.

Adams RJ, McKie VC, Nichols FT, Carl E, Zhang DL, McKie K, Figueroa R, Litaker M, Thompson W, Hess DC: The use of transcranial ultrasonography to predict stroke in sickle cell disease. N Engl J Med 1992;326:605–610.

Adams RJ, Nichols FT: Sickle cell anemia, sickle cell trait and thalassemia; in Vinken PJ, Bruyn GW, Klawans HL (eds): Handbook of Clinical Neurology, Vascular Diseases. III. Amsterdam, Elsevier, 1989, vol 11, pp 503–515.

Armstrong FD, Thompson RJ Jr, Wand W, Zimmerman R, Pegelow CH, Miller S, Moser F, Bello J, Hurtig A, Vass K: Cognitive functioning and brain magnetic resonance imaging in children with sickle cell disease. Neuropsychological Committee of the Cooperative Study of Sickle Cell Disease. Pediatrics 1996;97:864–870.

Balkaran B, Char G, Morris JS, Thomas PW, Serjeant BE, Serjeant GR: Stroke in a cohort or patients with homozygous sickle cell disease. J Pediatr 1992;120:360–366.

Brass L, Pavlakis S, DeVivo D, Piomelli S, Mohr J: Transcranial Doppler measurements of the middle cerebral artery. Effect of hematocrit. Stroke 1988;19:1466–1469.

Charache S, Lubin B, Reid C: Management and therapy of sickle cell disease. NIH Publ 91-2117. Washington, US Department of Health and Human Services, 1991, pp 22–24.

Cohen MJ, Branch WB, McKie VC, Adams RJ: Neuropsychological impairment in children with sickle cell anemia and cerebrovascular accidents. Clin Pediatr 1994;33:517–524.

El Gammal TE, Adams RJ, Nichols FT, McKie V, Milner P, McKie K, Brook BS: MR and CT investigation of cerebrovascular disease in sickle cell patients. Am J Neuroradiol 1986;7:1043–1049.

Frempong KO: Stroke in sickle cell disease: Demographic, clinical and therapeutic considerations. Semin Hematol 1991;28:213–219.

Frempong KO, Weiner SJ, Sleeper LA, Miller ST, Embury S, Moohr JW, Wethers DL, Pegelow CH, Gill FM: Cerebrovascular accidents in sickle cell disease: Rates and risk factors. Blood 1998;91:288–294.

Hariman LMF, Griffith ER, Hurtig AL, Keehn MT: Functional outcomes of children with sickle-cell disease affected by stroke. Arch Phys Med Rehabil 1991;72:498–502.

Hebbel RP: Adhesive interactions of sickle erythrocytes with endothelium. J Clin Invest 1997;100(suppl):83–86.

Houston PE, Rana S, Sekhsaria S, Perlin E, Kim KS, Castro OL: Homocysteine in sickle cell disease: Relationship to stroke. Am J Med 1997;103:192–196.

Moser FG, Miller ST, Bello JA, Pegelow CH, Zimmerman RA, Wang WC, Frempong KO, Schwartz A, Vichinsky EP, Gallagher D, Kinney TR: The spectrum of brain MR abnormalities in sickle cell disease: A report from the cooperative study of sickle cell disease. Am J Neuroradiol 1996;17:965–972.

Pavlakis SG, Bello J, Prohovnik I, Sutton M, Ince C, Mohr JP, Piomelli S, Hilal S, De Vivo DC: Brain infarction in sickle cell anemia magnetic resonance imaging correlates. Ann Neurol 1988;23:125–130.

Pegelow CH, Adams RJ, McKie V, Abboud M, Berman B, Miller ST, Olivieri N, Vichinsky E, Wang W, Brambilla D: Risk of recurrent stroke in patients with sickle cell disease treated with erythrocyte transfusions. J Pediatr 1995;126:896–899.

Pegelow CH, Colangelo L, Steinberg M, Wright EC, Smith J, Phillips G, Vichinsky E: Natural history of blood pressure in sickle cell disease: Risks for stroke and death associated with relative hypertension in sickle cell. Am J Med 1997;102:171–177.

Powars ER, Wilson B, Imbus C, Pegelow C, Allen J: The natural history of stroke in sickle cell disease. Am J Med 1978;65:461–471.

Rana S, Houston PE, Surana N: Discontinuation of long-term transfusion therapy in patients with sickle cell disease. J Pediatr 1997;131:757–760.

Russell MO, Goldberg HI, Hudson A, Kim HC, Halus RJ, Reivich M, Schwartz E: Effect of transfusion therapy on arteriographic abnormalities and on recurrence of stroke in sickle cell disease. Blood 1984;63:162–169.

Tam DA: Protein C and protein S activity in sickle cell disease and stroke. J Child Neurol 1997;12:19–21.

Touhy AM, McKie V, Manci EA, Adams RJ: Internal carotid artery occlusion in a child with sickle cell disease: Case report and immunohistochemical study. J Pediatr Hematol Oncology 1997;19:455–458.

Vichinsky EP, Lubin BH: A cautionary note regarding hydroxyurea in sickle cell disease. Blood 1994;83: 1124–1128.

Wang WC, Kovnar EH, Tonkin IL, Mulhern RK, Langston JW, Day SW, Schell MJ, Wilimas JA: High risk of recurrent stroke after discontinuance of five to twelve years of transfusion therapy in patients with sickle cell disease. J Pediatr 1991;118:377–382.

Zimmerman RA, Gill F, Goldberg HI, Bilaniuk LT, Hackney DB, Johnson M, Grossman RI, Hecht-Leavitt C: MRI of sickle cell cerebral infarction. Neuroradiology 1987;29:232–237.

Adeeb Ahmed, MD, Department of Neurology, Medical College of Georgia, Augusta, GA 30912 (USA)

Epidemiology and Primary Prevention

Gillum RF, Gorelick PB, Cooper ES (eds): Stroke in Blacks. Basel, Karger, 1999, pp 70–82

....

Epidemiology of Stroke in African Populations Outside of the United States

Ike S. Okosun[a], *Richard S. Cooper*[a], *Walinjom F. Muna*[b]

[a] Department of Preventive Medicine and Epidemiology, Loyola University Stritch School of Medicine, Maywood, Ill., USA
[b] General Hospital of Yaounde, Faculty of Medical and Biomedical Sciences, University of Yaounde, Cameroon

Stroke, the most common cerebrovascular disease (CVD) in many advanced countries and the third most common cause of mortality in the United States [1], is no longer regarded as a rare diagnostic oddity in Blacks outside the US. Until recently, the view had been that stroke was rare in Africa. In 1957 for example, Humphries [2] stated that in 14 years of work in South, Central and West Africa, he saw only very few cases. The demographic transformation from a traditional and rural life style to an urbanized and industrial pattern in countries occupied by Blacks outside the US is reshaping disease patterns. Thus, the spectrum and pattern of cerebrovascular disorders are rapidly becoming analogous to what is observed in the developed countries [3].

Stroke has now become a major public health problem, representing one of the most common causes of morbidity and mortality in Black populations outside the US [4–12]. However, some 20 years after the exhaustive reviews of stroke epidemiology by Akinkugbe [4] and Osuntokun [7], reliable data on stroke in African populations outside the US is still insufficient. Most of the studies from outside the US span a long time period and often do not meet standard criteria for comparative analysis. A comparative assessment of stroke epidemiology in Black populations outside the US must therefore be viewed against these limitations as well as against constraints in sample size, age ascertainment, lack of appropriate diagnostic technologies, strong cultural attitudes against postmortem examinations, and lack of qualified pathologists. Notwithstanding these limitations, a review of the distribution and determinants of stroke in these populations can contribute to overall knowledge worldwide.

Stroke is now common in sub-Saharan Africans [14, 15], among the Bantus of South Africa, and other cultural groups previously thought of as low risk [16–18]. In Jamaica, stroke is the leading cause of death [19] and is among the top causes in other Caribbean Island nations [19, 21, 22]. Between 1953–1957 and 1963–1967 in Trinidad and Tobago, stroke mortality increased by 32% in men but later declined by 34% between 1988 and 1992. In Trinidadian and Barbadian women, mortality increased by 24% in 1953–1957 and 1963–1967 but declined by 33% during 1988–1992 [26]. Stroke has also been shown to be a major cause of morbidity and mortality among Blacks residing in England and Wales [23–25]. Between 1983 and 1997, compared to other Black immigrants and natives living in England and Wales, mortality from stroke was highest in the Caribbean natives (standardized mortality ratio of 176 for men and 210 for women), followed by Africans [25]. A recent analysis of global burdens of cardiovascular diseases worldwide estimates almost three million strokes occur annually in the developing countries where most Blacks live [13].

Stroke in Blacks outside the US differs from that of the US Blacks in type and severity [27–32]. In Africa, cerebral atherosclerosis is less common and the frequencies of subarachnoid hemorrhage are higher among Africans than those reported for the US [29]. Pathologic investigation of West African patients dying from stroke shows less cerebral atheroma in those whose lipid composition differs from US Blacks [31, 32]. The factors associated with a stroke in Blacks outside the US are multiple and include hematological, infectious and cardiovascular diseases. Others have also noted snake bites as one of the causes of stroke in some African countries [33, 34].

Stroke Rates

Stroke incidence and mortality have shown a steady decline in the developed countries since the 1940s. Information on secular trends (mortality and incidence) is limited in Black populations outside the US. However, studies based on hospital data from Black communities in several countries in Africa suggest that stroke mortality has increased, despite the fact that it was previously believed to be uncommon. Most of the early work on stroke in Blacks outside the US was retrospective and based on hospital records. A review of hospital records of stroke patients (table 1) showed that cerebral infarction was the most commonly reported type of stroke. However, between 1952 and 1967 in Jamaica, 77% of 296 autopsies among patients with stroke demon-

Table 1. Relative frequencies of types of strokes in Blacks outside US

Country	Author(s)	Study date	Charac- teristics	Percentage frequencies				
				infarc- tion	hemor- rhage	subarach- noid	embo- lism	others
Nigeria	Osuntokun et al. [30]	1973–1975	all ages	46.2	15.7	11.3	2.5	–
	Osuntokun et al. [6]	1957–1963	all ages	55.6	17.0	8.7	3.2	15.5
	Dada et al. [38]	1961–1962	<11 years	57.6	22.3	13.6	4.9	1.6
	Bwala [15]	1989	all ages	63.0	37.0	–	–	–
	Nwosu et al. [39]	1992	16–45 years	58.2	17.9	11.9	7.5	–
Uganda	Billinghurst [40]	1968–1970	all ages	57.0	9.3	14.9	6.8	12.0
Zimbabwe	Matenga et al. [8]	1984–1985	all ages	62.0	29.0	2.0	13.0	7.0
South Africa	Rosman [41]	1979	<20 years	20.7	32.8	–	13.8	0.9
	Cosnett [17]	1969	8–40 years	–	30.0	13.0	23.0	–
Ethiopia	Abebe and Haimanot [42]	1983–1985	all ages	–	24.0	–	15.5	–
Jamaica	Cole and Cole [35]	1967	all ages	13.0	77.0	–	10.0	–

strated that they were hemorrhagic [35]. Nonfatal stroke occurs more frequently in people of Black ancestry than others [36]. Also, mortality from stroke is higher in Black migrants to the UK (Caribbeans and West Africans) than natives and other migrants [36]. In a recent retrospective review of cases of cerebrovascular attacks in the Bobo Dioulasso Hospital, Burkina Faso, stroke accounted for 15.1% of admissions for cardiovascular disorders [37]. Bantus living in Johannesburg, South Africa, have a stroke death rate similar to those among US populations [17].

Table 2 summarizes incidence and prevalence findings from different African populations. The prevalence of stroke ranged from 0.07% in a rural community of Nigeria to 25.8% in Ghana. Incidence rates and mortality from stroke tended to increase with age for males and females and should therefore increase further as the longevity of Africans increases [44]. In a report by Osuntokun et al. [30], the incidence of stroke in a large urban African city based on evaluation of the 1973–1975 Stroke Registry at Ibadan, Nigeria, was 74.8 per 100,000. Analysis of WHO stroke registries showed that age-specific incidence peaked in the 7th decade in men compared with the 8th decade for women [30]. In urban areas of South Africa, the annual incidence rate rose with age and peaked in the males at 65 to 74 years [41].

Rosman [41] using hospital admissions, monitored stroke incidence over a 12-month period in an urban Black population of Pretoria, South Africa. Out of a population at risk of 114,931, the overall incidence rate was 1.01

Table 2. Prevalence/incidence of stroke in Black populations outside US

Country	Year	Author(s)	Characteristics	Sample size	Rates, %
Nigeria	1973–1975	Osuntokun et al. [30]	Stroke Registry	318	0.07
Cameroon	1984–1990	Obama et al. [43]	historical, prospective	35	0.19
Ghana	1960–1968	Nyame et al. [10]	hospital-based	660	25.8
	1976–1983	Nyame et al. [10]	hospital-based	2,124	11.0
Ethiopia	1983–1985	Abebe and Haimanot [42]	retrospective	150	23.6
Zimbabwe	1991	Matenga [8]	cross-sectional, community-based	273	0.07
South Africa	1986	Rosman [41]	hospital-based	116	0.1
Burkina Faso	1994	Zabsonre et al. [37]	hospital population	193	15.1

admissions per 1,000 per year for those over age 20. The average annual pediatric incidence of stroke was estimated at 1.85 per 1,000 hospitalizations among those 5 months to 15 years of age [43]. In a recent community-based study in Harare, Zimbabwe, age-specific crude incidence ranged from 5.4/100,000 for the 15- to 24-year-old groups to 788.3/100,000 for the 75-year-old groups [8].

In a 1990 study by Abebe [42] investigating causes, risk factors, and outcomes of cerebrovascular accidents in 150 patients admitted to Tikur Anbessa Hospital, Addis Ababa, Ethiopia, cerebral thrombosis was the most common cause of stroke (50.6%), followed by cerebral hemorrhage (24%) and cerebral embolisms (15%).

Gradient of Risk Factors

The International Collaborative Study of Hypertension in Blacks (ICSHIB) provided risk profiles of Blacks in Nigeria, Cameroon, Jamaica, St. Lucia, Barbados and the US (table 3). The international comparative design of ICSHIB provided an opportunity to study the evolution of hypertension among populations with a common genetic heritage currently living in widely varied social conditions. In these populations, there was a trend toward increasing anthropometric variables (height, weight, body mass index, waist and hip circumference and waist to hip ratio) from West Africa to the US. Body mass index was collinear with the prevalence of stroke risk factors (obesity, high blood pressures and diabetes) in community cross-sections from rural West Africa, the Caribbean, and the US.

Table 3. Sex-specific mean level for anthropometric variables among Blacks of West African origin: The ICSHIB study, 1995

	n	Height, cm		Weight, kg		Body mass index, kg/m²		Waist, cm		Hip, cm		Waist-to-hip ratio	
		x̄	SD	x̄	SD	x̄	SD	x̄	SD	x̄	SD	x̄	SD
Males													
Nigeria	1,171	168.3	7.3	61.5	11.0	21.7	3.6	77.3	8.4	88.3	8.2	0.88	0.06
Cameroon													
Urban	612	172.3	7.2	74.5	12.1	25.1	3.6	83.3	9.1	96.8	8.1	0.86	0.06
Rural	745	170.1	7.0	68.1	10.4	23.5	3.1	80.4	7.1	90.7	6.7	0.89	0.05
Jamaica	524	172.1	6.9	70.6	13.7	23.8	4.3	80.8	11.9	95.8	8.3	0.84	0.07
St. Lucia	491	173.5	7.5	73.0	11.4	24.3	3.7	82.7	9.5	95.3	7.4	0.87	0.06
Barbados	330	171.9	7.4	76.4	13.2	25.9	4.3	86.2	11.3	97.8	7.7	0.88	0.07
USA (Maywood)	708	176.5	7.3	84.5	18.0	27.1	5.5	92.4	14.0	103.4	10.7	0.89	0.07
Females													
Nigeria	1,338	158.3	6.7	56.6	12.3	22.6	4.7	73.9	9.6	93.5	10.8	0.79	0.06
Cameroon													
Urban	749	162.1	5.7	71.0	13.6	27.0	4.7	82.5	9.8	102.5	11.0	0.81	0.07
Rural	722	160.7	6.6	60.6	11.9	23.5	4.3	80.9	9.2	92.6	9.3	0.87	0.06
Jamaica	733	160.7	6.5	72.2	17.7	27.9	6.6	83.2	12.9	104.3	13.0	0.80	0.06
St. Lucia	598	162.3	6.8	72.3	17.0	27.3	6.2	85.5	13.4	103.7	13.1	0.82	0.07
Barbados	483	160.1	6.4	75.2	16.3	29.4	6.4	87.1	12.6	106.7	12.8	0.82	0.07
USA (Maywood)	810	163.4	6.4	82.4	20.9	30.8	7.7	91.4	15.4	111.8	15.0	0.82	0.08

Globally, however, Blacks outside the US are of a predominantly lower risk, given the level of economic development in most of Africa and the Caribbean. Environmental factors associated with economic prosperity (obesity and the intake of sodium and potassium) vary consistently with disease prevalence across regions [45]. These findings demonstrate the determining role of social circumstances in the development of hypertension and diabetes risks and possibly their sequelae, which include stroke in these African populations.

Hypertension

Essential hypertension is a major contributor to stroke morbidity and mortality [46–48]. Stroke is a serious and frequent complication of hypertension in Black countries [48]. The overall frequency of hypertension among stroke patients is similar to what is generally found among US Blacks. This propensity toward high blood pressure is common in US Blacks of West African origin. Among Black populations outside the US, hypertension is a major risk factor for cerebral hemorrhage and infarction. Available data from African Blacks suggest that high blood pressure is vastly related to organ impairment in African Blacks [46, 49]. The clinical spectra of hypertensive cerebrovascular complications include transient ischemic attack and fatal and nonfatal stoke. In a study by Osuntokun et al. [30], 68% of stroke patients were evaluated to be hypertensive as defined by systolic blood pressure of greater than or equal to 160 mm Hg and diastolic pressure of greater than or equal to 100 mm Hg. In that study, hypertension was present in 80% of those with subarachnoid hemorrhage, 50% with nonembolic cerebral infarction and 76% in those with acute but ill-defined cerebrovascular disease.

Table 4 shows age and sex-adjusted prevalence of hypertension among six populations of West African origin. A consistent gradient of hypertension prevalence was observed, increasing from 16% in West Africa to 26% in the Caribbean and 33% in the United States. Although average blood pressures were comparable among persons from 25 to 34 years of age, increase in hypertension prevalence with age was twice as precipitous in the US as compared to Africa [52].

In a meta-analysis, Wilson et al. [53] showed that the rate of hypertension among 40- to 49-year-old sub-Sahara African stroke patients was greater than in East Africans. West African rural males are known to have higher blood pressures than those from central or southern African regions [53]. Regional differences in blood pressure may be attributable to differences in rates or frequencies of other predisposing factors in stroke pathogenesis, including heart diseases, or a combination of factors [54].

Table 4. Age-adjusted prevalence of hypertension by gender among Blacks of West African Origin: The ICSHIB Study, 1995

	Hypertension[1]			Hypertension[2]		
	males	females	total	males	females	total
West Africa	16.3	15.0	15.6	6.9	7.3	7.1
Nigeria	14.7	14.3	14.5	6.9	6.9	6.9
Cameroon	17.7	16.3	16.9	6.5	8.0	7.3
Urban	22.8	16.0	19.1	8.7	8.7	8.7
Rural	14.2	16.3	15.4	4.7	7.4	6.1
Caribbean	22.6	27.9	25.5	14.6	21.3	18.2
Jamaica	19.1	28.2	24.0	12.9	20.6	17.1
St. Lucia	24.1	27.4	25.9	13.9	20.8	17.6
Barbados	25.9	28.2	27.2	18.0	22.9	20.6
USA (Maywood)	31.3	33.6	32.6	23.1	28.2	25.8

[1] Systolic BP $\geq$ 140 or diastolic BP $\geq$ 90 or taking antihypertension medications.
[2] Systolic BP $\geq$ 160 or diastolic BP $\geq$ 95 or taking antihypertension medications.

In a case-control investigation of risk factors associated with cerebrovascular accidents in Nigeria, Danesi et al. [55] found that 67% of patients with nonembolic stroke had hypertension, as defined above. Rosman [41] also found Black adults with stroke living in urban areas in Pretoria, South Africa, with an overall 70% rate of hypertension. Among this group, the prevalence of cerebral hemorrhage, arterial thrombosis and lacunal infarction was 33, 32 and 21%, respectively. Joubert [56] also found an overall hypertension rate of 42% among Black Africans using a hospital-based sample in Ga-Rankuwa, Pretoria, South Africa. Analysis of the files on 545 hypertensive patents admitted to the same hospital 7 years earlier revealed a 54% incidence of stroke. Correlation between the incidence of stroke and hypertension was highest in the 60- to 70-year-old group.

Obesity

Obesity is one of the major risk factors for hypertension in a cross-cultural investigation, although the proportion of variance in blood pressure that it explains is consistently less than 20% [52]. The role of obesity in stroke is confounded by the close association between obesity and other risk factors for stroke, although the Framingham study suggests that obesity is an independent risk factor over a long period of exposure [57].

Obesity is associated with sedentarism, high serum triglycerides and low HDL-cholesterol. Results from ICSHIB show that obesity increases linearly across African nations along a socioeconomic slope and also along Westernization [58].

Cappuccio [36] investigated ethnicity and cardiovascular risk variations in people of African origin with respect to mortality from stroke. Cappuccio [36] found that Black migrants to the UK (Caribbeans and West Africans) had lower mortality from stroke than the natives and other immigrants. These Black migrants, however, tended to be obese and hyperinsulinemic, with low serum triglycerides and high HDL-cholesterol. They were also found to have higher rates of cigarette smoking than other migrants and natives. Although the pattern of mortality observed was found to be associated with a high prevalence of hypertension and diabetes, it is difficult to explain the low rates of stroke.

As demonstrated by Kaufman et al. [59] in African and Caribbean men and women from six nations age 25–74 years, the prevalence of overweight and obesity (defined by body mass index) fluctuated from 6 to 63%, and from 1 to 36%, respectively. In these populations, 6–29% of hypertension was attributable to overweight (BMI ≥ 27.8 for men and BMI ≥ 27.3 for women), and 0–16% to obesity (BMI ≥ 31.1 for men and BMI ≥ 32.3 for women). Compared with their rural African counterparts, US women and men were found to have 43 and 22% higher prevalence of hypertension attributable to overweight, respectively. Similarly, 14 and 11% differences in hypertension in US women and men were attributable to obesity compared to rural African women and men, respectively [59].

Diabetes

The prevalence of type 2 diabetes mellitus (non-insulin-dependent diabetes) is more common in urban than rural Blacks living outside the US [60]. To determine the contribution of diabetes mellitus to all-cause mortality and diabetes mortality rates in adults living in one urban and two rural areas of Tanzania (Dar es Salaam, Hai and Morogoro Rural Districts), McLarty et al. [61] surveyed three populations consisting of 307,912 persons. Using verbal autopsies conducted with the help of kindred of the deceased, a total of 4,299 deaths were recorded in children (aged < 15 years) and 8,054 in adults. In children there were no reported deaths associated with diabetes. The adult male mortality rates associated with diabetes were 34, 30, and 15 per 100,000 per year in Dar es Salaam, Hai and Morogoro Rural Districts, respectively. The mortality rates in women were 21, 18, and 4 per 100,000 per year, respectively. The percentages of all adult male deaths associated with diabetes were 2.6, 2.1 and 0.7%, in Dar es Salaam, Hai and Morogoro Rural Districts, respectively. In women the percentages were 1.7, 1.8, and 0.2% in Dar es Salaam, Hai and Morogoro Rural Districts, respectively. Infection, acute metabolic complications, and stroke each accounted for approximately 30% of all diabetic deaths.

Other Risk Factors

Data on smoking as a risk factor for stroke are limited for Black populations outside the US. In response to impeded opportunities and declining markets in Western countries, the tobacco industry has focused its marketing efforts in developing countries [62]. There is evidence that smoking is highly prevalent in urban affluent Blacks outside the US [56]. In a study by Joubert [56], 5.6% of the 304 patients diagnosed with stroke between 1986 and 1987 in Ga-Rankuwa hospital smoked more than 10 cigarettes a day.

Conclusions

This article has summarized data from different sources on the epidemiology of stroke and its risk factors among Black populations outside the US. Evidence shows that stroke is becoming a problem in populations of African descent living outside the US. Urban and affluent Blacks in these countries are experiencing far greater prevalence of hypertension, diabetes, and stroke as they become Westernized. Also, urban Africans suffer greater mortality from stroke than their rural counterparts, but less than Blacks living in the US and other Western countries. In contrast, rural Africans residing outside the US have a lower prevalence of hypertension, diabetes and stroke. This fits well with a migration study in Kenya where changes in rural to urban migration were associated with a rise in blood pressure [63] as well as with a study in Cape Peninsula, South Africa that found a clear association of urbanization with chronic diseases [64].

In Africa where stroke risk is low, the contribution of hypertension to risk may be restricted to individuals at the upper limits of blood pressure distribution. The imperative in the African frameworks might therefore be the management of blood pressure in the upper range rather than an attempt to achieve an optimal level such as 130 mm Hg, as proposed in the US [65]. In the absence of empirical data this inference is only speculative and defensible in as much as in the US the remarkable advantage of blood pressure control in reduction in stroke has been demonstrated [66].

The 'thrifty phenotype' hypothesis suggests that human fetuses in utero in order to adapt to a limited supply of nutrients have to permanently change their physiology and metabolism. These 'programmed' transformations may be the origins of chronic diseases in later life, including hypertension, diabetes, and stroke [67, 68]. The proposed nutritional basis of these links has been tested in an animal model [67]. If confirmed in humans, this may have special significance for Blacks residing outside the US. These populations will be at an increased risk because of the vast numbers of poorly nourished infants who have been born in the last decades. The steady improvement in child survival will lead to higher percentages of infants surviving to adulthood, when their hypothesized susceptibility to stroke may manifest itself. More detailed longitudinal and genetic studies are desired to determine the causes of stroke in Blacks outside the US.

In conclusion, in West Africa, the source of the African diaspora, the effect of Westernization has produced a group that suffers from lack of physical activity, high smoking rates, excess consumption of energy-rich foods, obesity, and associated chronic diseases. Unlike the US, high cost of medication, poor management strategy, the inability to monitor patient conformity, and the lack of resources for effective monitoring of ascertained and referred cases makes control complicated. These countries are overwhelmed by competing disease from infections and other health outcomes. With the present rates of Westernization the rates of hypertension, obesity, and diabetes will obviously increase. The incidence of stroke and other chronic diseases will approach or even surpass the rates among US Blacks.

References

1   National Center for Health Statistics: Advance Report of Final Mortality Statistics, 1993. Monthly Final Statistics Report. Hyattsville, Public Health Service, 1996, vol 44(7), suppl, DHHS Publ (PHS) 96–1120.
2   Humphries SV: Personal experience of a stroke. Cent Afr J Med 1982;28:203–204.
3   Muna WF: Cardiovascular disorders in Africa. World Health Stat Q 1993;46:125–133.
4   Akinkugbe OO: Epidemiology of hypertension and stroke in Africa; in Hatano S, Shigematsu I, Strasser T (eds): Hypertension and Stroke Control in the Community. Geneva, WHO, pp 28–42.
5   Osuntokun BO, Odeku EL, Adeloye RB: Cerebrovascular accidents in Nigerians. A study of 348 patients. West Afr Med J Niger Pract 1969;18:160–173.
6   Osuntokun BO, Odeku EL, Adeloye RB: Non-embolic ischaemic cerebrovascular disease in Nigerians. J Neurol Sci 1969;9:361–388.

7 Osuntokun OO: Stroke in the Africans. Afr J Med Sci 1977;6:39–53.
8 Matenga J: Stroke incidence rates among Black residents of Harare: A prospective community-based study. S Afr Med J 1997;87:606–609.
9 Matenga J, Kitai I: Iatrogenic strokes in hypertensive patients. Cent Afr J Med 1986;32:130–131.
10 Nyame PK, Bonsu-Bruce N, Amoah AG, Adjei S, Nyarko E, Amuah EA, Biritwum RB: Current trends in the incidence of cerebrovascular accidents in Accra. West Afr J Med 1994;13:183–186.
11 Matenga J, Kitai I, Levy L: Strokes among Black people in Harare, Zimbabwe: Results of computed tomography and associated risk factors. Br Med J 1986;292:1649–1651.
12 Fritz VU: Stroke incidence in South Africa. S Afr Med J 1997;87:584–585.
13 Murray CJT, Lopez AD: Mortality by cause for eight regions of the World: Burden of disease study. Lancet 1997;349:1269–1276.
14 Walker R: Hypertension and stroke in sub-saharan Africa. Trans R Soc Trop Med Hyg 1994;88:609–611.
15 Bwala SA: Stroke in a subsaharan Nigerian hospital: A retrospective study. Trop Doct 1989;19:11–14.
16 Wood CH, Jeans WD, Coakham HB: Moyamoya disease: An unusual cause of cerebral infarction. Clin Radiol 1986;37:289–292.
17 Cosnett JE: Strokes in young people: Experience in a Bantu hospital. S Afr Med J 1969;26:501–507.
18 Shnier MH, Isaacson C: Perinatal mortality in the Bantu. S Afr Med J 1965;39:676–679.
19 Cruickshant JK: An outline of cerebrovascular and renal disease; in Cruckshank JK, Beever DG (eds): Ethnic Factors in Health and Disease. London, Butterworth-Heinemann, 1989, pp 266–267.
20 Miller GJ, Kirkwood BR, Beckles GL, Alexis SD, Carson DC, Byam NT: Adult male all-cause, cardiovascular and cerebrovascular mortality in relation to ethnic group, systolic blood pressure and blood glucose concentration in Trinidad, West Indies. Int J Epidemiol 1988;17:62–69.
21 Wright-Pascoe R, Lindo JF: The age-prevalence profile of abdominal obesity among patients in a diabetes referral clinic in Jamaica. West Ind Med J 1997;46:72–75.
22 Maheswaran R, Elliott P, Strachan DP: Socioeconomic deprivation, ethnicity, and stroke mortality in Greater London and south east England. J Epidemiol Commun Health 1997;51:127–131.
23 Chaturvedi N, Jarrett J, Morrish N, Keen H, Fuller JH: Differences in mortality and morbidity in African Caribbean and European people with non-insulin dependent diabetes mellitus: Results of 20 year follow up of a London cohort of a multinational study. BMJ 1996;313:848–852.
24 Chaturvedi N, Fuller JH: Ethnic differences in mortality from cardiovascular disease in the UK: Do they persist in people with diabetes? J Epidemiol Commun Health 1996;50:137–139.
25 Balarajan R: Ethnic differences in mortality from ischaemic heart disease and cerebrovascular disease in England and Wales. BMJ 1991;302:560–564.
26 Gulliford MC: Epidemiological transition in Trinidad and Tobago, West Indies 1953–1992. Int J Epidemiol 1996;25:357–365.
27 Williams AO, Resch JA, Loewenson RB: Comparative study on cerebral atherosclerosis between an African (Nigerian) and American population groups (Caucasian and Negroes). East Afr Med J 1971;48:152–162.
28 Williams AO, Loewenson RB, Lippert DM, Resch JA: Cerebral atherosclerosis and its relationship to selected diseases in Nigerians: A pathological study. Stroke 1975;6:395–401.
29 Kuller LH: Epidemiology of stroke. Adv Neurol 1978;19:281–311.
30 Osuntokun BO, Bademosi O, Akinkugbe OO, Oyediran AB, Carlisle R: Incidence of stroke in an African City: Results from the Stroke Registry at Ibadan, Nigeria, 1973–1975. Stroke 1979;10:205–207.
31 Taylor GO, Barber JB, Jackson MA, Resch JA, Williams AO: Lipid composition of cerebral vessels in American Negroes, Caucasians and Nigerian Africans: A comparative study. Stroke 1975;6:298–300.
32 Resch JA, Williams AO, Lemercier G, Loewenson RB: Comparative autopsy studies on cerebral atherosclerosis in Nigerian and Senegal Negroes, American Negroes and Caucasians. Atherosclerosis 1970;12:401–407.
33 Mulley G: Letter: Stroke in Africa. Lancet 1976;ii:47.
34 Cole M: Cerebral infarct after rattlesnake bite. Arch Neurol 1996;53:957–958.

35   Cole FM, Cole HL: The pattern of fatal cerebrovascular disease in Jamaica. West Indian Med J 1969;18:202–209.

36   Cappuccio FP: Ethnicity and cardiovascular risk: Variations in people of African ancestry and South Asian origin. J Hum Hypertens 1997;11:571–576.

37   Zabsonre P, Yameogo A, Millogo A, Dyemkouma FX, Durand G: Risk and severity factors in cerebrovascular accidents in west african Blacks of Burkina Faso. Med Trop 1997;57:147–152.

38   Dada TO, Johnson FA, Araba AB, Adegbite SA: Cerebrovascular accidents in Nigerians: A review of 205 cases. West Afr Med J Niger Pract 1969;18:95–108.

39   Nwosu CM, Nwabueze AC, Ikeh VO: Stroke at the prime of life: A study of Nigerian Africans between the ages of 16 and 45 years. East Afr Med J 1992;69:384–390.

40   Billinghurst JR: Stroke. East Afr Med J 1970;47:653.

41   Rosman KD: The epidemiology of stroke in an urban Black population. Stroke 1986;17:667–669.

42   Abebe M, Haimanot RT: Cerebrovascular accidents in Ethiopia. Ethiop Med J 1990;28:53–61.

43   Obama MT, Dongmo L, Nkemayim C, Mbede J, Hagbe P: Stroke in children in Yaounde, Cameroon. Ind Pediatr 1994;31:791–795.

44   Bam WJ, Yako PM: Correlation between hypertension and cerebrovascular accidents in Black patients. S Afr Med J 1984;65:638–641.

45   Kaufman JS, Owoaje EE, James SA, Rotimi CN, Cooper RS: Determinants of hypertension in West Africa: Contribution of anthropometric and dietary factors to urban-rural and socioeconomic gradients. Am J Epidemiol 1996;143:1203–1218.

46   Mensah GA, Barkey NL, Cooper RS: Spectrum of hypertensive target organ damage in Africa: A review of published studies. J Hum Hypertens 1994;8:799–808.

47   Baddock DRW: Cerebrovascular accidents in Ghana. Trans R Soc Med. Hyg 1970;64:300–310.

48   Seedat YK: Perspectives of hypertension in Black patients: Black vs. White differences. J Cardiovasc Pharmacol 1990;16(suppl 7):S67-S70.

49   Bertrand E: Arterial hypertension, serious public health problem in Black Africa. Bull Soc Pathol Exot Filiales 1983;76:327–331.

50   Breslin DJ, Gifford RW, Fairbairn JF: Essential hypertension: A twenty-year follow-up study. Circulation 1966;33:87–97.

51   Failde I, Balkau B, Costagliola D, Moutet JP, Gabriel JM, Donnet JP, Eschwege E: Arterial hypertension in the adult population of Guadeloupe, and associated factors in subjects of African origin. Rev Epidemiol Sante Publique 1996;44:417–426.

52   Cooper R, Rotimi C, Ataman S, McGee D, Osotimehin B, Kadiri S, Muna W, Kingue S, Fraser H, Forrester T, Bennett F, Wilks R: The prevalence of hypertension in seven populations of west African origin. Am J Publ Health 1997;87:160–168.

53   Wilson TW, Hollifield LR, Grim CE: Systolic blood pressure levels in Black populations in sub-Sahara Africa, the West Indies, and the United States: A meta-analysis. Hypertension 1991; 18(3 suppl):187-191.

54   Lisk DR: Hypertension in Sierra Leone stroke population. East Afr Med J 1993;70:284–287.

55   Danesi MA, Oyenola YA, Ontiri AC: Risk factors associated with cerebrovascular accidents in Nigerians (a case-control study). East Afr Med J 1983;60:190–195.

56   Joubert J: The MEDUNSA Stroke Data Bank: An analysis of 304 patients seen between 1986 and 1987. S Afr Med J 1991;80:567–570.

57   Hubert HB, Feinleib M, McNamara PM, Castelli WP: Obesity as an independent risk factor for cardiovascular disease: A 26-year follow-up of participants in the Framingham Heart Study. Circulation 1983;67:968–977.

58   Wilks R, McFarlane-Anderson N, Bennett F, Fraser H, McGee D, Cooper R, Forrester T: Obesity in peoples of the African diaspora. Ciba Found Symp 1996;201:37–48.

59   Kaufman JS, Durazo-Arvizu RA, Rotimi CN, McGee DL, Cooper RS: Obesity and hypertension prevalence in populations of African origin: The investigators of the International Collaborative Study on Hypertension in Blacks. Epidemiology 1996;7:398–405.

60   Cooper RS, Rotimi CN, Kaufman JS, Owoaje EE, Fraser H, Forrester T, Wilks R, Riste LK, Cruickshank JK: Prevalence of NIDDM among populations of the African diaspora. Diabetes Care 1997;20:343–348.

61 McLarty DG, Unwin N, Kitange HM, Alberti KG: Diabetes mellitus as a cause of death in sub-Saharan Africa: Results of a community-based study in Tanzania. The Adult Morbidity and Mortality Project. Diabet Med 1996;13:990–994.

62 Peto R, Chen Z, Boreham J: Tobacco: The growing epidemic in China. JAMA 1996;275:1683–1684.

63 Poulter NR, Khaw KT, Mugambi M, Peart WS, Sever PS: Migration-induced changes in blood pressure: A controlled longitudinal study. Clin Exp Pharmacol Physiol 1985;12:211–216.

64 Steyn K, Kazenellenbogen JM, Lombard CJ, Bourne LT: Urbanization and the risk for chronic diseases of lifestyle in the Black population of the Cape Peninsula, South Africa. J Cardiovasc Risk 1997;4:135–142.

65 JNC V: The fifth report of the Joint National Committee on Detection, Evaluation and Treatment of High Blood Pressure. Arch Intern Med 1993;153:154–183.

66 Mariyama IM, Krueger DE, Stamler J: Cardiovascular Diseases in the United States. Cambridge, Harvard University Press, 1971, pp 175–225.

67 Barker DJ: Maternal nutrition, fetal nutrition, and disease in later life. Nutrition 1997;13:807–813.

68 Barker DJ: The fetal origins of coronary heart disease. Eur Heart J 1997;18:883–884.

Ike S. Okosun, MPH, PhD, Department of Preventive Medicine and Epidemiology,
Loyola University Stritch School of Medicine, 2160 South First Avenue,
Maywood, IL 60153 (USA)

Gillum RF, Gorelick PB, Cooper ES (eds): Stroke in Blacks. Basel, Karger, 1999, pp 83–93

....

Epidemiology of Stroke in Blacks

Richard F. Gillum

Centers for Disease Control and Prevention, Hyattsville, Md., USA

Stroke is the third leading cause of death in US Blacks [1]. It is an important cause of mortality and morbidity worldwide [2]. Since 1914, higher stroke mortality from stroke in US Blacks than Whites has been documented by vital statistics, with differentials maintained as diagnostic technology developed over the century [3–6]. In the 1960s, stroke death rates of US Blacks were among the highest in the world [3]; currently, they fall between the high rates of Eastern Europe and the low rates of North American Whites (fig. 1) [4, 7, 8]. Stroke is an important contributor to overall higher mortality in US Blacks than Whites [9]. Despite these facts, many questions remain regarding the etiology of stroke in Blacks and the basis for racial differences in stroke occurrence [4, 10]. Racial patterns and trends in stroke mortality (fig. 2), prevalence (fig. 3), and risk factors have been reviewed and reported at length elsewhere in the literature and in other chapters of this book [4–48]. This report examines data on stroke incidence, case fatality, medical care, and long-term survivorship from the US National Center for Health Statistics and reviews epidemiologic studies of stroke in Black populations in an attempt to critically examine the current state of knowledge and to suggest directions for future research and prevention.

Incidence

Cohort Studies
In the small number of biracial cohort studies available, incidence of completed stroke has been consistently higher in US Blacks than Whites [4, 10, 36–38, 49–52]. However, the incidence of transient ischemic attacks was reported to be almost twice as great in Whites as in Blacks in the Evans County study [36]. Estimates of stroke incidence in US Blacks have recently

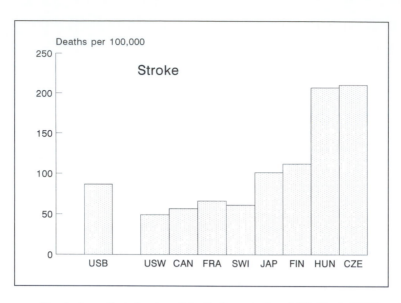

Fig. 1. Age-adjusted rates of death from stroke of US Black (USB) and US White (USW) men compared to men in selected industrialized countries (Canada, CAN; France, FRA; Switzerland, SWI; Japan, JAP; Finland, FIN; Hungary, HUN; former Czechoslovakia, CZE) in 1990. Reproduced with permission from Gillum [32].

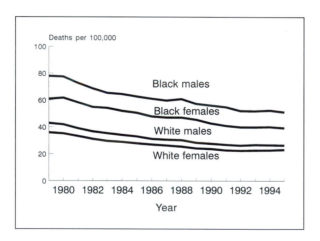

Fig. 2. Age-adjusted stroke mortality rates in the United States, 1979–1995. Reproduced with permission from Gillum [22].

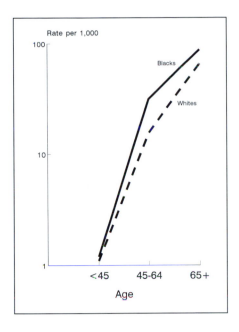

Fig. 3. Prevalence of self-reported stroke by race in the United States, 1990–1992. Reproduced with permission from Gillum and Wilson [5].

become available from a national cohort study of persons participating in a national health survey, the National Health and Nutrition Examination Survey I Epidemiologic Follow-up Study (NHEFS) [49]. During a follow-up period from 1971–1975 to 1987, Blacks were found to suffer higher rates of stroke incidence than Whites [49–51]. At 10 years, the age-adjusted relative risks (RR) was 1.8 in women and 1.3 in men (RR = 1.0 means no difference in risk between exposed and nonexposed groups). RR were higher in younger than older persons. This difference could only partially be explained statistically by controlling for major stroke risk factors in women (adjusted RR 1.4 in women and 1.1 in men). Black-White differences in incidence were greatest at age 35–44 (RR = 2.62, 95% confidence interval (CI) 1.23–5.57) and least at 65 and over (RR = 1.14, 95% CI 0.90–1.46) [51]. After adjustment for age, sex, education, history of heart disease, diabetes, systolic blood pressure, treatment for hypertension, Quetelet index, and serum hemoglobin and magnesium levels, the RR fell only to 2.07 in younger persons and to 0.82 in older persons. These findings confirmed results of an earlier analysis in which hypertension and diabetes were controlled for [50].

Hospitalization for cerebrovascular disease among 74,096 White and 33,041 Black persons in a prepaid health care program showed Blacks were at higher adjusted risk for hospitalization than Whites for hemorrhagic cerebrovascular disease (RR = 2.4, 95% CI 1.3–5.8), cerebral thrombosis (RR = 1.9,

95% CI 1.2–2.9), and nonspecific cerebrovascular disease (RR = 1.6, 95% CI 1.2–2.2) but at lower hospitalization risk for extracranial occlusive disease (RR = 0.4, 95% CI 0.2–0.7) [52]. Hence cohort studies are consistent with one another and with studies that used other methodologies in reporting higher incidence of stroke among Blacks. Further, some suggest the excess risk for Blacks is greater in women than men (in contrast to recent mortality rates) and in younger than older persons (consistent with mortality rates) and similar for hemorrhagic and thrombotic stroke.

Community Surveillance Studies

Several studies have reported higher rates of hospitalization for first acute stroke in Blacks than in Whites [49–65]. At all ages, rates per 100,000 in Blacks were 288 in Greater Cincinnati/Northern Kentucky and 233 at age 20 years and over in Northern Manhattan, New York City [53, 54]. One group used Medicare hospitalization data to estimate national trends in the incidence of stroke among African-Americans aged 70 years or older during 1985–1991 [56]. Blacks had consistently higher incidence rates (nearly 1,800 per 100,000 compared to 1,400 for Whites); no trends over time were found for Blacks whereas rates for Whites declined by nearly 7%. These and other studies consistently showed higher rates of first stroke, first hemorrhagic stroke and first thrombotic stroke in Blacks than Whites.

Other studies using administrative data, which were unable to effectively exclude persons with prior history, report higher rates of incident and recurrent stroke combined in US Blacks than Whites [4, 10, 14, 61–66]. For example, in Northern Manhattan, the age-adjusted hospitalization rate per 100,000 was 567 for Blacks, 306 for Hispanics, and 351 for Whites among men and 716, 361, and 326, respectively, among women [61]. In Medicare recipients, inconsistent trends in Blacks and steady declines in hospitalization rates in Whites produced widening racial gap between 1985 and 1990 [62]. More studies of trends in Blacks are needed. Population-based studies of Blacks outside North America are few and probably not comparable with those cited above, as discussed previously [4, 10, 64, 65].

Stroke Subtypes

Although of vital importance, studies of the incidence of stroke subtypes in Blacks are few. In the early part of this century, cerebral hemorrhage was thought to be the predominant cause of stroke mortality in Blacks and Whites in the US [3]. However, the number of deaths from cerebral hemorrhage in US vital statistics were inflated because coded 'cerebral vascular accident' was coded cerebral hemorrhage [3]. Wider access to hospital care, improved diagnostic techniques, and results of population-based studies of stroke morbidity revealed ischemic stroke to be the predominant type in Whites by the 1950s. Data accumulated since then has revealed this also to be the case for Blacks [4, 10, 66–72]. Available data indicate that compared to US Whites, US Blacks have greater incidence and mortality rates for every stroke subtype with the likely exception of cerebral infarction and transient cerebral ischemia due to extracranial carotid artery occlusion. Excess risk for cerebral infarction in blacks is similar to that for hemorrhage due to the high risk for lacunar infarcts which compensates for their reduced risk for extracranial occlusion.

Data on stroke subtypes from Africa are scarce and derive from case series [4, 65, 68–72]. Infectious etiologies of stroke syndromes, e.g. syphilis, HIV, tuberculosis, neurocysticercosis, remain important in young Black patients in developing countries. Cerebral infarction is the predominant pathology of stroke in Blacks in Africa as in America and presumably elsewhere, contrary to earlier speculation. Lacunar infarction seems to vary in frequency among Black populations, being common in the US and urban southern Africa but uncommon in rural southern Africa.

Survivorship

Case Fatality

Only limited population-based case fatality data for Blacks were found for cases that used hospital or administrative data [73–82]. In a series of ischemic stroke cases from Northern Manhattan, hospital case fatality was higher in younger Blacks and Hispanics than Whites [73]. Among patients discharged from US hospitals in 1988–1990 with the diagnosis of acute stroke (ICD-9 431–432, 434, 436), hospital case fatality rates for persons aged 65–74 were for Blacks 12.2% and for Whites 15.4%; for acute ischemic stroke (ICD-9 434–436) Blacks 8.9% and whites 12.3% [74]. However, these rates for blacks must be viewed with caution due to the small number of fatal cases in the sample. An analysis of data from the Maryland Health Services Cost Review Commission revealed higher incidence of coma, hospital death rate, and length of stay in Blacks than Whites hospitalized for acute hemorrhagic and occlusive stroke (with the exception of case fatality for hemorrhagic stroke) [75]. In a 1983–1986 series of 590 cerebral infarction patients in New York City, the 1-month mortality rate was similar in Whites and Blacks [79]. These limited data permit no firm conclusions to be drawn about relative case fatality in Blacks compared with Whites in the United States; they do, however, suggest that at least in some areas Blacks suffering from stroke may have a less favorable acute prognosis than Whites. No data on trends in case fatality for Blacks were found. Analyses of Medicare data would be helpful in shedding light on these questions.

Long-Term Survivorship

Few population-based studies of long-term survival after stroke in Blacks were found. Data from several hospital series indicate possibly poorer survivorship and functional recovery in Blacks [75, 79]. In among hospitalized stroke patients in Northern Manhattan, 2-year readmission rates, overall and for stroke, were similar in Blacks, Hispanics and Whites [61]. In a 1983–1986 series of 590 cerebral infarction patients in New York City, Whites had a slightly greater risk of recurrent stroke or death than Blacks until 6 months after infarction, when their risk stabilized, while the risk in Blacks continued to rise for the entire year of follow-up [73]. By 1 year, the rate of recurrent stroke or death was $34.8 \pm 4.2\%$ in Whites, $31.1 \pm 3.6\%$ in Blacks (p=0.04). Ethnic differences in stroke risk factors and infarct subtype explained the ethnic differences in outcome. An abnormal first electrocardiogram was a risk factor for stroke recurrence or death in Blacks and Whites. In a North Carolina county, physical and functional impairments after stroke were more severe in Blacks than Whites [81]. The epidemiology of late sequelae such as multi-infarct dementia will be discussed elsewhere in his book [82]. Rates of stroke recurrence, severe impairment, and death are high in Blacks and may be greater than in Whites in some populations.

Medical Care

Hospital statistics consistently show lower utilization of diagnostic and surgical procedures for CVD in US Blacks than Whites [4, 16, 83–87]. In 1980–1992, Whites had estimated rates of carotid endarterectomy procedures over four times higher than Blacks [83]. Whites also had higher rates of cerebral arteriography, but the disparity was not as great as for endarterectomy [83]. A study of utilization of stroke rehabilitations services at a university hospital in North Carolina failed to reveal racial disparities [86]. Discharge planning with African-American stroke patients and family members involved less use of nursing home care and more use of formal services in the home than planning with White patients and families [87]. The consistent observation of racial differences in utilization of procedures and other services deserve further study in richer administrative databases such as Medicare and in clinical epidemiology studies in health maintenance organizations (HMOs) and Veterans' Affairs hospitals.

Conclusions

Stroke is the third leading cause of death in US Blacks [1]. It is an important cause of mortality and morbidity worldwide. Despite these facts, many questions remain regarding the etiology of stroke in Blacks and the basis for racial differences in stroke occurrence. The third leading cause of death in Black women and the sixth in Black men in the US in 1995, stroke accounted for 10,526 deaths in women and 8,011 in men among Blacks in 1995, 7.96 and 5.20%, respectively, of the total [1]. Age-adjusted rates per 100,000 were Black women 39.9, White women 22.9, Black men 52.2, White men 26.6. The Black/White ratio of age-adjusted rates was 1.74 in women and 1.96 in men. Since the early 1980s a marked slow-down has occurred in the decline in US stroke mortality in Black and in White Americans. In the small number of biracial cohort studies available, incidence of completed stroke has been consistently higher in US Blacks than Whites. Available data indicate that compared to US Whites, US Blacks have greater incidence and mortality rates for every stroke subtype with the likely exception of cerebral infarction (and transient cerebral ischemia) due to extracranial carotid artery occlusion. Excess risk for overall cerebral infarction in blacks is similar to that for hemorrhage due to the high risk for lacunar infarcts which compensates for their reduced risk for extracranial occlusion. Limited data permit no firm conclusions to be drawn about relative case fatality in Blacks compared with Whites in the United States; they do, however, suggest that at least in some areas Blacks suffering from stroke may have a less favorable acute prognosis than Whites. Hospital statistics consistently show lower utilization of diagnostic and surgical procedures for stroke in US Blacks than Whites. The cause for this should be sought. In Blacks, advanced age, elevated blood pressure, diabetes, and smoking are the only common risk factors for stroke whose status is firmly established by published data. Thus, hypertension prevention and control, prevention of diabetes and risk factor management in diabetics, and smoking prevention and cessation are key to control of stroke in Black populations. Increased research on stroke in Blacks is needed to develop more effective strategies for primary and secondary prevention of stroke to reduce the high burden of premature mortality and morbidity.

References

1   National Center for Health Statistics: Health, United States, 1996–97 and Injury Chartbook. Hyattsville, Public Health Service, 1997.
2   Murray CJL, Lopez AD: Mortality by cause for eight regions of the world: Global Burden of Disease Study. Lancet 1997;349:1269–1276.

3   Moriyama IM, Kruger DE, Stamler J: Cardiovascular Diseases in the United States. Cambridge, Harvard University Press, 1971, pp 175–229.
4   Gillum RF: Stroke in Blacks. Stroke 1988;19:1–9.
5   Gillum RF, Wilson JB: The burden of stroke and its sequelae. Dis Management Health Outcomes 1997;1:84–94.
6   Gaines K, Burke G: Ethnic differences in stroke: Black-White differences in the United States population. Neuroepidemiology 1995;14:209–239.
7   Gillum RF: The epidemiology of hypertension in Black women. Am Heart J 1996;131:385–395.
8   Gillum RF: The epidemiology of cardiovascular disease in Black Americans. N Engl J Med 1996; 335:1597–1599.
9   Otten M, Teutsch S, Williamson D, Marks J: The effect of known risk factors on the excess mortality of Black adults in the United States. JAMA 1990;263:845–850.
10 Alter M: Black-White differences in stroke frequency: Challenges for research. Neuroepidemiology 1994;13:301–307.
11 Gillum RF: The epidemiology of cardiovascular disease: An American overview; in Livingston I (ed): Handbook of Black American Health: The Mosaic of Conditions, Issues, Policies, and Prospects. Westport, Greenwood Publishing, 1994, pp 3–23.
12 Morgenstern LB, Spears WD, Goff DC, Grotta JC, Nichaman MZ: African-Americans and women have the highest stroke mortality in Texas. Stroke 1997;28:15–18.
13 Morgenstern LB, Spears WD: A triethnic comparison of intracerebral hemorrhage mortality in Texas. Ann Neurol 1997;42:919–923.
14 Gillum, RF, Feinleib M: Cardiovascular disease in the United States: Mortality, prevalence, and incidence; in Kapoor AS, Singh BN (eds): Prognosis and Risk Assessment in Cardiovascular Disease. New York, Churchill-Livingstone, 1993, pp 49–59.
15 Neaton JD, Wentworth DN, Cutler J, Stamler J, Kuller L: Risk factors for death from different types of stroke. Ann Epidemiol 1993;3:493–499.
16 Gillum RF: Cerebrovascular disease morbidity in the United States, 1974–1983: Age, sex, race region and vascular surgery. Stroke 1986;17:656–661.
17 Feinleib M, Ingster L, Rosenberg H, Maurer J, Singh G, Kochanek K: Time trends, cohort effects, and geographical patterns in stroke mortality – United States. Ann Epidemiol 1993;3:458–465.
18 Howard G, Anderson R, Sorlie P, Andrews V, Backlund E, Burke GL: Ethnic differences in stroke mortality between non-Hispanic Whites, Hispanic Whites, and Blacks. The National Longitudinal Mortality Study. Stroke 1994;25:2120–2125.
19 Soltero I, Liu K, Cooper R, Stamler J, Garside D: Trends in mortality from cerebrovascular diseases in the United States, 1960 to 1975. Stroke 1978;9:549–558.
20 Cooper R, Sempos C, Hsieh SC, Kovar MG: Slowdown of the decline of stroke mortality in the United States, 1978–1986. Stroke 1990;21:1274–1279.
21 Howard G: Decline in stroke mortality in North Carolina: Description, predictions, and a possible underlying cause. Ann Epidemiol 1993;3:488–492.
22 Gillum RF: Secular trends in stroke mortality in African Americans: The role of urbanization, diabetes and obesity. Neuroepidemiology 1997;16:180–184.
23 Gillum RF, Sempos CT: The end of the long-term decline in stroke mortality in the United States? Stroke 1997;28:1527–1529.
24 Brown RD Jr, Whisnant JP, Sicks JD, O'Fallon WM, Wiebers DO: Stroke incidence, prevalence, and survival: Secular trends in Rochester, Minnesota, through 1989. Stroke 1996;27:373–380.
25 Sempos C, Cooper R, Kovar MG, McMillen M: Divergence of the recent trends in coronary mortality for the four major race-sex groups in the United States. Am J Publ Hlth 1988;78:1422–1427.
26 National High Blood Pressure Education Program: The Sixth Report of the Joint National Committee on Prevention, Detection, Evaluation, and Treatment of High Blood Pressure. National Institutes of Health. NIH Publ No 98–4080, Nov, 1997.
27 Pickle LW, Mungiole M, Jones GK, White AA: Atlas of United States Mortality. Hyattsville, National Center for Health Statistics, 1997.
28 Howard G, Evans GW, Pearce K, Howard VJ, Bell RA, Mayer EJ, Burke GL: Is the stroke belt disappearing? An analysis of racial, temporal, and age effects. Stroke 1995;26:1153–1158.

29 Casper ML, Wing S, Anda RF, Knowles M, Pollard RA: Changes in the geographic pattern of stroke mortality in the United States, 1962 to 1988. Stroke 1995;26:755–760.

30 Lanska DJ; Peterson PM: Comparison of additive and multiplicative models of regional variation in the decline of stroke mortality in the United States. Stroke 1996;27:1055–1059.

31 Pickle L, Mungiole M, Gillum RF: Geographic variation in stroke mortality in Blacks and Whites in the United States. Stroke 1997;28:1639–1647.

32 Gillum RF: The epidemiology of coronary heart disease and stroke in elderly African-Americans. Am J Geriatr Cardiol 1997;6:21–31.

33 Walker R: Hypertension and stroke in sub-Saharan Africa. Trans R Soc Trop Med Hyg 1994;88: 609–611.

34 Fang J, Madhavan S, Alderman MH: Association between birthplace and cardiovascular mortality in Black Americans in New York City. N Engl J Med 1996;335:1545–1551.

35 Blarajan R: Ethnic differences in mortality from ischemic heart disease and cerebrovascular disease in England and Wales. BMJ 1991;302:560–564.

36 Heyman A, Karp HR, Heyden S, Bartel A, Cassel JC, Tyroler HA, Cornoni J, Hames CG, Stuart W: Cerebrovascular disease in the bi-racial population of Evans County, Georgia. Stroke 1971;2:509–518.

37 Ostfeld AM: Heart disease and stroke in an elderly welfare population. Bull NY Acad Sci 1973; 49:458–465.

38 Stallones RA, Dyken ML, Fang HCH, Heyman A, Seltser R, Stamler J: Report of the Joint Committee for Stroke Facilities. Epidemiology for stroke facilities planning. Stroke 1972;3:359–371.

39 Centers for Disease Control and Prevention: Chronic Disease in Minority Populations. Atlanta, Centers for Disease Control and Prevention, 1992, pp 2-1–2-34.

40 Schoenberg BS, Anderson DW, Haerer AF: Racial differentials in the prevalence of stroke, Copiah County, Mississippi. Arch Neurol 1986;43:565–568.

41 Toole JF, Lefkowitz DS, Chambless LE, Wijnberg L, Paton CC, Heiss G: Self-reported transient ischemic attack and stroke symptoms – methods and base-line prevalence – the ARIC Study, 1987–1989. Am J Epidemiol 1996;144:849–856.

42 Collins JG: Prevalence of selected chronic conditions: United States, 1990–1992. National Center for Health Statistics. Vital Health Stat 1997;10:1-89.

43 Manolio TA, Burke GL, Psaty BM, Newman AB, Haan M, Powe N, Tracy RP, Oleary DH: Black-White differences in subclinical cardiovascular disease among older adults: The Cardiovascular Health Study. J Clin Epidemiol 1995;48:1141–1152.

44 Burke GL, Evans GW, Hutchinson R, Davis CE, Howard G, Higgins M, Heiss G: Racial differences in carotid wall thickness in middle-aged adults. Circulation 1994;89:939.

45 Burke GL, Evans GW, Riley WA, Sharrett AR, Howard G, Barnes RW, Rosamond W, Crow RS, Rautaharju PM, Heiss G: Arterial wall thickness is associated with prevalent cardiovascular disease in middle-aged adults: The Atherosclerosis Risk in Communities (ARIC) Study. Stroke 1995;26: 386–391.

46 Sacco RL, Roberts K, Boden-Albala B, Gu Q, Lin I, Kargman DE, Berglund L, Hauser WA, Shea S, Paik MC: Race-ethnicity and determinants of carotid atherosclerosis in a multiethnic population: The Northern Manhattan Stroke Study. Stroke 1997;28:929–935.

47 D'Agostino RB, Burke G, O'Leary D, Rewers M, Selby J, Savage PJ, Saad MF, Bergman RN, Howard G, Wagenknecht L, Haffner S: Ethnic differences in carotid wall thickness: The Insulin Resistance Atherosclerosis Study. Stroke 1996;27:1744–1749.

48 Prisant LM, Zermel PC, Nichols FT, Zemel MB, Sowers JR, Carr AA, Thompson WO, Bond G: Carotid plaque associations among hypertensive patients. Arch Intern Med 1993;153:501–506.

49 Gillum RF: Coronary heart disease, stroke and hypertension in a national cohort: The NHANES I Epidemiologic Follow-up Study. Ann Epidemiol 1996;6:259–262.

50 Kittner SJ, White LR, Losonczy KG, Wolf PA, Hebel JR: Black-White differences in stroke incidence in a national sample: The contribution of hypertension and diabetes mellitus. JAMA 1990;264: 1267–1270.

51 Giles WH, Kittner SJ, Heble JR, Losonczy KG, Sherwin RW: Determinants of Black-White differences in the risk of cerebral infarction: The National Health and Nutrition Examination Survey Epidemiologic Follow-up Study. Arch Intern Med 1995;155:1319–1324.

52   Klatsky AL, Armstrong MA, Friedman GD: Racial differences in cerebrovascular disease hospital-izations. Stroke 1991;22:299–304.

53   Broderick J, Brott T, Kothari R, Miller R, Khoury J, Pancioli A, Gebel J, Mills D, Minneci L, Shukla R: The Greater Cincinnati/Northern Kentucky Stroke Study: Preliminary first-ever and total incidence rates of stroke among blacks. Stroke 1998;29:415–421.

54   Sacco RL, Boden-Albala B, Gan R, Chen X, Kargman DE, Shea S, Paik MC, the Northern Manhattan Stroke Study Collaborators: Stroke incidence among White, Black, and Hispanic residents of an urban community. The Northern Manhattan Stroke Study. Am J Epidemiol 1998;147: 259–268.

55   Gross CR, Kase CS, Mohr JP, Cunningham SC, Baker WE: Stroke in south Alabama: Incidence and diagnostic features: A population-based study. Stroke 1984;15:249–255.

56   May DS, Kittner SJ: Use of Medicare claims data to estimate national trends in stroke incidence, 1985–1991. Stroke 1994;25:2343–2347.

57   Kittner SJ, McCarter RJ, Sherwin RW, Sloan MA, Stern BJ, Johnson CJ, Buchholz D, Seipp MJ, Price TR: Black-White differences in stroke risk among young adults. Stroke 1993;24(12 suppl): I13–I15.

58   Broderick JP, Brott T, Tomsick T, Huster G, Miller R: The risk of subarachnoid and intracerebral hemorrhages in blacks as compared with whites. N Engl J Med 1992;326:733–736.

59   Friday G, Lai SM, Alter M, Sobel E, LaRue L, Gil-Peralta A, McCoy RL, Levitt LP, Isack T: Stroke in the Lehigh Valley: Racial/ethnic differences. Neurology 1989;39:1165–1168.

60   Broderick J, Talbot GT, Prenger E, Leach A, Brott T: Stroke in children within a major metropolitan area: The surprising importance of intracerebral hemorrhage. J Child Neurol 1993;8:250–255.

61   Sacco RL, Hauser WA, Mohr JP: Hospitalized stroke in Blacks and Hispanics in Northern Manhat-tan. Stroke 1991;22:1491–1496.

62   Cerebrovascular disease mortality and Medicare hospitalization – United States, 1980–1990. MMWR 1992;41:477–480.

63   Heyman A, Fields WS, Keating RO: Joint study of extracranial arterial occlusion. VI. Racial differences in hospitalized patients with ischemic stroke. JAMA 1972;222:285–289.

64   Osuntokun BO, Bademosi O, Akinkugbe OO, Oyediran AB, Carlisle R: Incidence of stroke in an African city: Results from the Stroke Registry at Ibadan, Nigeria, 1973–1975. Stroke 1979;10:205–207.

65   Matenga J: Stroke incidence rates among Black residents of Harare: A prospective community-based study. S Afr Med J 1997;87:606–609.

66   Wityk RJ, Lehmann D, Klag M, Coresh J, Ahn H, Litt B: Race and sex-differences in the distribution of cerebral atherosclerosis. Stroke 1996;27:1974–1980.

67   Quereshi AI, Safdar K, Patel M, Janssen RS, Frankel MR: Stroke in young Black patients: Risk factors, subtypes and prognosis. Stroke 1995;26:1995–1998.

68   Joubert J: The MEDUNSA Stroke Data Bank: An analysis of 304 patients seen between 1986 and 1987. S Afr Med J 1991;80:567–570.

69   Rosman KD: The epidemiology of stroke in an urban Black population. Stroke 1986;17:667–669.

70   Matenga J, Kitai I, Levy L: Strokes among Black people in Harare, Zimbabwe: Results of computed tomography and associated risk factors. BMJ 1986;292:1649–1651.

71   Gilperalta A, Alter M, Lai SM, Friday G, Otero A, Katz M, Comerota AJ: Duplex Doppler and spectral flow-analysis of race differences in cerebrovascular atherosclerosis. Stroke 1990;21:740–744.

72   Mets TF: The disease pattern of elderly medical patients in Rwanda, Central Africa. J Trop Med Hyg 1993;96:291–300.

73   Sacco RL, Hauser WA, Mohr JP, Foulkes MA: One-year outcome after cerebral infarction in Whites, Blacks, and Hispanics. Stroke 1991;22:305–311.

74   Graves EJ: National Hospital Discharge Survey: Annual Summary, 1990. National Center for Health Statistics. Vital Health Stat 1992;13:1–63.

75   Kuhlemeier KV, Stiens SA: Racial disparities in severity of cerebrovascular events. Stroke 1994;25: 2126–2131.

76   Dennis GC, Welch B, Cole AN, Mendoza R, Morgan J, Epps J, Bernard E, St Louis P: Subarachnoid hemorrhage in the African-American population: A cooperative study. J Natl Med Assoc 1997;89: 101–108.

Gillum

77   Quereshi AI, Suri MA, Safdar K, Ottenlips JR, Janssen RS, Frankel MR: Intracerebral hemorrhage in Blacks: Risk factors, subtypes, and outcome. Stroke 1997;28:961–964.

78   Quereshi AI, Safdar K, Weil J, Barch C, Bliwise DL, Colohan AR, Mackay B, Frankel MR: Predictors of early deterioration and mortality in Black Americans with spontaneous intracerebral hemorrhage. Stroke 1995;26:1764–1767.

79   Sacco RL: Risk factors and outcomes for ischemic stroke. Neurology 1993;45:S10–S14.

80   Sacco RL: Ischemic stroke; in Gorelick PB, Alter M (eds): Handbook of Neuroepidemiology. New York, Marcel Dekker, 1994, pp 77–119.

81   Horner RD, Matchar DB, Divine GW, Feussner JR: Racial variations in ischemic stroke-related physical and functional impairments. Stroke 1991;22:1497–1501.

82   Gorelick PB, Brody J, Cohen D, Freels S, Levy P, Dollear W, Forman H, Harris Y: Risk factors for dementia associated with multiple cerebral infarcts: A case-control analysis in predominantly African-American hospital-based patients. Arch Neurol 1993;50:714–720.

83   Gillum RF: Epidemiology of carotid endarterectomy and cerebral arteriography in the United States. Stroke 1995;26:1724–1728.

84   Hsia DC, Moscoe LM, Krushat M: Epidemiology of carotid endarterectomy among Medicare beneficiaries. 1985–1996 update. Stroke 1998;29:346–350.

85   Maxwell JG, Rutherford EJ, Covington D, Clancy TV, Tacket AD, Robinson N, Johnson G: Infrequency of Blacks among patients having carotid endarterectomy. Stroke 1989;20:22–26.

86   Horner RD, Hoenig H, Sloane R, Rubenstein LV, Kahn KL: Racial differences in the utilization of inpatient rehabilitation services among elderly stroke patients. Stroke 1997;28:19–25.

87   Morrow-Howell N, Chadiha LA, Proctor EK, Hourd-Bryant M, Dore P: Racial differences in discharge planning. Health Soc Work 1996;21:131–139.

R.F. Gillum, MD, Office of Analysis, Epidemiology and Health Promotion,
Centers for Disease Control and Prevention, National Center for Health Statistics,
6525 Belcrest Road, Room 730, Hyattsville, MD 20782-2003 (USA)

Gillum RF, Gorelick PB, Cooper ES (eds): Stroke in Blacks. Basel, Karger, 1999, pp 94–105

....
Ethnic Differences in Cerebral Atherosclerosis

Gregory L. Burke, George Howard

Departments of Public Health Sciences and Neurology, Wake Forest University
School of Medicine, Winston Salem, N.C., USA

Cerebrovascular disease mortality is the third leading cause of death in the USA with overall stroke mortality rates higher in US Blacks than Whites. These ethnic differences in stroke mortality differ by age group. At age 45, stroke mortality is approximately 4 times greater in Black than White Americans, however this ethnic disparity in mortality decreases with increasing age, so that at age 75, Black and White Americans have similar stroke mortality rates [1, 2]. The primary etiology for the excess Black stroke mortality appears to be an increased *stroke incidence* among Blacks, with differences in case fatality playing a smaller role [3, 4]. Atherosclerosis in the carotid artery increases the risk of incident stroke both through thrombotic mechanisms [5] as well as serving as a source for artery-to-artery emboli [6]. As such, it is reasonable to examine ethnic differences in extracranial (and intracranial) atherosclerosis as a source of the observed ethnic differences in stroke mortality and morbidity.

Previous research studies describing ethnic differences in cerebral atherosclerosis can be divided into studies investigating atherosclerosis in symptomatic patient populations versus community-based studies. The literature in clinically symptomatic patients presenting with stroke or transient ischemic attack (TIA) symptoms has largely been reported by neurologists and neuroepidemiologists, while data on community-based (largely asymptomatic) populations has for the most part been described by pathologists and cardiovascular epidemiologists. This paper will provide an overview of the observed ethnic differences in atherosclerosis of both symptomatic and community-based populations. Differences and similarities in the descriptions of atherosclerosis between these groups will be discussed.

Table 1. Racial differences in extracranial atherosclerosis in stroke/TIA populations

Study	Sample Size (W/B)	Cut-point	White	Black
Heyman et al., 1972 [7]	3,925/535	Any angiographic stenosis	46%	36%
Gil-Pralta et al., 1990 [8]	45/61	>40% by Doppler	73%	44%
Gorelick et al., 1984 [9]	26/45	Any angiographic stenosis (ICA origin)	91%	63%
		>75% angiographic stenosis (ICA origin)	55%	0%
Tell et al., 1989 [20]	1,428/153 (77% referred for cerebrovascular symptoms)	Mean plaque score at bifurcation	2.1	1.6
Wityk et al., 1996 [11]	108/166	Extracranial carotid lesion >50% by angiography or duplex ultrasonography	33%	15%
Sacco et al., 1995 [12]	82/155	>60% by angiography or Duplex	11%	8%
Ryu et al., 1989 [13]	50/25	Mean B-mode score summing the near and far walls of the left and right low common, high common, and low internal carotid artery	13.7	13.1
Inzitari et al., 1990 [14]	1,058/86	Any angiographically defined stenosis	82%	64%

Cerebrovascular Atherosclerosis in Stroke/TIA Populations

There is general agreement that the extent of extracranial atherosclerosis is greater for Whites than for Blacks in the symptomatic stroke or TIA populations. These ethnic differences were first described in 1972 by the Joint Study of Extracranial Arterial Occlusion that observed angiographic evidence of carotid stenosis in 46% of White stroke victims compared to only 36% of Blacks [7]. At least six subsequent studies have also reported more extracranial atherosclerosis in White compared to Black stroke/TIA patients (table 1) [7–13]. In addition, although potentially distorted by the selection process required by a randomized clinical trial, 82% of the 1,058 White patients in the Extracranial/Intracranial Bypass Study had angiographically documented stenosis of the intracranial atherosclerosis, as compared to only 64% of the 86 Black patients [14]. Hence, it is clear that among stroke and TIA patients, White patients had a substantially greater burden of extracranial atherosclerosis than their Black counterparts.

This observed greater burden of extracranial atherosclerosis among Blacks has been offered as one potential underlying cause for the substantially greater use of angioplasty and endarterectomy among Whites as compared to Blacks [15–21]. For example, among 27,690 White and 6,526 Black veterans admitted with a stroke or TIA diagnosis, the odds of receiving an angiogram was only 46% as frequent for Blacks as compared to Whites, and the odds of having an endarterectomy was only 28% as frequent. These ethnic differences in the frequency of procedures was not substantially affected by adjustment for age, region of the USA, stroke versus TIA diagnosis, hypertension, and comorbidity index [16]. Likewise, the odds of having a carotid endarterectomy was estimated to be only 40% as frequent for Blacks than for Whites in the National Hospital Discharge Survey [17], 33% as frequent for Black Medicare enrollees [18], and 31–34% as frequent among Blacks than Whites discharged from acute care hospitals in Maryland [19] and Massachusetts [20]. Maxwell et al. [21] noted that among 2,256 patients having endarterectomy in 8 large North Carolina Hospitals, only 2.7% were substantially lower than the proportion of Blacks in the general North Carolina population (12.1%) or hospital discharges (12.0%). Again, it is clear that Whites have a greater use of angioplasty, and higher likelihood of endarterectomy than their Black counterparts. While a greater burden of extracranial atherosclerosis in stroke and TIA victims could clearly underlie the lower use of cerebrovascular procedures among Blacks, other potential explanations have been suggested including: (1) differential access to health care arising from ethnic differences in socioeconomic status, and (2) lower use of diagnostic testing introduced by the assumption of physicians that Blacks do not have extracranial atherosclerosis and therefore the tests/procedures are not warranted [15].

Because of the challenges of imaging intracranial vasculature, the literature describing ethnic differences in intracranial atherosclerosis among stroke and TIA populations is not as extensive. However, the available data appears to clearly suggest that Blacks have the greater burden of intracranial atherosclerosis (in contrast to their lesser burden of extracranial disease). Gorelick et al. [9] reported that 60% of Black patients had an angiographically detectable lesion in the right middle cerebral stem and 32% in the left middle cerebral stem, in stark contrast to the prevalence in Whites of 0 and 19%, respectively. Using transcranial Doppler testing, Sacco et al. [12] reported intracranial atherosclerosis in 6% of Black subjects, but in only 1% of White subjects. However, Wityk et al. [11] reported a marginally higher rate of intracranial atherosclerosis (established by any evidence on angiography, transcranial Doppler, or magnetic resonance angiography) in Whites (24%) as compared to Blacks (22%).

It would be difficult to reconcile the ethnic differences in extracranial atherosclerosis to ethnic differences in the prevalence of risk factors. Black men and women have a higher prevalence of hypertension, diabetes mellitus, and cigarette smoking than their White counterparts [22]. The ethnic differences in lipid profiles tend to be less dramatic, with Blacks having a more adverse lipid profile in some [11, 22], but not all [9, 12], studies. As such, the lower prevalence of extracranial atherosclerosis in Blacks in the presence of a more adverse risk factor profile is an anomaly. It could be logically argued that the more adverse risk factor profile in Blacks may underlie the greater burden of intracranial disease; however, differences in risk factors have failed to account for these differences [9, 12, 14]. As such, it appears that the ethnic differences in both extracranial and intracranial atherosclerosis in stroke populations must be attributed to factors other than ethnic differences in risk factors.

The subtyping of stroke diagnoses is largely dependent on the presence or absence of clinical data describing potential etiology of the stroke. Strokes are categorized as embolic if there are clear cardiac sources for the stroke (e.g. atrial fibrillation), atherothrombotic if there is clear evidence of extracranial atherosclerosis (e.g. carotid artery stenosis), and intracranial if there is evidence of intracranial atherosclerosis (e.g. middle cerebral artery stenosis). With this approach to stroke subtyping, and given the ethnic differences in the extracranial/intracranial disease burden, it is not surprising that there are dramatic ethnic differences in stroke subtypes, with Blacks being more likely to suffer strokes attributable to hemorrhagic, embolic or intracranial atherosclerosis; while Whites are more likely to suffer strokes attributable to extracranial atherosclerosis or extracranial etiologies [12, 23].

Cerebrovascular Atherosclerosis in Asymptomatic Populations

The studies of extracranial atherosclerosis among asymptomatic population stands in contrast to the studies among the symptomatic patients. These studies fall into two broad categories: (1) the autopsy reports of selected groups in populations from the International Atherosclerosis Project (IAP), or (2) ultrasound evaluation of epidemiologic (population-based) cohorts.

The IAP collected aortas, coronary, carotid, and intracranial arteries from 2,166 autopsied cases in New Orleans, Kingston (Jamaica), and Oslo (Norway) [24]. The New Orleans center is of particular interest to this report as it

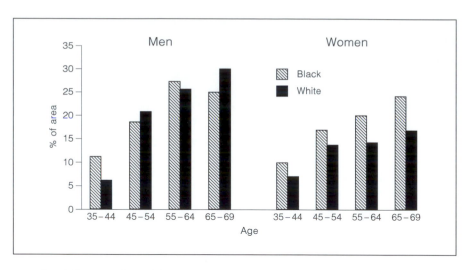

Fig. 1. Percent of carotid artery covered with raised lesions (IAP, New Orleans).

collected specimens from both US White and US Black individuals, allowing a direct ethnic comparison (while the Kingston center studied exclusively Black and the Oslo exclusively White, confounding geography and race). In these data from New Orleans there were 234 Blacks and 129 Whites with causes of death not attributed to atherosclerosis. Specifically, deaths from causes associated with atherosclerosis (myocardial infarctions, stroke, and other atherosclerotic causes) were not included in these analyses to remove bias created by selecting autopsies where the cause of death was related to the outcome of interest. The percent of the surface area covered by raised lesions was measured, and the average area covered by raised lesions calculated. In the carotid artery (fig. 1), among men there was no significant ethnic difference in the average area of raised lesions, with two of four age strata showing more advanced disease for Blacks than Whites and the other two showing the opposite trend. However, Black women showed greater carotid atherosclerosis in all four age strata, a difference that reached statistical significance in the oldest two strata (55–64 and 65–69). The IAP also offered the opportunity to assess racial differences in the percent of the area covered by raised lesions in the intracerebral bed (fig. 2). All eight gender-age strata Blacks showed greater atherosclerosis than their White counterparts (significant except for men aged 45–54). Hence, while the results of the IAP support the observation made in symptomatic patients that Blacks suffer a greater burden of intracranial atherosclerosis, it does not support the finding of greater extracranial atherosclerosis among Whites.

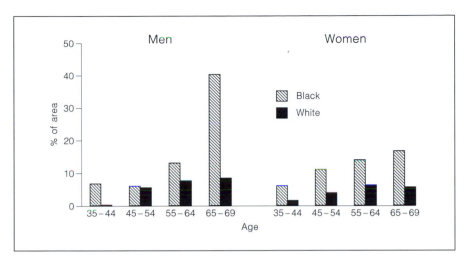

Fig. 2. Percent of intracranial arteries covered with raised lesions (IAP, New Orleans).

The advent of noninvasive imaging with high-resolution ultrasound has allowed the assessment of extracranial atherosclerosis among community-based populations. The intimal-medial thickness (IMT – a commonly used index of atherosclerosis) of the common and internal carotid artery has also been recently reported in four large epidemiologic studies (table 2). These data document the presence of atherosclerosis in these relatively asymptomatic populations and suggest that the extent of extracranial atherosclerosis was relatively similar across ethnic groups [25–28].

The Atherosclerosis Risk in Communities (ARIC) studied more than 9,000 Whites and 3,000 Blacks, aged 45–65, chosen at random from the general population of four cities in the USA. In general, a similar prevalence of atherosclerosis was observed in Black and White participants. The average IMT of the common carotid and carotid bifurcation was thicker among Black participants (by 0.01-0.05 mm), while the average thickness at the internal carotid artery was greater among White participants (0.02 mm in women and 0.06 mm in men) [25]. While these ethnic differences appear relatively small, the effects are similar to differences in IMT associated with major cardiovascular disease risk factors such as hypertension and diabetes (approximately 0.06 mm higher) [29]. Because atherosclerosis is more clinically significant in participants with the thickest carotid walls, differences in the estimated 95th percentile of wall thickness are of interest. Slightly greater ethnic differences were observed at the 95th compared to the mean with Black participants having thicker IMT at the common and bifurcation, and White participants having thicker IMT in the internal.

Table 2. Racial differences in extracranial atherosclerosis in asymptomatic populations: intimal-medial thickness in millimeters

Study	Sample size (W/B)	Cut-point or statistic	Women		Men	
			White	Black	White	Black
ARIC	9,789/3,610	Left CCA at age 55	0.64	0.67	0.71	0.73
		(mean/95th percentile)	0.91	0.96	1.00	1.07
		Left bifurcation at age 55	0.78	0.83	0.92	0.92
		(mean/95th percentile)	1.34	1.47	1.78	1.74
		Left ICA at age 55	0.66	0.64	0.76	0.70
		(mean/95th percentile)	1.21	1.12	1.53	1.29
CHS	4,926/244	Mean CCA	0.97	1.03	1.05	1.12
		Mean ICA	1.40	1.36	1.67	1.56

			Men + Women	
			White	Black
IRAS	219/281	Age- and sex-adjusted mean CCA thickness	0.81	0.87
		Age- and sex-adjusted mean ICA thickness	0.89	0.91
NOMASS	23% of 526/31% of 526	Maximum internal carotid plaque thickness	1.70	1.70

The Cardiovascular Health Study (CHS) assessed wall thickness and atherosclerosis in an elderly population-based cohort (age 65–100 years) randomly selected from four US communities. CHS found a similar pattern of ethnic differences in IMT as was observed in ARIC. Average IMT values in the common carotid of elderly Black participants were significantly thicker than for White participants (0.06 mm for women and 0.07 mm for men). Although there were no statistically significant ethnic differences in the internal carotid average IMT, there was a trend towards thicker IMT among White participants (0.04 mm greater for women and 0.11 mm greater for men).

The Insulin Resistance Atherosclerosis Study (IRAS) reported Black/White differences in the IMT of asymptomatic participants randomly selected from two California Kaiser Health Care populations (aged 40–70). In IRAS, the average common carotid IMT was significantly thicker among Black participants as compared to White participants (0.06 mm greater). While there was a nonsignificant trend for greater internal carotid IMT among Black participants, after adjustment for cardiovascular risk factors a nonsignificant trend of thicker ICA-IMT was observed among White participants.

In addition to identifying a cohort of stroke patients, the Northern Manhattan Stroke Study (NOMASS) selected 526 persons free of stroke by random-digit dialing as a control group, thus providing an opportunity to assess ethnic differences in an asymptomatic population. NOMASS reported the maximum internal carotid plaque thickness to be similar among Black and White participants (1.70 mm in both groups).

In summary, there appears to be a consistent pattern in these population-based studies with Black participants having greater IMT in the common carotid artery than White participants with inconsistent ethnic differences observed in the internal carotid artery (although trends indicate a slightly greater ICA-IMT in White participants).

In addition to assessing IMT, both ARIC and CHS data were also evaluated for the presence of a plaque or stenosis of the carotid artery. In ARIC, Whites proved to have only a slightly higher (and nonsignificant) prevalence of plaques than their Black counterparts (34.4 vs. 31.4%). In addition, the frequency of plaques with acoustic shadowing, likely reflecting calcification, was also slightly higher among Whites (6.9%) than among Blacks (5.0%). In CHS the proportion of the populations with a stenosis of greater than 50% was slightly higher in White (7.6%) than Black men (5.5%), and in White (5.4%) as compared to Black women (2.7%).

Discussion

Studies in both clinically symptomatic and free-living (asymptomatic) populations suggest that the US Blacks have more extensive intracranial atherosclerosis than their White counterparts. However, the population-based vs. clinically-based studies observed dramatically divergent pictures of the ethnic differences in extracranial atherosclerosis. Studies in clinical populations suggest that substantially greater atherosclerosis was observed in White compared to Black patients; however, in population-based studies there appears to be a similar extent of atherosclerosis across these two ethnic groups. There are at least three reasons that may underlie this observed difference.

First, the large excess Black stroke mortality is largely driven by differences in relatively young age strata (45–50 years). In this age group it is unlikely that atherosclerosis is playing the primary role underlying stroke etiology, but rather other causes (hemorrhage, intracranial disease, embolic, etc.) are relatively more important. It is reasonable to assume that these 'other' causes of stroke are at a relative excess at all ages among Black stroke patients (as compared to their White counterparts). Even under the assumption that there are no ethnic differences in the prevalence of, or implied risk of, extracranial atherosclerosis, this would enrich the population of Black stroke victims with individuals with stroke from causes other than atherosclerosis. This would have the impact of increasing the overall number of stroke victims, and under this hypothesis there would be as many Black stroke victims with atherosclerosis as White stroke victims with atherosclerosis; however, the proportion of strokes resulting from atherosclerosis in the Black population would be smaller. Hence, when the population prevalence of atherosclerosis is calculated for Black and White stroke victims, the prevalence of extracranial atherosclerosis would be smaller. As such, restricting analyses to stroke victims has the possibility of artificially making the prevalence of extracranial atherosclerosis smaller for Blacks relative to Whites.

Second, it is possible that there is differential susceptibility from extracranial atherosclerosis among the Black population. It is plausible to assume that Black populations may be at an overall greater risk of stroke due to the higher prevalence of major risk factors (e.g. cigarette smoking, diabetes, hypertension). Thus, there would be a higher likelihood of strokes in US Blacks at relatively lower levels of stenosis. This would tend to shift the distribution of the average level of atherosclerosis to lower levels in Black stroke victims, making the average level of atherosclerosis lower in Blacks as compared to their White counterparts. To the naive observer, this lower level of atherosclerosis among Blacks could be misinterpreted as indicating a lesser importance of extracranial atherosclerosis, when in fact it remains a very important factor.

Among these two hypotheses, we speculate the most likely reason is the first – that the denominator of stroke events is enriched by Blacks with non-atherogenic strokes. This hypothesis would seem to be consistent with the observation of excess mortality [1, 2] and incidence [3, 4] of stroke at relatively young ages where atherosclerosis seems unlikely. However, it is also possible that Blacks are differentially susceptible to extracranial atherosclerosis. In addition, ultrasound measures of carotid wall thickness have been shown to be strongly associated with atherosclerosis in vitro [31] and incident coronary events [32]. Thus, we are impressed with the quality and reliability of the IAP and believe that IMT is a reliable index of atherosclerosis and hence feel that it is unlikely that the observed population-based data can be ascribed to measurement error.

The hypothesis that the denominator of the Black stroke population is enriched with strokes of other causes does not imply that extracranial atherosclerosis is of lesser importance. The lower prevalence of extracranial atherosclerosis is most likely a product of differential susceptibility in Blacks and hence its importance should not be discounted. Thus these data support the importance of extracranial atherosclerosis in Blacks. Even though the clinical impression is that extracranial atherosclerosis is relatively rare in the Black population, it does not necessarily follow that it is not important.

Conclusion

Based on our review of the existing literature, a significant prevalence of both extracranial and intracranial atherosclerosis exist in both US Blacks and US Whites. Relying solely on studies done in clinical settings results in a suggestion that extracranial atherosclerosis is a disease primarily affecting US Whites. We have documented the potential biases that may artificially mediate the lower estimate of extracranial atherosclerosis in studies of patients with symptomatic cerebrovascular disease in US Blacks. However, community-based studies document the relatively high prevalence of extracranial athero-sclerosis in US Blacks and these finding are corroborated in autopsy series. Conversely, substantial evidence existing from autopsy studies corroborate the clinical findings of an increased burden from intracranial atherosclerosis observed in US Blacks. Given the burden of atherosclerosis in both White and Black populations, prevention efforts aimed at reducing the burden from cerebrovascular disease are certainly warranted. In fact we believe that efforts to prevent extracranial and intracranial atherosclerosis in US Blacks is especially important given the high prevalence of other cardiovascular disease risk factors.

References

1   Cooper ES: Clinical cerebrovascular disease in hypertensive Blacks. J Clin Hypertens 1987;3(suppl 3):79–84.
2   Howard G, Anderson R, Sorlie P, Andrews V, Backlund E, Burke GL: Ethnic differences in stroke mortality between non-Hispanic Whites, Hispanic Whites, and Blacks: The National Longitudinal Mortality Study. Stroke 1994;25:2120–2125.
3   Kittner SJ, White LR, Losonczy KG, Wolf PA, Hebel JR: Black-White differences in stroke incidence in a national sample: The contribution of hypertension and diabetes mellitus. JAMA 1990;264: 1267–1270.
4   Broderick J, Brott T, Kothari R, Miller R, Khoury J, Pancioli A, Gebel J, Mills D, Minneci L, Shukla R: The Greater Cincinnati/Northern Kentucky Stroke Study: Preliminary first-ever and total incidence rates of stroke among Blacks. Stroke 1998;29:415–421.
5   Mohr JP, Albers GW, Amareno P, Babikian VL, Biller J, Brey RL, Coull B, Easton JD, Gomez CR, Helgason CM, Kase CS, Pullicino PM, Turpie AGG: Etiology of stroke. Stroke 1997;28: 1501–1506.
6   Sacco RL, Benjamin EJ, Broderick JP, Dyken M, Easton JD, Feinberg WM, Goldstein LB, Gorelick PB, Howard G, Kittner SJ, Manolio TA, Whisnant JP, Wolf PA: Risk factors. Stroke 1997;28. 1507–1517.
7   Heyman A, Fields WS, Keafing RD. Joint Study of Extracranial Arterial Occlusion. VI. Racial differences in hospitalized patients with ischemic stroke. JAMA 1972;222:285–289.

8   Gil-Peralta A, Alter M, Lai S, Friday G, Otero A, Katz M, Comerota AJ: Duplex Doppler and spectral flow analysis of racial differences in cerebrovascular atherosclerosis. Stroke 1990;21:740–747.

9   Gorelick PB, Caplan LR, Hier DB, Parker SL, Patel D: Racial differences in the distribution of anterior circulation occlusive disease. Neurology 1984;34:54–59.

10 Tell GS, Howard G, McKinney WM: Risk factors for site-specific extracranial carotid artery plaque distribution as measured by B-mode ultrasound. J Clin Epidemiol 1989;42:551–559.

11 Wityk RJ, Lehman D, Klag M, Coresh J, Ahn H, Litt B: Race and sex differences in the distribution of cerebral atherosclerosis. Stroke 1996;27:1974–1980.

12 Sacco RL, Kargman DE, Gu Q, Zammanillo MC: Race-ethnicity and determinates of intracranial atherosclerotic cerebral infarction: The Northern Manhattan Stroke Study. Stroke 1995;26: 14–20.

13 Ryu JE, Murros KE, Espeland MA, Rubens J, McKinney WM, Toole JF, Crouse JF: Extracranial carotid atherosclerosis in Black and White patients with transient ischemic attacks. Stroke 1989; 20:1133–1137.

14 Inzitari D, Hachinski VC, Taylor DW, Barnett HJM: Racial differences in anterior circulation in cerebrovascular disease: How much can be explained by risk factors? Arch Neurol 1990;47: 1080–1084.

15 Horner RD, Oddone E, Matcar DB: Theories explaining racial differences in the utilization of diagnostic and therapeutic procedures for cerebrovascular disease. Milbank Q 1995;75:443–462.

16 Oddone EZ, Horner R, Monger M, Matchar DB: Racial variations in rates of carotid angiography and endarterectomy in patients with stroke and transient ischemic attacks. Arch Intern Med 1993; 153:2781–2786.

17 Elixhauser A, Harris DR, Coffey RM: Trends in hospital procedures performed in Black patients and White patients: 1980–87. US Public Health Service, AHCPR Publ No 94-0003, Rockville, Md, 1994.

18 Escarce JJ, Epstein KR, Colby DC, Schwartz JS: Racial differences in the elderly's use of medical procedures and diagnostic tests. Am J Public Health 1993;83:948–854.

19 Glittlesohn AM, Halpern J, Sanchez RL: Income, race, and surgery in Maryland. Am J Public Health 1991;81:1435–1441.

20 Mort EA, Weissman JS, Epstein AM: Physician discretion and racial variation in the use of surgical procedures. Arch Intern Med 1994;154:761–767.

21 Maxwell JG, Rutherford EJ, Covington D, Clancy TV, Tackett AD, Robinson N, Johnson G Jr: Infrequency of Blacks among patients having carotid endarterectomy. Stroke 1989;20:22–26.

22 Hutchinson RG, Watson RL, Davis CE, Barnes R, Brown S, Romm F, Spencer JM, Tyroler HA, Wu K: Racial differences in risk factors for atherosclerosis: The ARIC Study: Atherosclerosis Risk in Communities. Angiology 1997;48:279–290.

23 Klatsky AL, Armstrong MA, Friedman GD: Racial differences in cerebrovascular disease hospitalizations. Stroke 1991;22:229–304.

24 Solberg LA, McGarry PA. Cerebral atherosclerosis in Negroes and Caucasians. Atherosclerosis 1972;16:141–154.

25 Howard G, Sharrett AR, Heiss G, Evans GW, Chambless LE, Riley WA, Burke GL: Carotid artery intimal-medial thickness distribution in the general population as evaluated by B-mode ultrasound. Stroke 1993;24:1297–1304.

26 Manolio TA, Burke GL, Psaty BM, Newman AB, Haan M, Powe N, Tracy RP, O'Leary DH: Black-White differences in subclinical cardiovascular disease among older adults: The Cardiovascular Health Study. J Clin Epidemiol 1995;48:1141–1152.

27 D'Agostino RB Jr, Burke G, O'Leary D, Rewers M, Selby J, Savage PJ, Saad MF, Bergman RN, Howard G, Wagenknecht L, Haffner SM: Ethnic differences in carotid wall thickness: The Insulin Resistance Atherosclerosis Study. Stroke 1996;27:1744–1749.

28 Sacco RL, Roberts JK, Boden-Albala B, Gu Q, Lin I-F, Kargman DE, Berglund L, Hauser WA, Shea S, Paik MC: Race-ethnicity and determinates of carotid atherosclerosis in a multiethnic population: The Northern Manhattan Stroke Study. Stroke 1997;28:929–935.

29 Burke GL, Evans GW, Riley WA, Sharrett AR, Howard G, Barnes RW, Rosamond W, Crow RS, Rautaharju PM, Heiss G: Arterial wall thickness is associated with prevalent cardiovascular disease in middle-aged adults. The Atherosclerosis Risk in Communities (ARIC) Study. Stroke 1995;26: 386–391.

30 Li R, Duncan BB, Metcalf PA, Crouse JR III, Sharrett AR, Tyroler HA, Barnes R, Heiss G: B-mode-detected carotid artery plaque in a general population. Stroke 1994;25:2377–2383.

31 Pignoli P, Longo T: Evaluation of atherosclerosis with B-mode ultrasound imaging. J Nucl Med Allied Sci 1988;32:166–173.

32 Chambless LE, Heiss G, Folsom AR, Rosamond W, Szklo M, Sharrett AR, Clegg LX: Association of coronary heart disease incidence with carotid arterial wall thickness and major risk factors: The Atherosclerosis Risk in Communities (ARIC) Study, 1987–1993. Am J Epidemiol 1997;146:483–494.

Gregory L. Burke, MD, Departments of Public Health Sciences and Neurology,
Wake Forest University School of Medicine,
Medical Center Blvd, Winston Salem, NC 27157 (USA)

Gillum RF, Gorelick PB, Cooper ES (eds): Stroke in Blacks. Basel, Karger, 1999, pp 106–117

Stroke Incidence, Comorbid Conditions, Health Care Utilization, and Poststroke Mortality in Black and White Medicare Beneficiaries

National Patterns and Trends

Wayne H. Giles [a], *Janet B. Croft* [a], *Michele L. Casper* [a], *Joan K. Miller* [b]

[a] Cardiovascular Health Branch and the
[b] Community Health and Program Services Branch, Division of Adult and Community Health, National Center for Chronic Disease Prevention and Health Promotion, Centers for Disease Control and Prevention, Atlanta, Ga., USA

Stroke is the third leading cause of death and the leading cause of serious disability among US adults [1]. In 1995, approximately 150,000 persons died from stroke, and over 600,000 persons were hospitalized with a stroke. The vast majority of stroke cases occur in adults aged ≥ 65, and 95% of adults in this age group are enrolled in Medicare [2]. Thus analysis of Medicare data offers a unique opportunity to examine national trends in morbidity associated with stroke (stroke is currently the fourth leading cause of hospitalization among Medicare beneficiaries) [3].

In this chapter, data from the Health Care Financing Administration's Medicare Provider Analysis and Review (MEDPAR) files are used to describe national trends in incidence, comorbid conditions, and health care utilization among persons hospitalized for incident stroke during 1990–1995. The data are also used to describe racial differences in poststroke mortality and the correlates of mortality among Medicare beneficiaries. The analysis was limited to persons over the age of 67 years in order to exclude Medicare beneficiaries who had been hospitalized with a stroke during the preceding 2 years. May and Kittner [2] have previously reported that most recurrent hospitalizations for stroke occur within 2 years of the index hospitalization.

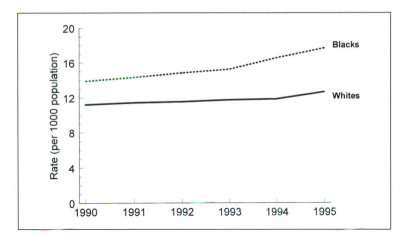

Fig. 1. Age-adjusted stroke incidence rates for Medicare beneficiaries aged ≥67 years, by race: United States, 1990–1995. The incidence rates are standardized to the 1980 US population. Blacks, dotted lines; Whites, solid lines. Incident case was defined as first hospital admission in each year for which the principal diagnosis was acute stroke (ICD-9-CM code 430-433 or 436-437); each subject had not been admitted for stroke in the previous 2 years.

Stroke Incidence

Most previous studies examining stroke incidence have included relatively few Black subjects and have been limited to community studies (e.g. Mayo Clinic [4] medical records linkage system for Rochester, Minn. and the Minnesota Heart Survey [5] for Minneapolis-St. Paul). Previous estimates of national trends in stroke incidence have relied on data from the National Hospital Discharge Survey, which does not distinguish between incident and recurrent stroke cases [6]. Studies that have included many Black participants (Georgia [7], Southern Alabama [8], and Mississippi [9]) were performed more than 20 years ago before the widespread use of computed tomography (CT scans) and magnetic resonance imaging (MRI). Relatively few recent studies have examined racial differences in stroke incidence [10, 11].

Recently, investigators have used Medicare records to track enrollees over time and to distinguish between incident and recurrent cases so that national trends in stroke incidence can be examined [2]. Between 1990 and 1995, age-adjusted stroke incidence rates were higher among Black than White Medicare enrollees, and the Black-White difference increased over time (fig. 1). Among both Black and White Medicare enrollees, stroke incidence rates increased slightly between 1990 and 1993, and increased more dramatically between 1993 and 1995. These findings contrast with previous findings from Medicare

Table 1. Age-adjusted[1] stroke incidence[2] (per 1,000 population) among Medicare beneficiaries aged ≥ 67 years by gender and race

Year	Men		Women		B/W ratio	
	White	Black	White	Black	Men	Women
1990	11.6	14.2	11.0	14.5	1.22	1.32
1991	11.8	14.5	11.2	14.6	1.23	1.31
1992	11.9	14.7	11.3	14.8	1.24	1.31
1993	12.1	15.0	11.4	15.3	1.24	1.34
1994	12.4	16.5	11.7	16.9	1.33	1.44
1995	13.1	17.0	12.3	17.6	1.30	1.43

[1] Standardized to the 1980 US population.

[2] Incident case was defined as first admission in each year for which the principal diagnosis was acute stroke (ICD-9-CM code 430-433 or 436-437); each subject had not been admitted for stroke in the previous 2 years.

data, in which Whites experienced a 7.5% decline in stroke incidence from 1985 to 1989 and then a slight increase between 1990 and 1991 [2]. Among Blacks, stroke incidence during the late 1980s and early 1990s changed very little [2].

For each year during 1990–1995, Black women experienced the highest incidence rate, followed by Black men, White men, and White women (table 1). The Black-White incidence ratio increased from 1.22 in 1990 to 1.30 in 1995 among men and from 1.32 to 1.43 among women. This widening difference in stroke incidence continued a trend that was originally noted in the late 1980s; the trend has also been observed for other cardiovascular diseases, including coronary heart disease and acute myocardial infarction [1].

Between 1990 and 1995, stroke incidence rates among Medicare beneficiaries were higher among Blacks than Whites for ischemic, ill-defined, and hemorrhagic strokes (fig. 2). Among both Blacks and Whites the rate for hemorrhagic stroke increased only slightly over the 6 years, whereas the rates for ill-defined and ischemic strokes increased substantially. These findings are consistent with data from Lehigh Valley, for which the rates of hemorrhagic stroke were higher among Blacks than Whites [13]. In addition, data from Kaiser Permanente indicated higher rates of intracerebral and subarachnoid hemorrhage among Black patients [14]. The higher rates of ischemic, ill-defined, and hemorrhagic stroke may be secondary to higher rates of stroke risk factors among Black adults. However, data from the First National Health and Nutrition Examination Survey (NHANES I) Epidemiologic Follow-Up

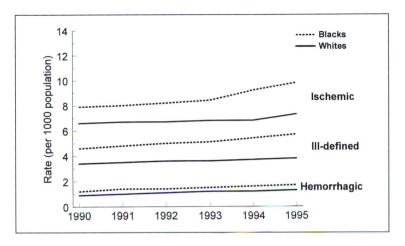

Fig. 2. Age-adjusted stroke incidence rates for Medicare beneficiaries aged ≥67 years, by race and stroke type: United States, 1990–1995. Incidence rates are standardized to the 1980 US population. Blacks, dotted lines; Whites, solid lines. Incident case was defined as first hospital admission in each year for which the principal diagnosis was acute stroke (ICD-9-CM code 430-433 or 436-437); each subject had not been admitted for stroke in the previous 2 years.

Study indicated that the higher rates of ischemic stroke among Black adults may have been only partly explained by the differences in the prevalence of stroke risk factors [11]. Additional adjustment for access to medical care, measures of wealth, and racism may more fully explain the excess stroke risk experienced by Black Americans.

The reasons for the recent rise in stroke incidence among Blacks and Whites are not clearly understood. The observed trend may reflect a true increase in the incidence rate for stroke secondary to the increasing prevalence of stroke risk factors, including uncontrolled hypertension, obesity, and diabetes mellitus. Data from NHANES III indicated that the proportion of US adults who had their blood pressure treated and adequately controlled declined during the late 1980s and early 1990s (treatment decreased from 55.0 to 53.6%; control decreased from 29.0 to 27.4%) [15]. Another explanation for the increasing stroke incidence may be ascertainment bias: the increasing use of radiographic imaging techniques (CT scans and MRIs) [16] could lead to an increased diagnosis of milder strokes. If the increasing stroke incidence is indeed due to the diagnosis of milder strokes, poststroke mortality might be expected to decline. Indeed, Medicare data from the late 1980s suggested that the 2-year poststroke mortality declined 4% between 1986 and 1989 [17].

Table 2. Comorbid conditions and health care utilization among Medicare beneficiaries aged ≥67 years, hospitalized for acute stroke, 1995[1]

	Whites (n = 360,264)	Blacks (n = 44,373)
Mean age, years	79.0	77.6
Hypertension, %	49.5	60.8
Diabetes mellitus, %	21.2	30.6
Coronary heart disease, %	23.9	15.2
Atrial fibrillation, %	19.6	11.1
Heart failure, %	10.8	10.6
Computed tomography, %	74.0	75.9
Carotid endarterectomy, %	18.1	2.1
Mean length of stay, days	9.7	12.2
Discharge outcomes, %		
Home	48.8	46.3
Skilled nursing facility	20.5	17.2
Transferred to another hospital	8.2	12.0
Other	22.5	24.5
In-hospital mortality, %	10.2	10.9

[1] Limited to incident cases defined as the first admission in each year for which the principal diagnosis was acute stroke (ICD-9-CM code 430-433 or 436-437); each subject had not been admitted for stroke in the previous 2 years.

Comorbid Conditions and Utilization of Health Care

In 1995, 360,264 White and 44,373 Black Medicare beneficiaries were hospitalized for incident stroke (table 2). Blacks who were hospitalized for incident stroke tended to be younger than their White counterparts. Data from the NHANES I Epidemiologic Follow-Up Study also indicated that Blacks who had had a stroke were younger than their White counterparts [11].

Comorbid conditions were highly prevalent among Black and White stroke patients (table 2). Blacks had higher prevalences of hypertension and diabetes mellitus and lower prevalences of coronary heart disease and atrial fibrillation. A previous report also documented a higher rate of hypertension and a lower rate of cardiac arrhythmias among Black stroke patients [18]. The prevalence of heart failure was similar in the two race groups (table 2).

Three-fourths of Black and White stroke patients underwent a CT scan during their hospitalization, but the proportion of patients who underwent carotid endarterectomy (CEA) differed markedly by race (table 2): White

Medicare beneficiaries were substantially more likely to undergo CEA (18.1%) than were their Black counterparts (2.1%). Hsai et al. [19] reported a 15.4% absolute difference in the rates of CEA among Black and White Medicare beneficiaries (over 91.6% of those undergoing CEA had a principal diagnosis of cerebrovascular disease). The racial differences in the rate of CEA is not new; during the 1980s Gillum [20] reported that the CEA rate among Blacks was 40% that of Whites.

The lower rate of CEA among Blacks may be partially explained by differences in the distribution of vascular pathology. The distribution of atheromatous involvement in the cerebrovascular tree (as demonstrated by cerebral angiography) has been observed to differ significantly between Blacks and Whites [21]. Black patients have also been observed to have more severe occlusive disease involving the middle cerebral artery, whereas White patients have more severe disease involving the internal carotid artery [22]. In addition, autopsy studies have reported more intracranial disease among Blacks and more extracranial disease among Whites [23]. However, many of these studies are subject to a referral bias. In the Northern Manhattan Stroke Study [24], B-mode ultrasound of the internal carotid was performed in a population-based sample of middle-aged adults; the researchers were unable to document lower rates of internal carotid atherosclerosis among Black participants. Finally, a large body of evidence documents lower rates of invasive cardiovascular procedures among Blacks suffering from cardiovascular disease [25–29], and it is possible that CEA may be yet another invasive cardiovascular procedure that Black patients are substantially less likely to undergo than are their White counterparts.

Horner et al. [18] reported that the use of inpatient rehabilitation services among Medicare beneficiaries did not differ significantly by race. Overall, 66.0% of Black stroke patients and 55.8% of White stroke patients received inpatient occupational or physical therapy (Black-White adjusted odds ratio for inpatient occupational or physical therapy was 1.06; p=0.42). The median time to initiation of inpatient rehabilitation services was 5.6 days for Blacks and 6.6 days for Whites (p=0.22), and the median duration of inpatient physical or occupational therapy was 7.6 days for Blacks and 8.2 days for Whites (p=0.34) [18].

Mean length of hospital stay was slightly longer among Blacks than Whites in the Medicare population (table 2). Similarly, Kuhlemeier and Steins [21] reported that Black stroke victims from Maryland stayed 3 days longer on average than their White counterparts. In-hospital mortality was also slightly higher among the Black than the White Medicare beneficiaries (table 2). These findings are consistent with data from other studies that noted higher poststroke mortality among Black adults, including data from the Northern

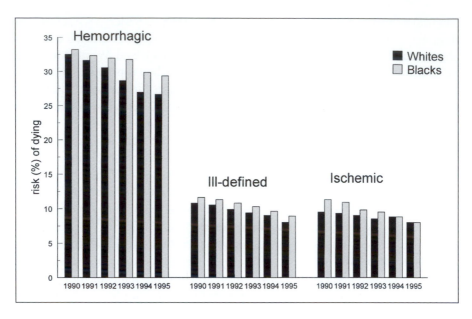

Fig. 3. Risk for in-hospital mortality among Medicare beneficiaries, aged ≥67 years, hospitalized for stroke, by race and stroke type: United States, 1990–1995. Blacks, shaded bars; Whites, solid bars. Incident case was defined as first hospital admission in each year for which the principal diagnosis was acute stroke (ICD-9-CM code 430-433 or 436-437); each subject had not been admitted for stroke in the previous 2 years.

Manhattan Stroke Study [10], Duke University [30], and Mississippi [31, 32]. The increased in-hospital mortality and lengths of stay among Blacks suggest that Black adults may be suffering from more severe strokes. Horner et al. [30] reported that Blacks suffered from more severe strokes as manifested by higher in-hospital mortality and a longer recovery time. In addition, Kuhlemeir and Steins [21] reported that the proportion of stroke victims who were admitted to the hospital in a coma was substantially higher among Black than White stroke victims.

National Trends in Poststroke Mortality

Between 1990 and 1995, in-hospital mortality among Medicare beneficiaries declined in both Blacks and Whites for hemorrhagic, ill-defined and ischemic stroke (fig. 3). For ischemic stroke, there were no racial differences in case fatality for the years 1994 and 1995. For hemorrhagic and ill-defined stroke, in all years, Blacks had higher case fatality during hospitalization than did their White counterparts in all years. May et al. [17] also reported higher poststroke mortality rates among Blacks than Whites. In both our study and the study of May et al., the greatest declines in poststroke mortality occurred among patients suffering from hemorrhagic stroke.

May et al. [17] found that 2-year poststroke survival was low among both Black and White Medicare beneficiaries; only 54% of Black and 58% of White Medicare beneficiaries survived 2 years after their initial hospitalization for stroke. Between 1985 and 1989, this survival increased slightly, with the greatest increase in survival observed for hemorrhagic stroke and minimal increases observed for ill-defined and ischemic stroke [17]. A potential explanation for the increases in survival may be the increased detection of milder strokes through the increased use of CT scans and MRI [16]. Supporting this hypothesis is the finding that the segments of the population that have experienced the greatest improvements in poststroke survival (Blacks and older adults) are the same segments that have experienced the greatest increases in the use of CT scans and MRI [16]. Another possible explanation is an overall shift in the distribution of stroke severity toward less severe stroke. Data from the Framingham Study [33], which examined secular trends in stroke severity, suggested that the frequency of mild strokes increased from 14 to 44% and the frequency of severe strokes decreased from 37 to 16%. Recent advancements in the treatment of stroke may also help explain the declines in stroke mortality. Improvements in care (such as the use of aspirin to prevent recurrent stroke, acute control of blood pressure, and an increased emphasis on physical therapy) may have affected poststroke survival. In addition, the increased use of specialized stroke units rather than general medical units to treat stroke patients may have further improved patient survival. The benefits associated with stroke units reflect the integrated approach of linking acute treatment with early mobilization and rehabilitation and with active participation by both the patient and family. The increasing use of stroke teams and thrombolytic therapy for the acute treatment of stroke, will likely also affect poststroke survival.

Factors associated with poststroke mortality among Medicare beneficiaries were also assessed (table 3). Persons aged ≥ 85 years were 75% more likely to die than were persons aged 67–74 years after adjustment for differences in age, gender, race, hypertension, diabetes mellitus, coronary heart disease, heart failure, atrial fibrillation, stroke type and length of stay. Differences in poststroke survival by gender and race were minimal. Persons with hypertension were 34% less likely to die, persons with heart failure were 2.3 times more likely to die, and persons with atrial fibrillation were 76% more likely to die than were those without each condition. The results for atrial fibrillation are similar to risk estimates for poststroke mortality from the Framingham Study [34], which reported an odds ratio of 1.84 and the Copenhagen Stroke Study

Table 3. Correlates of in-hospital mortality among Medicare beneficiaries aged ≥67 years, admitted for stroke, 1995[1]

Characteristic	Mortality rate[1]	Odds ratio[2]	95% confidence interval
Age group, years			
67–74	8.4	1.00	Referent
75–84	10.7	1.26	1.23–1.29
≥85	14.4	1.75	1.70–1.80
Gender			
Women	11.0	1.00	Referent
Men	10.7	0.97	0.95–0.99
Race			
White	10.9	1.00	Referent
Black	10.2	1.11	1.08–1.15
Hypertension			
No	11.2	1.00	Referent
Yes	9.6	0.66	0.65–0.68
Diabetes mellitus			
No	11.2	1.00	Referent
Yes	9.6	1.06	1.04–1.09
Coronary heart disease			
No	11.0	1.00	Referent
Yes	10.3	0.99	0.97–1.02
Heart failure			
No	10.9	1.00	Referent
Yes	20.3	2.31	1.84–2.91
Atrial fibrillation			
No	9.8	1.00	Referent
Yes	15.3	1.76	1.72–1.80
Stroke type			
Ischemic	8.0	1.00	Referent
Ill-defined	8.8	0.98	0.95–1.00
Hemorrhagic	29.0	4.63	4.51–4.75
Length of stay, days			
<7	9.3	1.00	Referent
≥7	12.1	1.82	1.78–1.87

[1] Limited to incident cases defined as the first admission in each year for which the principal diagnosis was acute stroke (ICD-9-CM code 430-433 or 436-437); each subject had not been admitted for stroke in the previous 2 years.
[2] Odds ratios are adjusted for age, gender, race, hypertension, diabetes mellitus, coronary heart disease, heart failure, atrial fibrillation, stroke type, and length of stay.

[35], which reported an odds ratio of 1.7. Because stroke is usually the initial manifestation of embolism in atrial fibrillation, preventing the formation of embolism through the use of anticoagulants is crucial to reducing disability and mortality associated with stroke.

No substantial differences in the risk for in-hospital mortality were observed among stroke victims defined by either diabetes mellitus or coronary heart disease (table 3). Minimal differences in mortality were observed between persons who suffered an ischemic stroke and those whose stroke was ill-defined stroke; persons who suffered a hemorrhagic stroke were almost 5 times more likely to die than were persons who suffered an ischemic stroke. Finally, persons who were hospitalized ≥ 7 days were 82% more likely to die than were those hospitalized for < 7 days.

Conclusion

Incidence rates for ischemic, ill-defined, and hemorrhagic stroke were substantially higher among Blacks than Whites and the Black-White difference increased from 1990 to 1995. The racial difference in stroke incidence was greater among women than men. Black Medicare beneficiaries hospitalized for stroke tended to be younger and were more likely to have hypertension and diabetes; their White counterparts were more likely to have coronary heart disease and atrial fibrillation. The racial differences in the use of CT scans and inpatient rehabilitation services were minimal, but Black stroke victims were substantially less likely to undergo CEA. Poststroke mortality was higher among Blacks than Whites, and the largest racial difference in mortality occurred among those who suffered a hemorrhagic stroke. Several factors were correlated with poststroke mortality, including advanced age, the presence of heart failure and atrial fibrillation, longer hospital stays, and a diagnosis of hemorrhagic stroke.

References

1   National Center for Health Statistics: Health, United States, 1996–1997 and Injury Chartbook. Hyattsville, US Department of Health and Human Services, 1997.
2   May DS, Kittner SJ: Use of Medicare claims data to estimate national trends in stroke incidence, 1985–1991. Stroke 1994;25:2343–2347.
3   Health Care Financing Administration: Health Care Financing Review: Medicare and Medicaid Statistical Supplement, 1997. HCFA Publication No. 03399. Baltimore, US Department of Health and Human Services; 1997.
4   Broderick JP, Phillips SJ, Whinsant JP, O'Fallon WM, Bergstraln EJ: Incidence rates of stroke in the eighties: The end of the decline in stroke? Stroke 1989;20:577–582.

5   McGovern PG, Burke GL, Sprafka MH, Xue S, Folsom AR, Blackburn H: Trends in mortality, morbidity, and risk factor levels for stroke from 1960 through 1990: The Minnesota Heart Survey. JAMA 1992;268:753–759.

6   Modan B, Wagener DK: Some epidemiological aspects of stroke: Mortality/morbidity trends, age, sex, race, socioeconomic status. Stroke 1992;23:1230–1236.

7   Heyman A, Karp HR, Hayden S, Bartel A, Cassel JC, Tyroler HA, Hames CG: Cerebrovascular disease in the biracial population of Evans County, Georgia. Arch Intern Med 1971;128:949–955.

8   Gross CR, Kase CS, Mohr JP, Cunningham SC, Baker WE: Stroke in south Alabama: Incidence and diagnostic features in population-based study. Stroke 1984;15:249–255.

9   Schoenberg BS, Anderson DW, Haerer AF: Racial differentials in the prevalence of stroke. Copiah County, Mississippi. Arch Neurol 1986;43:565–568.

10 Sacco RL, Hauser WA, Mohr JP: Hospitalized stroke in Blacks and Hispanics in northern Manhattan. Stroke 1991;22:1491–1496.

11 Giles WH, Kittner SJ, Hebel JR, Losonczy KG, Sherwin RW: Determinants of Black-White differences in the risk of cerebral infarction. The National Health and Nutrition Examination Survey Epidemiologic Follow-Up Study. Arch Intern Med 1995;155:1319–1324.

12 Haerer AF, Woolsey PC: Prognosis and quality of survival in a hospitalized stroke population from the south. Stroke 1975;6:543–548.

13 Friday G, Lai SM, Alter M, Sobel E, LaRue L, Gil-Peralta A, McCoy RL, Levitt LP, Isack T: Stroke in Lehigh Valley: Racial/ethnic differences. Neurology 1989;39:1165–1168.

14 Klatsky AL, Armstrong MA, Friedman GD: Racial differences in cerebrovascular disease hospitalizations. Stroke 1991;22:299–304.

15 Joint National Committee on Prevention, Detection, Evaluation, and Treatment of High Blood Pressure. The Sixth Report of the Joint National Committee on Prevention, Detection, Evaluation, and Treatment of High Blood Pressure. DHHS Publ No 98-4080. Bethesda, US Department of Health and Human Services, 1997.

16 Boutwell RC, Mitchell JB: Diffusion of new technologies in the treatment of the Medicare population: Implications for patient access and program expenditures. Int J Technol Assess Health Care 1993; 9:62–75.

17 May DS, Casper ML, Croft JB, Giles WH: Trends in survival after stroke among Medicare beneficiaries. Stroke 1994;25:1617–1622.

18 Horner RD, Hoenig H, Sloane R, Robenstein LV, Kahn KL: Racial differences in the utilization of inpatient rehabilitation services among elderly stroke patients. Stroke 1997;28:19–25.

19 Hsai DC, Moscoe LM, Krushat WM: Epidemiology of carotid endarterectomy among Medicare beneficiaries. Stroke 1998;29:346–350.

20 Gillum RF: Cerebrovascular disease morbidity in the United States, 1970–1983: Age, sex, region, and vascular surgery. Stroke 1986;17:656–661.

21 Kuhlemeier KV, Steins SA: Racial disparities in severity of cerebrovascular events. Stroke 1994;25: 2126–2131.

22 Gorelick PB, Caplan LR, Hier DB, Parker SL, Patel D: Racial differences in the distribution of anterior circulation disease. Neurology 1984;34:54–59.

23 Williams AO, Resch JA, Loewenson BR: Cerebral atherosclerosis – A comparative autopsy study between Nigerian Negroes and American Negroes and Caucasians. Neurology 1969;19:205–210.

24 Sacco RL, Roberts JK, Boden-Albala B, Gu Q, Lin IF, Kargman DE, Berglund L, Hauser WA, Shea S, Paik MC: Race-ethnicity and determinants of carotid atherosclerosis in a multiethnic population. The Northern Manhattan Stroke Study. Stroke 1997;28:929–935.

25 Giles WH, Anda RF, Casper ML, Escobedo LG, Taylor HA: Race and sex differences in the rates of invasive cardiac procedures in US hospitals: Data from the National Hospital Discharge Survey. Arch Intern Med 1995;155:318–324.

26 Franks AL, May DS, Wenger DK, Blount SB, Eaker ED: Racial differences in the use of invasive coronary procedures after acute myocardial infarction in Medicare beneficiaries. Ethn Dis 1993;3: 213–220.

27 Feinleib M, Havlik RJ, Gillum RF, Pokras R, McCarthy E, Moien M: Coronary heart disease and related procedures: National Hospital Discharge Survey Data. Circulation 1989;79:I12-I18.

28   Ayanian JZ, Udvarhelyi IS, Gastonis CA, Pashos CL, Epstein AM: Racial differences in the use of revascularization procedures after coronary angiography. JAMA 1993;269:2642–2646.
29   Ford E, Cooper R, Castaner A, Simmons B, Mar M: Coronary arteriography and coronary bypass surgery among Whites and other racial groups relative to hospital-based incidence rates for coronary artery disease: Findings from NHDS. Am J Public Health 1989;79:437–440.
30   Horner RD, Matcher DB, Divine GW, Feussner JR: Racial variations in ischemic stroke-related physical and functional impairments. Stroke 1991;22:497–501.
31   Gaines K, Burke G: Ethnic differences in stroke: Black-White differences in the United States population. Neuroepidemiology 1995;14:209–239.
32   Gaines K: Regional and ethnic differences in stroke in the southeastern United States population. Ethn Dis 1997;7:150–164.
33   Wolf PA, D'Agostino RB, O'Neal MA, Sytkowski CS, Kase CS, Belanger AJ, Kannel WB: Secular trends in stroke incidence and mortality. The Framingham Study. Stroke 1992;23:1551–1555.
34   Lin HJ, Wolf PA, Kelly-Hayes M, Beiser AS, Kase CS, Benjamin EJ, D'Agostino RB: Stroke severity in atrial fibrillation. The Framingham Study. Stroke 1996;27:1760–1764.
35   Jorgensen HS, Nakayama H, Reith J, Raaschou HO, Olsen TS: Acute stroke with atrial fibrillation. The Copenhagen Stroke Study. Stroke 1996;27:1765–1769.

Wayne H. Giles, MD, Cardiovascular Health Branch,
4770 Buford Hwy, MS K47, Atlanta, GA 30341 (USA)

Gillum RF, Gorelick PB, Cooper ES (eds): Stroke in Blacks. Basel, Karger, 1999, pp 118–128

....

Risk Factor Identification and Primary Prevention of Stroke in African-American Populations

Clinical Trials, Community Trials, and Their Applications in Patient Management

Wallace R. Johnson, Jr.

Division of Hypertension, Department of Medicine, University of Maryland
School of Medicine, Baltimore, Md., USA

Although cerebrovascular disease mortality rates have fallen significantly over the past 50 years, African-Americans continue to lag behind Whites in the degree of reduction seen. In terms of stroke the overall prevalence is expected to rise as the population continues to live longer. Age is the single most important risk factor for stroke but obviously not a modifiable factor (table 1). Therefore, for primary prevention of first stroke the emphasis is placed on risk factors such as hypertension, diabetes, dyslipidemia, obesity, smoking and excessive alcohol intake.

There are three different strategies used to approach primary prevention: (1) a population-based or mass approach and (2) a targeted strategy dealing with high-risk individuals or (3) a combination of the previous two methods. In population-based strategies the objective is to achieve even a small decrease in the average blood pressure in the population. In a large population a very small reduction such as a 2-mm Hg drop in systolic blood pressure could potentially result in a substantial decline in hypertension prevalence and cardiovascular risk [9]. This chapter will explore methods to improve primary prevention of stroke including community intervention programs and medical modification of stroke risk factors.

Hypertension

Hypertension is a contributing factor in approximately 70% of strokes. While increasing age is the single most important risk factor for stroke, hyper-

Table 1. Modifiable risk factors for first ischemic stroke

Strong evidence-based risk factors	Less well-documented risk factors
Hypertension	Obesity
Cigarette smoking	Diabetes
Transient ischemic attacks	Dyslipidemia (including Lp(a))
Asymptomatic carotid stenosis	Oral contraceptives
Sickle cell disease	Heavy alcohol use
Cardiac disease	Use of illicit drugs
Atrial fibrillation	Physical inactivity
Infectious endocarditis	Elevated hematocrit
Recent large myocardial infarction	Dietary factors
Mitral stenosis	low fish intake
Diabetes	low fruit and vegetable intake
Hyperhomocysteinemia	low potassium intake
Left ventricular hypertrophy	low folate intake
	Hyperinsulinemia and insulin resistance
	Acute triggers (stress)
	Migraine headaches
	Socioeconomic features
	Hypercoagulable states
	Cardiac disease
	Cardiomyopathy
	Segmental wall motion abnormalities
	Mitral valve prolapse

tension is the single most important modifiable risk factor for ischemic stroke. It is estimated that hypertension gives a relative stroke risk of 4 when systolic blood pressure is ≥160 mm Hg and diastolic blood pressure is ≥95 mm Hg. A summary of seven studies assigning a relative risk of 1 for mild high blood pressure or what was then called borderline hypertension (≥140/90) determined the relative risk to be about 0.5 at a blood pressure of 136/84 mm Hg and about 0.35 for a blood pressure of 123/76 mm Hg [1, 4]. Although hypertension is still an important risk factor in the elderly, its importance decreases with age, the odds ratio is 4 at age 50 and decreases to 1 by age 90 [2].

Hypertension promotes stroke by aggravating atherosclerosis in the aortic arch and cervicocerebral arteries, while causing arteriosclerosis and lipohyalinosis in the small-diameter, penetrating end arteries of the cerebrum [3, 5]. Treatment of hypertension has repeatedly been proven to be effective in preventing stroke in all age groups. In the elderly, two large trials, the SHEP

(Systolic Hypertension in the Elderly Program) and SYS-EUR (Systolic Hypertension in Europe) studies showed the benefit of antihypertensive therapy in lowering the risk of stroke [6, 7]. Although any antihypertensive therapy which brings hypertension down to a goal blood pressure of < 140/90 will reduce the stroke risk, certain populations may respond better to a particular class of drug. In general, hypertension in African-Americans is more responsive to monotherapy with diuretics and long-acting calcium channel blockers. The elderly with isolated systolic hypertension respond well to thiazide diuretics and long-acting dihydropyridine calcium channel blockers [6, 7] as well.

Overall, hypertension is a very modifiable risk factor for the occurrence of stroke in Blacks and other ethnic groups. The Joint National Committee on Prevention, Detection, Evaluation, and Treatment of High Blood Pressure – Sixth Report is different from the Fifth Report in that it uses the word prevention in its title, indicating there is a growing feeling that the best way to deal with hypertension and its complications is to take a large-scale approach towards preventing it [8]. Accordingly, the National Heart, Lung and Blood Institute has been studying the idea of primary prevention of hypertension by lifestyle changes such as weight loss, sodium restriction, increasing physical activity and eliminating excessive alcohol intake [9].

Noninsulin-Dependent Diabetes

It has been concluded, based on both clinical and epidemiologic data, that type II diabetics have a prevalence of risk factors for cardiovascular disease such as hypertension, obesity and dyslipidemia which is higher than nondiabetics [16]. Despite this association, observational studies have shown diabetes to be an independent risk factor for stroke with a relative risk of 1.8–3.0 for both diabetic men and women. The population-attributable risk due to diabetes is between 2 and 5% for strokes of all types [17–19]. The degree of glucose intolerance also seems to have a positive association with an increased risk of ischemic stroke [5, 18]. Hyperinsulinemia and insulin resistance were both shown to be risk factors for ischemic stroke among patients with normal glucose status [21]. Increased insulin secretion is also associated with increased atherosclerosis of the carotid arteries, independent of glucose status, insulin levels or other cardiovascular risk factors [22].

The greatest reduction in risk for stroke would probably come by modifying the risk factors for the incidence of type II diabetes itself, such as adiposity (both total fat and centrally distributed body fat) [23] and sedentary lifestyle. The effect of strict glycemic control on stroke risk in diabetics remains uncertain. Data on type I diabetes in the DCCT trials did not specifically deal with reducing the incidence of stroke by strict glycemic control [25]. Information from large long-term trials, like the DCCT for type II diabetes, is lacking. Hopefully, the emergence of 'insulin sensitizers' like metformin and troglitazone will give doctors the possibility of preventing or delaying the onset of diabetes. Since African-Americans have a higher prevalence and more complications from diabetes than Whites, it would be wise to institute risk reduction with exercise, diet and drug therapy to delay the onset of diabetes and to aggressively treat associated risk factors like hypertension and dyslipidemia in these patients. Presently, exercise, weight loss, vasodilating antihypertensive drugs (especially ACE inhibitors) and certain lipid-lowering drugs appear to have a favorable effect on metabolic disturbances like higher peripheral insulin levels and insulin resistance [26]. Also, it is important to remember in diabetics the goal blood pressure should at the very least be <130/85 [8] and to follow the new American Diabetes Association guidelines for the early diagnosis and treatment of diabetes [25].

Cigarette Smoking

Cigarette smoking was found to increase the risk of ischemic stroke by about two-fold in a large number of studies. The prevalence of smoking is higher in men than in women (27.8 vs. 23.3%) and in Blacks than in Whites (33.7 vs. 27.7%) [12]. Smoking also seems to be inversely related to the level of education [20]. The Framingham Study concluded that cessation of smoking led to a prompt reduction in stroke with a major risk reduction occurring within 2–4 years [4].

Physicians and public health workers certainly understand that they need to prevent smoking and help smokers quit smoking in order to improve their cardiovascular health, but the question is how? The most effective public health education strategies for reducing cigarette consumption included giving information on the dangers of second-hand smoke as well as industry manipulation which involves portraying the tobacco industry as dishonest and manipulative [46]. Physicians should repeatedly advise smokers to quit, and use more aggressive intervention strategies detailed in materials from the National Cancer Institute and American Lung Association. Pharmacologic therapies (e.g. nicotine patch or gum) are also available but they also seem to be most effective when patients make a true commitment to quitting.

Blood Lipids

Multiple studies have shown hyperlipidemia to be an important modifiable risk factor for coronary heart disease, but the association between increased lipids and stroke remains uncertain [22, 28]. One could certainly make an argument for an indirect link based on the fact there is a clear positive relationship between the total and LDL cholesterol and extracranial carotid atherosclerosis [29].

Data from several studies seems to support the use of HMG-CoA reductase inhibitors to prevent stroke [31, 32, 34]. In a meta-analysis of four clinical trials involving the reductase inhibitor pravastatin, a 62% decrease in the risk for stroke of borderline significance (p=0.054) was noted [30].

What specific statements can you make about African-Americans and lipid-lowering therapy? If one accepts the idea that Blacks have more intracranial lesions versus extracranial lesions as a cause for stroke then one might conclude that lipid reduction would have a lessened impact on Blacks versus Whites [33]. Very little data is available on this subject. In spite of any controversy that might exist, it seems clear that lipid lowering, especially with HMG-CoA reductase inhibitors, would certainly be recommended unless there were strong contraindications. As far as the level is concerned, the NCEP guidelines are the standard of care for patients meeting criteria for drug treatment of the National Cholesterol Education Program – Adult Treatment Panel [24].

Diet and the Prevention of Stroke and Hypertension

Both doctors and many lay people are aware of the fact that Americans consume too much salt (an average of 12 g/day). In many African-American communities, high-sodium diets are particularly troublesome because of the high prevalence of salt-sensitive hypertension in comparison to their Caucasian counterparts.

Some studies suggest that stringent sodium restriction (10–20% of our average consumption of 12 g) may worsen carbohydrate tolerance and activate neurohormonal systems [13]. In the African-American community the best initial approach is probably to aim for modest dietary salt avoidance (particularly highly processed foods and table salt) which should result in 20–30% reduction in salt consumption. A 2- to 3-gram sodium diet is probably an appropriate goal based on the available information.

Recently, the DASH Diet, published in the 1997 *New England Journal of Medicine* [14], was shown to lower blood pressure and thus may help to prevent the onset of high blood pressure. The diet (table 2) is rich in fruits and

Table 2. The DASH Diet, National Institutes of Health – the eating plan is from the 'Dietary Approaches to Stop Hypertension' (DASH) clinical study (the DASH eating plan shown is based on 2,000 cal/day)

Food group	Daily servings	Serving size	Examples and notes	Significance of each food group to the dash diet pattern
Grains and grain products	7–8	1 slice bread 1/2 cup dry cereal 1/2 cup cooked rice, pasta or cereal	Whole wheat bread, English muffin, pita bread, bagel, cereals, grits, oatmeal	Major sources of energy and fiber
Vegetables	4–5	1 cup raw leafy vegetable 1/2 cup cooked vegetable 6 oz vegetable juice	Tomatoes, potatoes, carrots, peas, squash, broccoli, turnip greens, collards, kale, spinach, artichokes, beans, sweet potatoes	Rich sources of potassium, magnesium, and fiber
Fruits	4–5	6 oz fruit juice 1 medium fruit 1/4 cup dried fruit 1/4 cup fresh, frozen, or canned fruit	Apricots, bananas, dates, grapes, oranges, orange juice, mangoes, melons, peaches, pineapples, prunes, raisins, strawberries, tangerines	Important sources of potassium, magnesium, and fiber
Low-fat or nonfat dairy foods	2–3	8 oz milk 1 cup yogurt 1.5 oz cheese	skim or 1% milk, skim or low-fat buttermilk, nonfat or low-fat yogurt, part-skim mozzarella cheese, nonfat cheese	Major sources of calcium and protein
Meats, poultry, and fish	2 or less	3 oz cooked meats, poultry, or fish	Select only lean; trim away visible fats; broil, roast, or boil, instead of frying; remove skin from poultry	Rich sources of protein and magnesium
Nuts, seeds, and legumes	4–5/week	1.5 oz or 1/3 cup nuts 1/2 oz or 2 table spoons seeds 1/2 cup cooked legumes	Almonds, filberts, mixed nuts, peanuts, walnuts, sunflower seeds, kidney beans, lentils	Rich sources of energy, magnesium, potassium, protein, and fiber

vegetables as well as low-fat dairy foods. It is called the 'combination diet' because it emphasizes low-fat, low-cholesterol food, while at the same time the diet is high in dietary fiber, potassium, calcium and magnesium.

Animal studies have suggested that dietary potassium may protect against stroke. A retrospective analysis of the data from the Northern Manhattan Stroke Study [15] showed that Blacks, Whites, and Hispanics were all found to have a lower risk of stroke with the higher serum levels of potassium. The most protection (60% risk reduction) occurred in Blacks. Although potassium supplementation has been correlated with lower blood pressure in other studies, the link between serum potassium and stroke was independent of blood pressure levels [47].

As far as eating polyunsaturated fatty acids derived from fish oils (n-3 fatty acids) is concerned, most of the evidence seems to favor an inverse relation between fish intake and the risk of stroke [41, 42]. One study on Blacks showed a 50% lower incidence of all strokes in persons who ate fish compared to those who did not [10]. Although this finding requires confirmation, consuming fish once a week may be a prudent health practice.

Supplemental vitamins B_6, B_{12} and folic acid seem to reduce plasma homocysteine levels. Epidemiologic studies have shown a strong correlation between higher homocysteine levels and atherosclerotic disease. Ongoing studies to see if vitamin B_6, B_{12} and folic acid can decrease stroke risk should be published soon [4].

Physically Active Lifestyle

The relationship between strokes and physical activity has not been extensively evaluated. However, the results from available studies are consistent with an inverse relation between physical activity and the risk of stroke in men and women [35–38]. A recent study found that leisuretime physical activity in participants aged 70 and over was associated with a reduction in the risk of ischemic stroke [40], with African-Americans having a 67% reduction versus 56% in Whites and 73% in Hispanics. Thus, for stroke prevention the promotion of exercise may be an important first step.

Alcohol

The Framingham data indicate a J-shaped relation between alcohol consumption with the moderate to heavy drinkers (> 3 drinks/day) having a high risk for ischemic stroke and light drinkers (1–2 drinks/day) having a lower risk than nondrinkers [43]. Hemorrhagic stroke on the other hand appears to have an increased incidence at all levels of alcohol intake. Since many of these types of studies have at least partial reliance on patient recall it is not surprising to find that methodologic problems have hampered this research.

Alcoholism is a major health problem in African-Americans and acute alcohol withdrawal can be a major cause of morbidity and mortality if not appropriately diagnosed and managed. It also seems that the J-shaped association curve for moderate alcohol consumption and risk of ischemic stroke was most consistent in White populations with little or no association noted for Japanese and possibly Black populations [4]. Therefore, it does not seem advisable to recommend drinking alcohol even in small quantities.

Postmenopausal Estrogen Replacement Therapy, Oral Contraceptives and Low-Dose Aspirin

A closer look at stroke risk and postmenopausal estrogen replacement therapy shows a relative risk of 0.96 in meta-analysis data [45]. In contrast, higher dose formulations of oral contraceptives were found to increase stroke in women, especially smokers, hypertensives and those with a history of migraine headaches [5]. The manufacturers responded by providing low-dose oral contraceptives with substantially lower amounts of estrogen and progesterone, but further study is needed to better determine the stroke risk of these newer formulations.

It remains unclear whether aspirin is beneficial in the primary prevention of stroke [4, 44]. However, it is useful in secondary prevention for patients with a diagnosis of cerebrovascular disease or coronary heart disease.

Community Prevention

The Stroke Belt Initiative is an example of a program set up to address the disproportionately high stroke rate in the Southeastern United States (i.e. the Stroke Belt) [27]. The NHLBI (National Heart Lung Blood Institute) funded the project which used various community-based and prevention programs to lower the risk of stroke. Several important lessons learned from the project include (1) to work in churches you must have strong support from the clergy as well as involvement with the health care ministry or team; (2) church-based programs must be flexible in their approach and have a lot of time and patience; (3) community-based programs that can be integrated into the health center's basic services and have buy-in from both physicians and support staff are likely to be sustained, and (4) quality control audits and automated equipment can improve hypertension detection and control efforts.

Conclusion

Despite recent advances in the treatment on acute stroke, primary prevention of first stroke will continue to be a major point of emphasis especially in a health care system where cost is always a consideration. Modifiable risk factors like hypertension which contributes to about 70% of strokes [5] will have to be aggressively treated according to the Joint National Committee VI Guidelines [8].

When looking at primary prevention of stroke one must certainly pay particular attention to increasing prevalence of diabetes and obesity in Blacks. Overall, the most potentially powerful method of primary prevention of type II diabetes is the use of weight loss, exercise and insulin sensitizers (i.e. metformin, troglitazone, etc.) to delay or even avoid clinically overt diabetes in high-risk populations.

Because of limited resources in many lower socioeconomic groups within the African-American community, a large part of stroke prevention in the African-American neighborhoods will have to be done by volunteers in churches and community health centers.

Acknowledgment

With acknowledgment to Richard F. Gillum, MD, MSPH, FACC, Elijah Saunders, MD, FACC, Steven Kittner, MD, and B. Waine Kong, PhD, JD.

References

1   MacMahon S, Rodgers A: The epidemiological association between blood pressure and stroke: Implications for primary and secondary prevention. Hypertens Res 1994;17(suppl):523–532.
2   Whisnant JP: Effectiveness versus efficacy of treatment of hypertension for stroke prevention. Neurology 1996;46:301–307.
3   Phillips SJ, Whisnant JP: Hypertension and the brain: The National High Blood Pressure Education Program. Arch Intern Med 1992;152:938–945.
4   Sacco RL, Benjamin EJ, Broderick JP, Dyken M, Easton JD, Feinberg WM, Goldstein LB, Gorelick PB, Howard G, Kittner SJ, Manolio TA, Whisnant JP, Wolf PA: American Heart Association Prevention Conference IV: Prevention and Rehabilitation of Stroke. Stroke 1997;28:1498–1526.
5   Bronner L, Kanter D, Manson J: Primary prevention of stroke. N Engl J Med 1995;333:1392–1400.

6   SHEP Cooperative Research Group: Prevention of stroke by antihypertensive drug treatment in older persons with isolated systolic hypertension: Final results of the Systolic Hypertension in the Elderly Program (SHEP). JAMA 1991;256:3255–3264.

7   Staessen JA, Fagard R, Thijs L, Celis H, Arabidze GG, Birkenhager WH, Bulpitt CJ, de Leeuw PW, Dollery CT, Fletcher AE, Forette F, Leonetti G, Nachev C, O'Brien ET, Rosenfeld J, Rodicio JL, Tuomilehto J, Zanchetti A, for the Systolic Hypertension-Europe (SYS-EUR) Trial Investigators. Morbidity and mortality in the placebo-controlled European Trial on Isolated Systolic Hypertension in the Elderly. Lancet 1997;360:757–764.

8   Joint National Committee on Prevention, Detection, Evaluation, and Treatment of High Blood Pressure: The Sixth Report of the Joint National Committee on Prevention, Detection, Evaluation, and Treatment of High Blood Pressure (JNC VI). Arch Intern Med 1997;157:2413–2446.

9   Lenfant C, Rocella EJ: The First Goal of the NHBPEP: Primary Prevention. Hypertension Watch: Pursing the Advantage 1995;1(June/July):1–3.

10   Gillum RF, Mussolino ME, Madans JH: The relationship between fish consumption and stroke incidence. The NHANES I epidemiologic follow-up study (National Health and Nutrition Examination Survey). Arch Intern Med 1996;156:537–542.

11   Cook NR, Cohen J, Herbert PR, Taylor JO, Hennekens CH: Implications of small reductions in diastolic blood pressure for primary prevention. Arch Intern Med 1995;155:701–709.

12   Fingerhut LA, Warner M: Injury Chartbook. Health, United States, 1996–97. Hyattsville, National Center for Health Statistics, 1997.

13   Alderman MN, Madhavan S, Cohen H, Sealy JE, Laragh JH: Low urinary sodium is associated with greater risk of myocardial infarction among treated hypertensive men. Hypertension 1995;62: 740–745.

14   Appel LJ, Moore TJ, Obarzanck E, Vollmer WM, Svetkey LP, Sacks FM, Bray GA, Vogt TM, Cutler JA, Windhauser MM, Lin PH, Karanja N, for the DASH Collaborative Research Group: A clinical trial of the effects of dietary patterns on blood pressure. N Engl J Med 1997;336(16): 1117–1124.

15   Borden-Ablala B, Gu Q, Kargman DE, Lipset C, Shea S, Hauser WA, Paik M, Sacco RL: Increased stroke incidence in Blacks and Hispanics: The Northern Manhattan Stroke Study. Neurology 1995; 45(suppl 4):A300.

16   American Diabetes Associations: Role of cardiovascular risk factors in prevention and treatment of macrovascular disease in diabetes. Diabetes Care 1989;12:573–579.

17   Wolf PA, Cobb JL, D'Augustino RB: Epidemiology of stroke; in Barnett HJM, Mohr JP, Stein BM, Yatsu FM (eds): Stroke: Pathophysiology, Diagnosis, and Management, ed 2. New York, Churchill Livingstone, 1992, pp 3–27.

18   Burchfiel CM, Curb JD, Rodriquez BL, Abbott RD, Chiu D, Yano K: Glucose intolerance and 22-year stroke incidence: The Honolulu Heart Program. Stroke 1994;25:951–957.

19   Manson JE, Colditz GA, Stampfer MJ, Willett WC, Krolewski AS, Rosner B, Arky RA, Speizer FE, Hennekens CH: A prospective study of maturity-onset diabetes mellitus and risk of coronary heart disease and stroke in women. Arch Intern Med 1991;151:1141–1147.

20   Wolf PA, D'Agostino RB, Kannel WB, Bonita R, Belanger AJ: Cigarette smoking as a risk factor for stroke: The Framingham Study. JAMA 1988;259:1025–1029.

21   Shinozaki K, Naritomi H, Shimizu T, Suzuki M, Ikebuchi M, Sawada T, Harano Y: Role of insulin resistance associated with compensatory hyperinsulinemia in ischemic stroke. Stroke 1996;27: 37–43.

22   Howard G, O'Leary DH, Zaccaro D, Haffner S, Rewers M, Hamman R, Selby JV, Saad MF, Savage P, Bergman R: Insulin sensitivity and atherosclerosis: The Insulin Resistance Atherosclerosis Study (IRAS) Investigators. Circulation 1996;93:1459–1817.

23   National Research Council, Diet and Health: Implications for Reducing Chronic Disease Risk. Washington, National Academy Press, 1989.

24   Summary of the National Cholesterol Education Program (NCEP) Adult Treatment Panel II Report. JAMA 1993;269:3015–3023.

25   Report of the Expert Committee on the Diagnosis and Classification of Diabetes mellitus. Diabetes Care 1997;20:1183–1197.

26 Ketchen TA: Attenuation of hypertension by insulin-sensitizing agents. Hypertension 1996;28:219–223.

27 Okwumabua JO, Martin B, Clayton-Davis J, Pearson CM: Stroke Belt Initiative: The Tennessee Experience. J Health Care Poor Underserved 1997;8:292–299.

28 Iso H, Jacobs DR Jr, Wentworth D, Neaton JD, Cohen JD: Serum cholesterol levels and six-year mortality from stroke in 350,977 men screened for the multiple risk factor intervention trial. N Engl J Med 1989;320:904–910.

29 Welin L, Suardsudd K, Wilhelmsen L, Larsson B, Tibblin G: Analysis of risk factors for stroke in a cohort of men born in 1913. N Engl J Med 1987;317:521–526.

30 Crouse JR: Reductase inhibitor monotherapy reduces stroke in patients with CHD. Today Med 1997;11:18.

31 Crouse JR, Byington RP, Hoen HM, Furberg CD: Reductase inhibitor monotherapy and stroke prevention. Arch Intern Med 1997;157:1305–1310.

32 Bucher HC, Griffith LE, Guyatt GH: Effect of HMG-CoA reductase inhibitors on stroke. Ann Intern Med 1998;128:89–95.

33 Gillum RF: Stroke in Blacks. Stroke 1988;19:1–9.

34 Douglass PL: Controlling cardiovascular risk factors for strokes. ABC Digest of Urban Cardiology 1995(July/August):8–16.

35 Abbott RD, Rodriquez BL, Burchfiel CM, Curb JD: Physical activity in older middle-aged men and reduced risk of stroke: The Honolulu Heart Program. Am J Epidemiol 1994;139:881–893.

36 Wannamethee G, Shaper AG: Physical activity and stroke in British middle-aged men. BMJ 1992; 304:597–601.

37 Kiely DK, Wolf PA, Cupples LA, Beiser AS, Kannel WB: Physical activity and stroke risk: The Framingham Study. Am J Epidemiol 1994;140:608–620. (Erratum, Am J Epidemiol 1995;141:178.)

38 Manson JE, Stampfer MJ, Willett WC, Colditz GA, Speizer FE, Hennekens CH: Physical activity and incidence of coronary heart disease and stroke in women (abstract). Circulation 1995;91:927.

39 Public Health Service: Healthy People 2000 Review. DHHS Publ No (PHS)94-1223-1. Washington, Government Printing Office, 1993.

40 Kher Unmesh: Physical activity helps prevent ischemic strokes in elderly. Med Trib 1998;39:12.

41 Keli SO, Feskens JM, Kromhout D: Fish consumption and risk of stroke: The Zutphen Study. Stroke 1997;25:328–332.

42 Hirai A, Terano T, Saito H, Tamura Y, Yoshida S: Clinical and epidemiological studies of eicosapentaenoic acid in Japan; in Lands WEM (ed): Polyunsaturated Fatty Acids and Eicosanoids. Champaign, American Oil Chemists' Society, 1987, pp 9–24.

43 Camargo CA Jr: Moderate alcohol consumption and stroke: The epidemiologic evidence. Stroke 1989;20:1611–1626.

44 Steering Committee of the Physicians' Health Study Research Group: Final report on the aspirin component of the ongoing Physicians' Health Study. N Engl J Med 1989;321:129–135.

45 Grady D, Rubin SM, Petitti DB, Fox CS, Black D, Ettinger B, Ernster VL, Cummings SR: Hormone therapy to prevent disease and prolong life in postmenopausal women. Ann Intern Med 1992;117: 1016–1037.

46 Goldman LK, Glantz SA: Evaluation of antismoking advertising campaigns. JAMA 1998;279: 772–777.

47 Boden-Albala B: High serum potassium protects against stroke and hypertension. Mod Med 1998; 66:33–36.

Wallace R. Johnson, Jr., MD, Assistant Clinical Professor, Division of Hypertension,
Department of Medicine, University of Maryland School of Medicine,
419 W. Redwood St., Suite 620, Baltimore, MD 21201-1734 (USA)

Gillum RF, Gorelick PB, Cooper ES (eds): Stroke in Blacks. Basel, Karger, 1999, pp 129–141

....

Atrial Fibrillation, Heart Disease, and Ischemic Stroke in Blacks

Richard F. Gillum[a], John Thomas[b], Charles L. Curry[c]

[a] Centers for Disease Control and Prevention, Hyattsville, Md.;
[b] Meharry Medical College, Nashville, Tenn., and
[c] Howard University College of Medicine, Washington, D.C., USA

Worldwide, heart disease and stroke are now the leading causes of death, accounting for 21% of the 50 million deaths in 1990 [1, 2]. In US Blacks, heart disease is the leading cause of death and stroke is the third leading cause of death [3, 4]. In 1995, 38,389 Black men and 40,254 Black women died of heart disease. It has long been recognized that US Blacks suffer mortality from heart disease and stroke at rates far in excess of those of Whites (fig. 1) [3, 4]. Age-adjusted heart disease death rates per 100,000 were higher in Black men (259.2) than White men (184.5) and in Black women (159.8) than White women (96.7). Heart disease death rates of US Blacks have been among the highest in the world (fig. 2). Self-reported prevalence of heart disease in the National Health Interview Survey was similar and self-reported prevalence of coronary heart disease lower in Blacks than Whites, perhaps reflecting racial differences in access to care as well as population prevalence (fig. 3) [6]. Thanks to recent declines, stroke death rates of US Blacks fall between the high rates of Eastern Europe and the low rates of North American Whites [3, 5–9]. Heart disease, especially atrial fibrillation, is an established risk factor for ischemic stroke in populations of European descent [10–13]. Mechanisms of cerebral embolism of cardiac origin have been discussed at length elsewhere [12, 13]. It is important to confirm this association in populations of African descent. Many questions remain regarding the cardiac etiology of stroke in Blacks and the role of differing patterns in heart disease as a basis for racial differences in stroke occurrence [14]. This report reviews studies of stroke in Blacks with heart disease in an attempt to answer these questions and to suggest directions for future research. Because of limitation of data sources, only the most common types of cardiac disease associated with stroke will be discussed here.

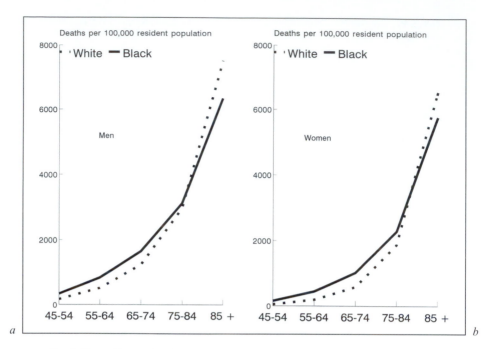

Fig. 1. Heart disease death rates by race and age in men (*a*) and women (*b*) in 1989–91. Adapted from Gillum [76].

Atrial Fibrillation

Prevalence and Incidence in Blacks

The epidemiology of atrial fibrillation (AF) in persons of European ancestry has been reviewed elsewhere [15–17]. Published data on population prevalence of AF in Black populations are few. Among 244 Blacks aged 65 and over in the Cardiovascular Health Study, self-reported AF was reported for 1.5% of men and 3.6% of women [18]. AF by electrocardiogram was reported in 1.1% of men and 0.7% of women compared to 4.0% and 2.7%, respectively, in Whites (nonsignificant racial difference). In data from one large US hospital case series, the age-adjusted odds ratio comparing European with African-Americans was 2.0 (95% confidence interval (CI) 1.79–2.27, $p < 0.001$) [19]. In the USA in 1988–1990, there were 186,673 hospital discharges with any diagnosis of AF in Blacks aged 35 years and over [20]. Among patients with acute myocardial infarction (AMI) in a clinical trial, the frequency of AF prior to randomization seemed lower in Blacks but was not significantly different in Blacks (1.8%) and Whites (6.7%) [21]. The only report of AF

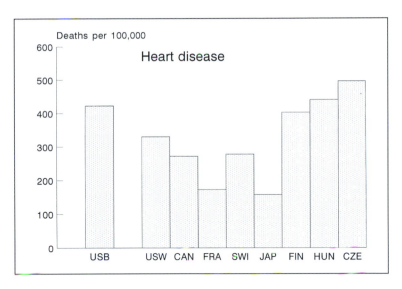

Fig. 2. Age-adjusted rates of death from heart disease of US Black (USB) and US White (USW) men compared to men in selected industrialized countries (Canada, CAN; France, FRA; Switzerland, SWI; Japan, JAP; Finland, FIN; Hungary, HUN; former Czechoslovakia, CZE) in 1990. From Gillum [6].

incidence in Blacks is from the Cardiovascular Health Study. In persons 65 and over, incidence was lower in Blacks than others (12 vs. 19.5/1,000 person-years, p > 0.10). The difference became significant after controlling for multiple variables in subjects without cardiovascular disease at baseline (relative risk 0.21, 95% CI 0.05–0.86) and nearly so in all subjects (relative risk (RR) 0.47, 0.22–1.01) [22]. Thus, the limited available data suggest lower prevalence rates of AF in Blacks than Whites in the USA. Given the higher heart disease and stroke mortality in Blacks, lower AF prevalence in Blacks may reflect poorer survival in Blacks with AF as well as lower incidence. Further studies of larger samples are needed for estimation of racial differences in prevalence, incidence, and prognosis.

Association of AF with Ischemic Stroke

In persons of European descent, AF is a potent risk factor for stroke [10]. However, with one exception, data are lacking to determine whether it carries the same risk in persons of African descent. A study of 4 million Medicare recipients followed 4 years revealed that compared to those without AF, Black men and women with AF had 1.4 and 1.7 times the risk of nonem-

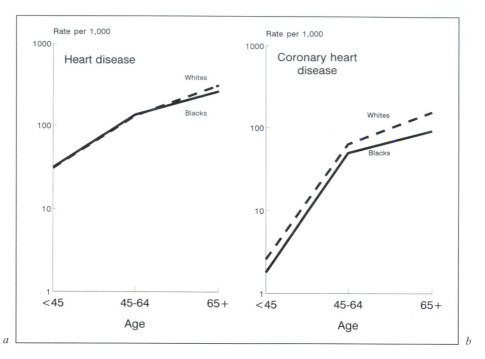

Fig. 3. Prevalence of self-reported heart disease (*a*) and CHD (*b*) by race and age in 1990–92. From Gillum [6].

bolic stroke and 4.3 and 7.3 times the risk of embolic stroke (table 1) [23]. Four-year risks were highest in Black women with AF (21.3% for nonembolic and 3.28% for embolic stroke). The association was similar in Whites. In the USA in 1988–1990, of 327,428 discharges with any diagnosis of acute cerebrovascular disease, International Classification of Diseases, Clinical Modification (ICD9-CM) 430–437, in Blacks aged 35–74 years 21,844 (6.67%) had an associated diagnosis of AF (ICD9-CM 427.3) (table 2). The comparable percentage in Whites was 8.00% [20]. In a series of 430 hospitalized stroke patients with acute ischemic stroke in New York City, AF was less prevalent in Blacks (11%) than Whites (29%); the mean age was 70 in Blacks and 80 in Whites; age-adjusted results were not presented [24a]. In a series of Blacks from urban South Africa, cerebral embolism was diagnosed in 13.8% of stroke cases, AF being the presumed cause of cerebral embolism in 6.9% of patients [24b]. No prospective cohort studies or case-control studies were found that assessed the relative risk of stroke in Black persons with and without AF. Also associated with stroke in Whites [13], sick sinus syndrome has not been

Table 1. Sex-specific incidence (%) of developing stroke over a 4-year follow-up period in African-American Medicare recipients hospitalized with and without AF in 1985 (n = 30,850) [adapted from 23]

	Patients with AF		Patients without AF	
	rate	95% Cl	rate	95% Cl
Nonembolic stroke				
Men	16.5	(15.3–17.7)	11.9	(11.2–12.6)
Women	21.3	(20.2–22.4)	12.9	(12.3–13.5)
Embolic stroke				
Men	2.55	(2.03–3.07)	0.59	(0.42–0.76)
Women	3.28	(2.80–3.76)	0.45	(0.33–0.57)

studied in relation to stroke in Blacks. Possible associations of other cardiac rhythm disorders with embolic stroke has been discussed elsewhere [12]. Could increased heart rate predispose to stroke in Blacks? Blacks with a high pulse rate had twice the risk of stroke was seen in Blacks with a low pulse rate (table 3) [25]. No significant association of pulse rate and stroke was seen in Whites. Numerous clinical trials have demonstrated the effectiveness of antithrombotic and antiplatelet therapy in reducing the risk of stroke in AF [26]. However, no clinical trial of antithrombotic or antiplatelet therapy has included sufficient Blacks for subgroup analysis, e.g. of the 1,330 patients in the Stroke Prevention in Atrial Fibrillation Study (SPAF), 6% were Black [26]. In the absence of adequate clinical and epidemiologic data in Blacks with AF, clinicians must extrapolate results obtained from Whites to Black patients, i.e. that AF is a powerful risk factor for ischemic stroke. However, well-designed case-control studies are urgently needed to confirm the validity of such generalizations [27].

Coronary Heart Disease

In developed countries such as the USA, coronary heart disease (CHD) is now the leading cause of death in Blacks with age-adjusted death rates now exceeding those of Whites in both women and men [28–34]. Although rates of first AMI remain lower in Blacks than Whites, prognosis may be similar or poorer in Blacks [28–34]. Despite its importance, few data have been published on acute or chronic CHD as a risk factor for stroke in Blacks. In

Table 2. Hospital discharges with stroke diagnosis associated with AMI or AF diagnosis in persons aged 35 years and over in the National Hospital Discharge Survey 1988–1990

Diagnosis	Blacks			Whites		
	discharges[1]	SE	%	discharges	SE	%
Any AMI	145	28	100	1,865	212	100
Any AMI with stroke[2]	9	6	6	79	19	4
Any stroke	327	49	100	2,636	293	100
Any stroke with AF	22	9	7	296	45	11

AMI = Acute myocardial infarction, ICD-9 code 410; Stroke = ICD-9 codes 430–437; AF = atrial fibrillation, ICD-9 code 427.3; SE = standard error (thousands).

[1] Discharges in thousands.

[2] Estimate for Blacks must be used with caution due to small number of cases in sample.

Table 3. Resting pulse rate and stroke incidence in African-Americans aged 45–74 years in the NHANES I Epidemiologic Follow-Up Study, 1971–1987

Pulse rate, beats/min	Age- and sex-adjusted			Risk-adjusted[1]		
	RR	95% Cl		RR	95% Cl	
<74	1.00			1.00		
75–84	1.67	1.04	2.70	1.59	0.98	2.58
>84	2.14	1.31	3.51	2.07	1.25	3.43

[1] Adjusted for age, sex, smoking, diabetes, history of heart disease, education, systolic blood pressure, serum cholesterol, body mass index, and hemoglobin.

analyses of risk of cerebral infarction in the NHANES I Epidemiologic Follow-up Study [35a], there was a significant interaction of race with history of heart disease (p = 0.01), indicating a different effect on risk in Blacks than Whites. Blacks with and without history of heart disease had a similar risk of cerebral infarction while Whites with history of heart disease had a much greater risk than those without [35a]. However, this result is based on a very small number of events and on self-reports of heart disease and must be confirmed in other studies. In the USA in 1988–1990, of 144,615 discharges with any diagnosis of AMI (ICD9-CM 410) in Blacks aged 35 years and over, 8,531 (5.90%) had an associated diagnosis of acute stroke (ICD9-CM 430–437) (table 2). The comparable percentage in Whites was 4.22% [20]. Results of other studies were also inconclusive [24a, 35b, 36]. Thus, while CHD and AMI are presumptive risk factors for ischemic stroke in Blacks based on studies of Whites, the results of the few available studies are conflicting.

Heart Failure and Hypertensive Heart Disease

Myocardial disease and congestive heart failure (CHF) are more common in Blacks than Whites in the USA [37–40]. However, data are few on their role as risk factors for stroke in Blacks [24a]. The epidemiology of hypertension and hypertensive heart disease, both more common in Blacks, has been reviewed at length elsewhere [5, 37, 41–48]. The relationship of left ventricular hypertrophy (LVH) to stroke in Blacks has been little studied. In the North Manhattan Study case series, ECG LVH was more frequent in Black (20%) than White (9%) stroke cases [24a]. Antecedent electrocardiographic abnormalities were associated with only slightly increased risk of stroke in Blacks in the Evans County study [49]. Approximate age-adjusted relative risks were for Black men 1.3, for White men 1.9, for Black women 1.3, and for White women 1.3. Thus, although an association of CHF and myocardial disease with stroke is presumed, the question has not been studied in Blacks. The few available data suggest a different mode of action for this risk factor in Blacks than in Whites, perhaps related to greater prevalence of hypertension and greater susceptibility to the effects of hypertension in Blacks.

Valvular Heart Disease

Studies in Whites have linked valvular heart disease to increased risk of ischemic stroke in Whites [10–13]. Rheumatic heart disease and infective endocarditis remain serious problems in less developed nations [12, 50]. Mitral valve prolapse reportedly occurs with similar frequencies in Blacks and Whites in the USA [51–54]. Mobile, filamentous strands on the mitral or aortic valves were associated with stroke in a case-control study (odds ratio 2.0, 0.4–9.3) in Blacks; associations were even stronger in Hispanics and Whites with large numbers [55]. Thus, while studies of valvular heart disease in Blacks are lacking, Blacks with these conditions are likely at increased risk for embolic stroke.

Other Heart and Vascular Causes

Dissecting aneurysm, more common in Blacks than Whites [56], may also cause stroke. A number of studies have shown that US Blacks have higher rates of fatal cardiac arrest than Whites and poorer outcomes after cardiac arrest among survivors [57, 58]. Studies are needed of racial differences in global cerebral ischemia and focal deficits in Black survivors of cardiac arrest. Proximal aortic atheromas occurred with similar frequency in Black and White stroke cases [59]. Because of the high prevalence of hypertension, Blacks treated for AMI with thrombolysis might be at increased risk for complicating intracerebral hemorrhage [60, 61]. Since it was first reported in 1982 [28], many studies have documented lower rates of coronary artery bypass grafting in US Blacks compared to Whites, that cannot be fully explained by coronary anatomy or ability to pay [62–64]. The frequency of stroke complicating these procedures in Blacks might be examined further in large data sets such as those of Medicare. Patent foramen ovale was a risk factor for ischemic stroke in Whites and Hispanics but not in Blacks [65]. Case series from southern Africa reveal that cardiac embolism is a not uncommon cause of stroke in Black Africans [24b, 66, 67].

Future Research Needs

Case-control studies should be performed to estimate the relative odds of ischemic stroke associated with the more common types of heart disease discussed above in African-Americans and other Blacks. The largest population-based cohort studies may also be able to provide data on risk associated with LVH, and history of any heart disease [68]. Data from national registries of AMI, other diseases, and cardiac surgery and from Medicare may also be valuable resources for analysis in the USA. Meta-analyses should be performed of all studies of antiplatelet therapy in the setting of heart disease for combined results for Blacks.

Implications for Clinical Practice

Until adequate data become available in Black populations, clinicians must assume that diseases of the heart which are proven risk factors for stroke in Whites also increase the risk of stroke in Blacks. Current guidelines for the prevention of stroke in the setting of heart disease found in standard texts and elsewhere should be followed in caring for the Black patient with heart disease [68–75]. Care must be individualized, weighing likely risks and benefits. While the use of therapies such as warfarin which require intensive follow-up must be considered carefully in patients with financial and educational barriers to care, they must not be denied out of hand. Provisions should be made to provide extra support and educational services to such patients whenever possible. Because of their low cost and once-daily regimens, antiplatelet agents such as aspirin should be used more widely in Black patients with heart disease at increased risk for ischemic stroke. Noncardiac risk factors for stroke such as hypertension and smoking should be assessed and vigorously controlled in cardiac patients.

Conclusion

In developed countries, heart disease is the leading cause of death in Blacks and may have similar prevalence in Blacks and Whites. In developing countries, heart disease and stroke are growing problems. Heart disease is an established risk factor for stroke in populations of European descent; however, few studies have addressed this question in Blacks. AF may be less prevalent in US Blacks than Whites. A powerful risk factor for stroke in Whites, its role in stroke in Blacks has been inadequately studied. Similarly, little is known about coronary disease and CHF as stroke risk factors in Blacks. In series of stroke patients, Blacks tended to have less AF and coronary disease and similar frequency of heart failure. In one cohort, a history of heart disease was a significant risk factor for stroke in Whites but not in Blacks. The effectiveness of antithrombotic and antiplatelet therapy for AF or other forms of heart disease has not been studied in Blacks. Until further research is conducted, clinicians in developed countries should follow established guidelines for stroke prevention in Black as well as White patients. In Black patients with heart disease, special attention should be given to the control of noncardiac risk factors for stroke and to removing financial, educational, and cultural barriers to the effective utilization of therapies such as warfarin. Antiplatelet agents should be more widely used and their efficacy evaluated further in Black patients with heart disease.

References

1   Murray CJ, Lopez AD: Mortality by cause for eight regions of the world: Global burden of disease study. Lancet 1997;349:1269–1276.
2   Murray CJ, Lopez AD: Global mortality, disability, and the contribution of risk factors: Global burden of disease study. Lancet 1997;349:1436–1442.
3   National Center for Health Statistics. Health, United States, 1996–97 and Injury Chartbook, Hyattsville, 1997.
4   Gillum RF, Feinleib M: Cardiovascular disease in the United States: Mortality, prevalence, and incidence; in Kapoor AS, Singh BN (eds): Prognosis and Risk Assessment in Cardiovascular Disease. New York, Churchill Livingstone, 1993, pp 49–59.
5   Gillum RF: The epidemiology of hypertension in Black women. Am Heart J 1996;131:385–395.
6   Gillum RF: The epidemiology of heart disease and stroke in African-American elders. Am J Geriatr Cardiol 1997;6:21–31.
7   Gaines K, Burke G: Ethnic differences in stroke: Black-White differences in the United States population. Neuroepidemiology 1995;14:209–239.
8   Gillum RF: The epidemiology of cardiovascular disease in Black Americans. N Engl J Med 1996; 335:1597–1599.
9   Francis CK: Hypertension and cardiac disease in minorities. Am J Med 1990;88:S3–S8.
10   Sacco RL: Ischemic stroke; in Gorelick PB, Alter M (eds): Handbook of Neuroepidemiology. New York, Dekker, 1994, pp 77–119.
11   Kannel WB, Abbott DR, Savage DD, McNamara PM: Epidemiologic features of chronic atrial fibrillation. N Engl J Med 1982;306:1018–1022.
12   Salgado ED, Furlan AJ, Conomy JP: Cardioembolic sources of stroke; in Furlan AJ (ed): The Heart and Stroke. Exploring Mutual Cerebrovascular and Cardiovascular Issues. London, Springer, 1987, pp 47–61.
13   Caplan LR: Stroke: A Clinical Approach. Boston, Butterworth-Heinemann, 1993.
14   Gillum RF: Stroke in Blacks. Stroke 1988;19:1–9.
15   Camm AJ, Obel OA: Epidemiology and mechanism of atrial fibrillation and atrial flutter. Am J Cardiol 1996;78:3–11.
16   Reardon M, Camm AJ: Atrial fibrillation in the elderly. Clin Cardiol 1996;19:765–775.
17   Wolf PA, Benjamin EJ, Belanger AJ, Kannel WB, Levy D, D'Agostino RB: Secular trends in the prevalence of atrial fibrillation: The Framingham Study. Am Heart J 1996;131:790–795.
18   Manolio TA, Burke GL, Psaty BM, Newman AB, Hann M, Powe N, Tracy RP, O'Leary DH: Black-White differences in subclinical cardiovascular disease among older adults: The Cardiovascular Health Study. J Clin Epidemiol 1995;48:1141–1152.
19   Ali AS, Fenn NM, Zarowitz BJ, Niemyski P, Vitarelli A, Gheorghiade M: Epidemiology of atrial fibrillation in patients hospitalized in a large hospital. Panminerva Med 1993;35:209–213.
20   Graves EJ: National Hospital Discharge Survey: Annual Summary, 1990. National Center for Health Statistics. Vital Health Stat 1992;13(112).
21   Haywood LJ: Coronary heart disease mortality/morbidity and risk in Blacks. I. Clinical manifestations and diagnostic criteria: The experience with the Beta Blocker Heart Attack Trial. Am Heart J 1984;108:787–793.
22   Psaty BM, Manolio TA, Kuller LH, Kronmal RA, Cushman M, Fried LP, White R, Furberg CD, Rautaharju PM: Incidence of and risk factors for atrial fibrillation in older adults. Circulation 1997; 96:2455–2461.
23   Yuan Z, Bowlin S, Einstadter D, Cebul RD, Conners AR Jr, Rimm AA: Atrial fibrillation as a risk factor for stroke: A retrospective cohort study of hospitalized Medicare beneficiaries. Am J Public Health 1998;88:395–400.
24a   Sacco RL, Kargman DE, Zamanillo M: Race-ethnic differences in stroke risk factors among hospitalized patients with cerebral infarction – The Northern Manhattan Stroke Study. Neurology 1995;45:659–663.
24b   Rosman KD: The epidemiology of stroke in an urban Black population. Stroke 1986;17:667–669.

25   Gillum RF, Mussolino ME, Ingram DD: Physical activity and stroke incidence in women and men: The NHANES I Epidemiologic Follow-up Study. Am J Epidemiol 1996;143:860–869.
26   Stroke Prevention in Atrial Fibrillation Investigators: Stroke Prevention in Atrial Fibrillation Study: Final Results. Circulation 1991;84:527–539.
27   National Heart Lung and Blood Institute: Report of the Working Group on Research in Coronary Heart Disease in Blacks. Bethesda, National Institutes of Health, 1994, pp 1–94.
28   Gillum RF: Coronary heart disease in Black populations. 1. Mortality and morbidity. Am Heart J 1982;104:839–851.
29   Gillum RF: Trends in acute myocardial infarction and coronary heart disease death in the United States. J Am Coll Cardiol 1994;23:1273–1277.
30   Gillum RF, Mussolino ME, Madans JH: Coronary heart disease incidence and survival in African-American women and men: The NHANES I Epidemiologic Follow-Up Study. Ann Intern Med 1997;127:111–118.
31   Curry CL, Crawford-Green C: Coronary artery disease in Blacks: Past perspectives and current overview; in Saunders E (ed): Cardiovascular Diseases in Blacks. Philadelphia, Davis, 1991, pp 197–204.
32   Curry CL: Coronary artery disease in Blacks; in Livingston IL (ed): Handbook of Black American Health. Westport/Conn, Greenwood Press, 1994, pp 24–32.
33   Curry CL: Coronary artery disease in African-Americans. Circulation 1991;83:1474–1475.
34   Curry CL, Oliver J, Mumtaz FB: Coronary artery disease in Blacks: Risk factors. Am Heart J 1984;108:653–657.
35a   Giles WH, Kittner SJ, Heble JR, Losonczy KG, Sherwin RW: Determinants of Black-White differences in the risk of cerebral infarction: The National Health and Nutrition Examination Survey Epidemiologic Follow-Up Study. Arch Intern Med 1995;155:1319–1324.
35b   Burke GL, Evans GW, Riley WA, Sharrett AR, Howard G, Barnes RW, Rosamond W, Crow RS, Rautaharju PM, Heiss G: Arterial wall thickness is associated with prevalent cardiovascular disease in middle-aged adults. The Atherosclerosis Risk in Communities (ARIC) Study. Stroke 1995;26: 386–391.
36   Friday G, Lai SM, Alter M, Sobel E, LaRue L, Gil-Peralta A, McCoy RL, Levitt LP, Isack T: Stroke in the Lehigh Valley: Racial/ethnic differences. Neurology 1989;39:1165–1168.
37   Gillum RF: Cardiovascular disease in the United States: An epidemiologic overview; in Saunders E (ed): Cardiovascular Diseases in Blacks. Philadelphia, Davis, 1991, pp 3–16.
38   Gillum RF: Epidemiology of heart failure in the United States. Am Heart J 1993;126:1042–1047.
39   Gillum RF: Idiopathic cardiomyopathy in the United States, 1970–1982. Am Heart J 1986;111: 752–755.
40   Gillum RF: The epidemiology of cardiomyopathy in the United States. Prog Cardiol 1989;2:11–21.
41   Flack JM, Wiist WH: Epidemiology of hypertension and hypertensive target-organ damage in the United States. J Assoc Acad Minor Phys 1991;2:143–150.
42   Cooper ES, Caplan LR: Cerebrovascular disease in hypertensive Blacks. Cardiovasc Clin 1991;21: 145–155.
43   Thomas J, Semenya K, Thomas DJ, Neser WB, Pearson TA, Gillum RF: Precursors of hypertension in Black compared to White medical students. J Chron Dis 1987;40:721–727.
44   Thomas J, Semenya K, Neser WB, Thomas JN, Green DR, Gillum RF: Risk factors and the incidence of hypertension in Black physicians: The Meharry Cohort Study. Am Heart J 1985;110: 637–645.
45   Thomas J, Semenya K, Neser WB, Thomas DJ, Green DR, Gillum RF: Precursors of hypertension in Black medical students: The Meharry Cohort Study. J Natl Med Assoc 1984;76:111–21.
46   Thomas J, Thomas DJ, Pearson T, Klag M, Mead L: Cardiovascular disease in African-American and White physicians: The Meharry Cohort and Meharry-Hopkins Cohort Studies. J Health Care Poor Underserved 1997;8:270–283.
47   Aronow WS, Ahn C, Kronzon I, Koenigsberg M: Congestive heart failure, coronary events, and atherothrombotic brain infarction in elderly Blacks and Whites with systemic hypertension and with and without echocardiographic and electrocardiographic evidence of left ventricular hypertrophy. Am J Cardiol 1991;67:295–299.

48   Gillum RF, Thomas J, Salam A, Thomas J: White blood cell count and hypertension. J Clin Epidemiol 1996;49:392–393.
49   Heyman A, Karp HR, Heyden S, Bartel A, Cassel JC, Tyroler HA, Cornoni J, Hames CG, Stuart W: Cerebrovascular disease in the bi-racial population of Evans County, Georgia. Stroke 1971;2: 509–518.
50   Gillum RF: Trends in acute rheumatic fever and chronic rheumatic heart disease – A national perspective. Am Heart J 1986;111:430–432.
51   Savage DD, Devereux RB, Donahue R: Mitral valve prolapse in Blacks. J Natl Med Assoc 1982; 74:895–900.
52   Savage DD, Garrison RJ, Castelli WP, McNamara PM, Anderson SJ, Kannel WB, Feinleib M: Prevalence of submitral (annular) calcium and its correlates in general population-based sample (The Framingham Study). Am J Cardiol 1983;51:1375–1378.
53   Lauzier S, Barnett HJM: Cerebral ischemia with mitral valve prolapse and mitral annulus calcifica-tion; in Furlan AJ (ed): The Heart and Stroke. Exploring Mutual Cerebrovascular and Cardiovas-cular Issues. London, Springer, 1987, pp 63–100.
54   Gillum RF: Nonrheumatic valvular heart disease in the United States. Am Heart J 1993;125: 915–918.
55   Roberts JK, Omarali I, Di Tullio MR, Sciacca RR, Sacco RL, Homma S: Valvular strands and cerebral ischemia: Effect of demographics and strand characteristics. Stroke 1997;28:2185–2188.
56   Gillum RF: Epidemiology of aortic aneurysm in the United States. J Clin Epidemiol 1995;48: 1289–1298.
57   Gillum RF: Sudden coronary death in the United States, 1980–1985. Circulation 1989;79:756–765.
58   Gillum RF: Sudden cardiac death in Hispanic-Americans and African Americans. Am J Public Health 1997;87:1461–1466.
59   Di Tullio MR, Sacco RL, Gersony D, Nayak H, Weslow RG, Kargman DE, Homma S: Aortic atheromas and acute ischemic stroke: A transesophageal echocardiographic study in an ethnically mixed population. Neurology 1996;46:1560–1566.
60   Sane D, Califf R, Topol E, Stumpf D, Mark D, Greenberg C: Bleeding during thrombolytic therapy for acute myocardial infarction: Mechanisms and management. Ann Intern Med 1989;11:1010–1022.
61   Gaines KJ, Chesney C, Zwaag RV, Cape C: Racial differences in coagulation studies in stroke. Neurol Res 1992;14:103–108.
62   Gillum RF, Gillum BS, Francis CK: Coronary revascularization and cardiac catheterization in the United States: Trends in racial differences. J Am Coll Cardiol 1997;29:1557–1562.
63   Gillum RF: Coronary artery bypass surgery and coronary angiography in the United States, 1979–1983. Am Heart J 1987;113:1255–1260.
64   Furlan AJ, Jones SC: Central nervous system complications related to open heart surgery; in Furlan AJ (ed): The Heart and Stroke. Exploring Mutual Cerebrovascular and Cardiovascular Issues. London, Springer, 1987, pp 287–304.
65   Di Tullio MR, Sacco RL, Sciacca R, Savoia MT, Nahar T, Boden-Albala B, Mendoza L, Thompson E, Homma S: Patent foramen ovale as a risk factor for ischemic stroke in a multiethnic population. Stroke 1998;29:277.
66   Joubert J: The MEDUNSA Stroke Data Bank. An analysis of 304 patients seen between 1986 and 1987. S Afr Med J 1991;80:567–570.
67   Matenga J, Kitai I, Levy L: Strokes among black people in Harare, Zimbabwe: Results of computed tomography and associated risk factors. Br Med J 1986;292:1649–1651.
68   Sempos CT, Bild DE, Manolio TA: Overview of the Jackson Heart Study: A study of cardiovascular diseases in African American men and women. Am J Med Sci 1998; in press.
69   Prystowsky EN, Benson DW Jr, Fuster V, Hart RG, Myerburg RJ, Naccarelli GV, Wyse DG: Management of patients with atrial fibrillation. A Statement for Health Care Professionals from the Subcommittee on Electrocardiography and Electrophysiology, American Heart Association. Circulation 1996;93:1262–1277.
70   Francis CK: Hypertension, cardiac disease, and compliance in minority patients. Am J Med 1991; 91:S29–S36.

71   National High Blood Pressure Education Program: The Sixth Report of the Joint National Commit-
     tee on Prevention, Detection, Evaluation, and Treatment of High Blood Pressure. National Institutes
     of Health, NIH Publ No 98-4080, Nov 1997.
72   Bonner LL, Kanter DS, Manson JE: Primary prevention of stroke. N Engl J Med 1995;333:
     1392–1400.
73   Pearson TA, Criqui MH, Luepker RV, Oberman A, Winston M: Primer in Preventive Cardiology.
     Dallas, American Heart Association, 1994.
74   Ryan TJ, Anderson JL, Antman EM, Braniff BA, Brooks MH, Califf RM, Hillis LD, Hiratzka
     LF, Rapaport E, Riegel BJ, Russel RO, Smith EE Jr, Weaver WD: ACC/AHA guidelines for the
     management of patients with acute myocardial infarction. A report of the American College of
     Cardiology/American Heart Association Task Force on Practice Guideline (Committee on Manage-
     ment of Acute Myocardial Infarction). J Am Coll Cardiol 1996;28:1328–1428.
75   Guidelines for the Evaluation and Management of Heart Failure. Report of the American College
     of Cardiology/American Heart Association Task Force on Practice Guideline (Committee on Evalu-
     ation and Management of Heart Failure). J Am Coll Cardiol 1995;26:1376–1398.
76   Gillum RF: Epidemiology of stroke in Hispanic Americans. Stroke 1995;26:1707–1712.

R.F. Gillum, MD, Office of Analysis, Epidemiology and Health Promotion,
Centers for Disease Control and Prevention, National Center for Health Statistics,
6525 Belcrest Road, Room 730, Hyattsville, MD 20782-2003 (USA)

Gillum RF, Gorelick PB, Cooper ES (eds): Stroke in Blacks. Basel, Karger, 1999, pp 142–155

··························

Improving Survival after Ischemic Stroke and Prevention of Recurrent Ischemic Stroke in African-Americans: Medical and Surgical Intervention

Gary H. Friday[a], *Edward S. Cooper*[b], *Harold L. Mignott*[b]

[a] Clinical Research, Astra USA, Inc., Westborough, Mass. and
[b] University of Pennsylvania School of Medicine, Philadelphia, Pa., USA

This chapter deals with the management of ischemic stroke and the prevention of recurrent stroke with an emphasis on special concerns for African-Americans. Since the management of intracranial hemorrhage and ischemic stroke is markedly different, it is important to differentiate between these two types of stroke [1]. The reader is directed to pp. 29–35 for a discussion of hemorrhagic stroke.

Acute and Subacute Treatment following Ischemic Stroke: Neurological Perspective

Emergency Evaluation and Neurological Complications
Emergency medical evaluation, neurological diagnosis and management, and prevention of neurological complications in ischemic stroke are covered in detail in a number of publications [1–6] and also are reviewed in standard texts on stroke [7]. For the patient who has suffered an acute stroke, rapid clinical evaluation and initiation of treatment measures are critical [2]. Such measures will reduce the likelihood of stroke-related morbidity and mortality. Table 1 lists the routine tests for emergency evaluation of stroke and table 2 lists common neurological complications of acute stroke. The medical complications of stroke are discussed on pp. 180–187. Echocardiography, transcranial Doppler, MRI, magnetic resonance angiography, cerebral angiography, tests for coagulopathy, dysproteinemia, sickle cell anemia, arteritis, bacterial

Table 1. Emergency tests for patients with acute ischemic stroke

CT of brain, noncontrast
ECG
CXR
Hematologic studies
   Complete blood count
   Platelet count
   Prothrombin time
   Partial thromboplastin time
Serum electrolytes
Blood urea nitrogen/creatinine
Liver function tests
Blood glucose
Lateral cervical spine (if head or cervical spine trauma is suspected)
EEG (if seizures are suspected)

Table 2. Neurological complications of acute ischemic stroke

Cerebral edema
Hydrocephalus
Increased intracranial pressure
Hemorrhagic transformation
Seizures

endocarditis, sepsis, AIDS, substance abuse and others are reserved for selected patients for whom an etiology is not detected after the initial workup.

There may be important racial differences in the distribution of occlusive vascular lesions in ischemic stroke. African-Americans may have more severe disease of the large intracranial arteries and a higher incidence of lacunar strokes [8]. This partially reflects a higher prevalence of diabetes mellitus and hypertension in African-Americans. Cerebral angiography [8] and transcranial Doppler are useful for detecting lesions of the intracranial vessels [9] and therefore may be more likely to be used in the evaluation of African-American patients. A detailed discussion of special techniques in assessing cerebrovascular disease in African-American patients is presented on pp. 36–61.

African-Americans with stroke have been found to have a higher prevalence of hypertension which was often untreated, with higher mean admission systolic and diastolic blood pressures and a higher frequency of LVH by ECG criteria. On the other hand, cardiac disease (atrial fibrillation, myocardial infarction, and angina) was found to be less prevalent in African-Americans [10]. Therefore, hypertension requires special consideration in the acute treatment of stroke in African-Americans. The management of medical complications, including hypertension and cardiac arrhythmias, is reviewed on pp. 180–187.

In a population study of hospitalized stroke in Northern Manhattan which included 235 African-Americans and 590 Whites, the overall in-hospital mortality rate was similar between the two groups [11]. This same result was also found in a community hospital-based study from North Carolina, Oregon and New York of 4,109 stroke patients of whom 628 were non-White ($>95\%$ African-American) [12]. However, in the Northern Manhattan study, the mortality rate in the younger stroke group (age 40–69) was higher in African-Americans (24.6 vs. 7.9%). This may have been due to more severe strokes and neurological complications or more severe associated medical morbidity in the younger African-Americans with stroke.

In a population study of ischemic stroke in Durham County, North Carolina (146 patients), 41 (28%) were African-American, and it was found that African-Americans had slower recovery of activities of daily living and physical function [13]. This could result in a higher risk of complications of stroke such as contractures, decubitus ulcer, stiff joints, pneumonia, deep vein thrombosis and pulmonary embolus. In that same study although the mortality rate was the same for both groups, deaths tended to occur earlier for African-Americans (6 of 7, vs. 10 of 20 deaths within 90 days) suggesting a different pattern and etiology for mortality; stroke is the leading cause of death in the acute phase (first week), with pulmonary embolism and pneumonia the leading causes in the subacute phase (up to 3 months) and cardiac disease after 3 months [14].

Antiplatelet Agents and Anticoagulants

Treatment with aspirin (within 48 h) has recently been shown to improve outcome modestly after an acute ischemic stroke [15]. This effect was partially due to a reduction of recurrent stroke. In this same study, low- or high-dose (5,000 or 12,500 IU bid) subcutaneous heparin, however, did not show an advantage for outcome at 6 months. A randomized study from Hong Kong of subcutaneous low-molecular-weight heparin initiated within 48 h of stroke onset showed a benefit at 6 months for death or dependency [16]. However, a positive result was not seen for the primary outcome of neurological recovery and performance of activities of daily living at 3 months in a clinical trial from the USA of intravenous low-molecular-weight heparinoid [17]. In that study, 290 (23%) of 1,275 patients were African-American. There was a favorable outcome in a secondary analysis of the subgroup of patients with large artery atherosclerosis (18% of total). In this study, patients with severe stroke (NIHSS score >15) were excluded due to increased risk of intracranial hemorrhage.

In patients with recent myocardial infarction complicated by cerebral embolism, anticoagulation reduces the incidence of recurrent embolism [18]. In these patients and those with atrial fibrillation and acute embolic stroke, it is generally recommended to wait 7–10 days before starting anticoagulant therapy for recurrent stroke prevention, as there is risk of conversion of a bland cerebral infarct to a hemorrhagic infarction or frank cerebral hemorrhage. If the stroke is mild, a shorter interval before introduction of anticoagulant therapy may suffice.

Low-dose subcutaneous heparin to prevent deep venous thrombosis is recommended in immobilized patients [5]. Typically, the dose should not exceed 5,000 IU bid. Further discussion of antiplatelet and anticoagulation treatment is presented on pp. 156–179.

Thrombolysis

In 1996 the US Food and Drug Administration (FDA) approved the use of recombinant tissue plasminogen activator (tPA) for the treatment of acute ischemic stroke. This approval was based on the results of a two-part study conducted by the National Institute of Neurological Disorders and Stroke (NINDS) [19]. A total of 624 patients was enrolled, of which approximately 30% were African-American. The high percentage of African-Americans was a result of the inclusion of study centers with large numbers of African-American patients. Outcome was based on the National Institutes of Health Stroke Scale (NIHSS, a measure of neurological deficit), the Barthel Index (a measure of activities of daily living), the Rankin Scale (a global measure of disability) and the Glasgow Outcome Scale (a handicap scale). Complete or near complete recovery was 11–13% more common with tPA than with placebo across all outcome measures. An important inclusion criterion for the study was treatment within 3 h of stroke onset. Patients with a high risk of bleeding were excluded as were patients with difficult to control and elevated blood pressure (>185 mm Hg systolic or >110 mm Hg diastolic on repeated measures).

Symptomatic intracerebral hemorrhage was a major thrombolytic treatment complication and occurred within 36 h of treatment in 6.4% of patients given tPA as compared with 0.6% of those given placebo. Deaths due to hemorrhage within 36 h of treatment occurred in 2.9 and 0.3% of tPA- and placebo-treated patients, respectively. However, the overall mortality rate at 3 months was not substantially different between the two groups (17% for tPA and 21% for placebo).

In a post hoc subgroup analysis, which included race as a study variable, a beneficial effect of tPA was noted [20]. This was a post hoc analysis, however, and the results may not be given the same importance as a predefined outcome measure.

In a study of 30 patients treated with tPA at a university and two community hospitals in Houston, Texas, 11 of 30 patients were African-American [21]. Patient outcomes were similar to those of the NINDS tPA study. Race was found to have no significant effect on outcome. In a European tPA study, the European Cooperative Acute Stroke Study (ECASS) [22], intention-to-treat analysis showed no significant benefit for tPA. A wider time window to treatment (6 h), a higher dose of tPA (1.1 vs. 0.9 mg/kg), less emphasis on blood pressure control, and inclusion of patients who already had early signs of infarction on the initial CT scan may have contributed to a less favorable result and higher rate of hemorrhagic complications [23]. This finding has led to the recommendation that tPA not be used within 3 h of stroke onset in patients who have evidence of extensive acute ischemic changes on the baseline CT scan [24].

Three trials using streptokinase were stopped prematurely as there was excessive mortality in the active treatment group. The possible reasons for the failure of this therapy were similar to those given for the ECASS study (i.e. too long a time window to inclusion, too high a dose of the thrombolytic, and lack of adequate control of blood pressure) [25].

Thrombolytic administration beyond 3 h of stroke onset is not recommended and patients who have elevated blood pressure (i.e. $>180/110$ mm Hg on repeated measures) that does not respond to treatment with antihypertensive medication (e.g. labetalol) should not receive thrombolysis. Blood pressure should be monitored carefully after tPA infusion. Guidelines for the use of tPA developed by the American Heart Association (AHA) [26] and the American Academy of Neurology [27] should be reviewed and followed [25]. Use of tPA in clinical practice has fueled a debate among stroke experts [28].

Use of thrombolytics would require presentation to the hospital within less than 3 h. This greatly reduces the number of patients who may be eligible from this treatment. In the NINDS study, only 3% of patients screened were eligible for treatment mainly due to late time of presentation. In a study of 67 patients who presented with stroke in 1995 at Indiana University Medical Center in Indianapolis, of whom 24 (36%) were African-American, race was not a factor in time to presentation [29]. In that study, arrival via ambulance and severity of stroke were found to predict early (i.e. <3 h) arrival, whereas knowledge of stroke warning signs did not predict early arrival. In the TOAST study [17] where treatment with a low-molecular-weight heparin was initiated within 24 h of ischemic stroke, White race was associated with a longer time from stroke onset to arrival at the hospital. These studies suggest that many African-American acute stroke patients could arrive at the hospital during a time frame whereby they would be eligible for treatment with tPA. African-Americans, however, have a higher prevalence of hypertension and more severe hypertension which could make them ineligible for tPA therapy.

Other therapies for stroke, such as carotid endarterectomy, have been underutilized in African-Americans. Although the reason is not clear, possible explanations include access to or financing of medical care, bias on the part of physicians in offering this option to the patient, or differences in patient willingness to undergo the procedure [30]. Also, it is possible that some health workers do not establish rapport as readily with minority patients, especially when there is no physician advocate to intercede on the behalf of the patient.

Intra-arterial thrombolysis has been performed in a small number of patients [31]. Many of the studies were carried out without a control group. In a placebo-controlled study of intra-arterial recombinant prourokinase (rpro-UK) in acute thrombotic/thromboembolic stroke, it was shown that the MCA could be recanalized with active treatment [32]. In this study, 40 patients were treated with rpro-UK (n = 26) or placebo (n = 14). Ten of the 40 (25%) patients were non-White. Hemorrhagic transformation with neurologic deterioration was seen in 15.4% of those treated with rpro-UK and 7.1% of the placebo-treated patients. The difference was not statistically significant. There was a trend, however, toward better neurologic and functional outcome in the rpro-UK-treated patients. More studies are needed before intra-arterial thrombolysis can be recommended for clinical use.

Increasing Collateral Circulation by Pharmacological Means

Vasodilating agents have been used to try to improve cerebral blood flow in ischemic areas. These include papaverine, hydergine, nicotinic acid and cyclandelate [33, 34]. None have proved effective. Various calcium channel blockers remain under study. CO_2 inhalation is no longer used for its cerebrovascular dilatory effect as there may be an accompanying rise in systemic arterial blood pressure that could be dangerous and also a possible 'steal' phenomenon, i.e. the shunting of blood away from the already maximally dilated vessels in infarcted zones [35].

Neuroprotective Agents

Neuroprotective agents have not yet been approved for the acute treatment of stroke. Agents shown to be effective in animal models of stroke include free radical scavengers, granulocyte inhibitors, glutamate antagonists and γ-aminobutyric (GABA) agonists [36]. A number of clinical trials to assess the safety and efficacy of these agents are ongoing or have been recently completed. Many of these studies have been conducted in the USA and have enrolled African-Americans. A study of the free radical scavenger tirilizad was conducted in North America, and involved 660 ischemic stroke patients of whom 146 (22%) were non-White. There was no evidence of an effect on functional outcome after 3 months of follow-up [37]. In a study of GM_1 ganglioside, an agent that is thought to act via protection against glutamate toxicity or through potentiation of growth factors, 287 patients were enrolled of whom about 18% were African-American [38]. An improvement in functional outcome was not demonstrated in that study. Lubeluzole, a neuroprotective agent believed to possibly act via inhibition of nitrous oxide production, was studied in 721 patients with ischemic stroke of whom 64 (9%) were African-American. In this study in a secondary analysis there was a favorable outcome in functional status in the lubeluzole treatment group compared to placebo treatment [39]. Although the FDA does not require that efficacy be proven in different race-ethnic groups such as African-Americans, it does encourage the reporting of results by subgroup. However, even though the percentage of African Americans in acute stroke studies in the USA is close to the proportional representation in the overall population, the numbers are still too small to be able to draw firm conclusions about efficacy of treatment. It is estimated that more than a hundred patients are needed to clearly demonstrate a benefit in stroke trials [40] and with neuroprotective agents even larger numbers may be necessary [41]. Perhaps the strategy used in the NINDS tPA study of including study centers with high numbers of African-American patients should be used in other stroke trials to increase the number of African-American patients.

Stroke Units

Stroke units are associated with improvement in outcome after stroke. For example, randomized clinical trials have shown that stroke units reduce mortality, institutionalization and dependency [42]. A meta-analysis of data from 19 randomized trials shows a reduction of death within a median follow-up of 1 year with an odds ratio of 0.83 (95% CI 0.69–0.98), combined outcome of death or dependency (odds ratio 0.69 (95% CI 0.59–0.82)) and death or institutionalization (odds ratio of 0.75 (95% CI 0.65–0.87)). The definition of a stroke unit in these 19 studies was variable and included acute care stroke units, rehabilitation stroke units to which patients were sent after acute care, and a combination of the latter two. Only 2 of the 19 randomized trials were conducted in the USA, one in Chicago, Ill. [43] and one in New York City, N.Y. [44]. Neither of these studies emphasized the race-ethnic mix of the patients. The latter two studies were published in the 1960s and compared rehabilitation units with regular medical care. A detailed discussion of stroke rehabilitation in African-American patients is on pp. 198–209. The AHA Stroke Council recommends early admission of stroke patients to a unit whose staff has specialized interest in the treatment of cerebrovascular disease [5]. Studies of the effect of stroke unit care in African-Americans are needed.

Prevention of Recurrent Stroke and Stroke after Transient Ischemic Attack (TIA)

Carotid Endarterectomy

Two randomized clinical trials, the North American Symptomatic Carotid Endarterectomy Trial (NASCET) [45] and the Veterans Administration Symptomatic Trial (VAST) [46] have shown the benefit of carotid endarterectomy in symptomatic patients with high-grade carotid stenosis when compared to medical management. The NASCET study enrolled 659 patients (3% African-American) with carotid artery stenosis and ipsilateral recent hemispheric or retinal TIA or nondisabling stroke. In patients with 70–99% stenosis, risk of stroke over 2 years was 26% in medically treated patients and 9% in surgical patients. The VAST study which included 193 men had similar results.

Carotid endarterectomy is recommended for surgical candidates with TIA and for patients with mild stroke within a 6-month interval with carotid stenosis of 70% or greater [47, 48]. A preliminary report from the NASCET study indicates a beneficial effect of carotid endarterectomy in symptomatic patients with 50–69% stenosis [49].

The Asymptomatic Carotid Atherosclerosis Study (ACAS) included 1,662 patients (3% African-American) with asymptomatic carotid artery stenosis [50]. In patients with 60% or more stenosis, there was an estimated 5-year risk of ipsilateral stroke and any perioperative stroke or death of 11.0% vs. 5.1% in medically treated patients and those receiving carotid endarterectomy, respectively.

The AHA guidelines for carotid endarterectomy set a surgical complication rate of less than 6% (i.e. combined death and/or stroke associated with the procedure) as a maximum acceptable risk in symptomatic patients [48] and less than 3% in asymptomatic patients [51]. In a retrospective analysis of surgical risk for endarterectomy at 12 academic medical centers which included 36 non-White patients out of a total of 697 patients, race was not associated with increased surgical risk [52]. However, a complication rate of 7.3% for death and stroke was reported in that study. In a study of carotid endarterectomy among Medicare beneficiaries in Georgia in 1993, an outcome of severe stroke or death within 30 days after operation occurred in 3.3% of 184 non-White patients, of whom half were classified as African-American, compared with 2.9% in 1,761 White patients [53]. In a study of carotid endarterectomy among Medicare beneficiaries in the USA from 1985 to 1996, the perioperative mortality rate ranged from 3.0% in 1985 to 1.3% in 1996. Although the perioperative mortality rate was 0.8% higher in African-Americans than Whites during this period, the rates converged over time with less of a difference in 1996 [54].

The small number of African-Americans in the NASCET and ACAS studies may relate to multiple factors. African-Americans may have a lower incidence of TIAs, which was one of the inclusion criteria for the NASCET study [55]. In addition, while African-Americans have been underrepresented in clinical trials [56], it is believed that they may less frequently harbor extracranial carotid disease [57]. However, other studies have not shown this [58]. Overall, African-Americans receive endarterectomy at a lower rate than Whites. In 1985 and 1986, 188,000 carotid endarterectomies were performed in the USA and only 2.7% of the patients were African-American [59]. In a study of carotid endarterectomy among Medicare beneficiaries in Georgia in 1993, it was found that only 4.8% of the patients were African-American while the racial distribution of all Medicare beneficiaries was approximately 22% African-American [53]. Additional explanations for this trend could include access to or financing of medical care, bias on the part of physicians in offering this option to the patient, or differences in patient willingness to undergo the procedure [30]. In a study of patient perceptions, among patients hospitalized with stroke or TIA, African-Americans expressed more aversion to carotid endarterectomy than Whites [60].

Percutaneous Transluminal Angioplasty (PCTA)

PCTA is a popular method for treatment of coronary and other arterial stenosis. The procedure usually involves the use of a balloon catheter that is placed within the lumen of the artery and then inflated. PCTA with or without stenting is being used to treat intra- and extracerebral arterial stenosis [61]. Complication rates are higher for intracranial angioplasty. Complications include thromboemboli, vessel rupture and restenosis. Stents are sometimes used to prevent emboli and restenosis. Currently, stents are not approved for use in the extracranial or intracranial cerebral vessels. PCTA is currently being compared with medical therapy in the Carotid and Vertebral Artery Transluminal Angioplasty Study, CAVATAS [62]. Since this is an international study, the percentage of African-Americans is not expected to be high. Although carotid angioplasty and stenting have become popular, many experts have recommended against the use of this procedure outside of well-controlled clinical trials [63].

Antiplatelet Agents and Anticoagulants

Aspirin offers protection from major vascular events after cerebral ischemia [64]. Other antiplatelet agents have also been shown to reduce risk. These include ticlopidine [65], dipyridamole [66] and clopidogrel [67] (see pp. 167–179).

Long-Term Prevention of Recurrent Stroke

Modifiable risk factors for primary prevention of stroke include hypertension, heart disease, diabetes, hyperlipidemia, carotid stenosis, cigarette smoking and alcohol abuse. A discussion of treatment of risk factors for initial stroke is presented on pp. 118–141. Further studies are needed to clarify the role of these factors in recurrent stroke; however, control of these risk factors is recommended for the prevention of recurrent stroke. In a population-based study of risk factors for recurrent stroke in a cohort of 323 with cerebral infarction of whom 40% were African-American, hypertension requiring discharge medication, elevated blood sugar within 48 h of stroke and ethanol abuse were independent predictors of recurrence [68]. No interactions by race were found indicating that these risk factors for recurrent stroke were applicable to African-Americans in the study. Studies from largely homogeneous White populations have given different results. In a study from Rochester, Minnesota [69], hypertension was not an independent risk factor for recurrent stroke. However, in the Framingham study [70] and the Lehigh Valley study [71] hypertension was a risk factor for recurrent stroke. Control of hypertension was found to reduce stroke recurrence in the Lehigh Valley study but not in the Rochester study. In a prospective randomized clinical trial in 452 patients with stroke or TIA and mild to moderate hypertension of whom 80% were African-American, no effect on stroke recurrence was seen in the treated compared to the placebo group [72]. However, in a analysis of the subgroup of patients without LVH on ECG, a reduction in the rate of recurrent stroke was seen. Diabetes has been found to be a risk factor for recurrent stroke in studies from predominately White populations [69]. Alcohol use has not been well studied as a risk factor for recurrent stroke, thus it is difficult to make any firm conclusions about this factor.

Conclusion

In the acute treatment of stroke, tPA has been shown to be effective in two clinical trials in the USA that included a substantial number of African-Americans and where a beneficial effect was demonstrated in a subgroup analysis. Careful selection of patients is required when contemplating administration of tPA to reduce the risk of intracerebral hemorrhage. Admission of the stroke patient to an acute stroke unit has been shown to improve outcome. This finding is based mainly on controlled studies carried out in Europe. There is probably a benefit yet little risk for management of African-Americans in acute care stroke units.

Carotid endarterectomy has been shown to be effective in symptomatic patients with stenosis $\geq 50\%$ as well as in asymptomatic patients with stenosis $> 60\%$. The risk of surgical complications currently does not appear to be much greater in African-Americans based on a small number of studies, yet African-Americans are less likely to receive this procedure.

Studies of risk factors suggest that control of hypertension may be helpful in reducing recurrent stroke in African-Americans. Observational epidemiologic studies suggest that glucose control may also reduce the risk of recurrent stroke. The paucity of information on treatment of stroke in African-Americans both from an acute perspective and in secondary prevention points to the need to include this group of patients in future stroke treatment research initiatives.

References

1   Caplan LR: What's wrong with Mr. Jones, a 58-year-old man with cerebrovascular disease? Heart Dis Stroke 1992;1:252–254.
2   Adams RJ: Management issues for patients with ischemic stroke. Neurology 1995;45(suppl 1):15–18.
3   Bentson JR: Present status of imaging of acute strokes. J Stroke Cerebrovasc Dis 1997;6:200–203.
4   Saver JL, Starkman S: State-of-the-art medical management of acute ischemic stroke. J Stroke Cerebrovasc Dis 1997;6:189–184.
5   Adams HP, Brott TG, Crowell RM, Furland AJ, Gomez CR, Grotta J, Helgason CM, Marler JR, Woolson RF, Zivin JA, Feinberg W, Mayberg M: Guidelines for the management of patients with acute ischemic stroke. A statement for health care professionals from a special writing group of the Stroke Council, American Heart Association. Stroke 1994;25:1901–1914.
6   Biller J, Patrick JT: Management of medical complications of stroke. J Stroke Cerebrovasc Dis 1997;6:217–220.
7   Caplan LR, Stein RW: Stroke: A Clinical Approach, Boston, Buttterworth, 1986.
8   Caplan LR, Cooper ES: Cerebrovascular disease in Blacks. J Natl Med Assoc 1987;79:33–36.
9   Petty GW, Wiebers DO, Meissner I: Transcranial Doppler ultrasonography: Clinical applications in cerebrovascular disease. Mayo Clin Proc 1990;65:1350–1364.
10 Sacco RL, Kargman DE, Zamanillo MC: Race-ethnic differences in stroke risk factors among hospitalized patients with cerebral infarction: The Northern Manhattan Stroke Study. Neurology 1995;45:659–663.
11 Sacco RL, Hauser WA, Mohr JP: Hospitalized stroke in Blacks and Hispanics in Northern Manhattan. Stroke 1991;22:1491–1496.
12 Becker C, Howard G, McLeroy KR, Yatsu FM, Toole JF, Coull B, Feibel J, Walker MD: Community hospital-based stroke programs: North Carolina, Oregon, and New York. II. Description of study population. Stroke 1986;17:285–293.
13 Horner RD, Matchar DB, Divine GW, Feussner JR: Racial variation in ischemic stroke-related physical and functional impairments. Stroke 1991;221:1497–1501.
14 Viitanen M, Winblad B, Asplund K: Autopsy verified causes of death after stroke. Acta Med Scand 1987;222:410–408.
15 International Stroke Trial Collaborative Group: International Stroke Trial (IST): A randomised trial of aspirin, subcutaneous heparin, both, or neither among 19,435 patients with acute ischaemic stroke. Lancet 1997;349:1569–1581.
16 Kay R, Wong KS, Yu YL, Chan YW, Tsoi TH, Ahuja AT, Chan FL, Fong KY, Law CB, Wong A: Low-molecular-weight heparin for the treatment of acute ischemic stroke. N Engl J Med 1995; 333:1588–1593.

17   The Publications Committee for the Trial of ORG 10172 in Acute Stroke Treatment (TOAST) Investigators: Low molecular weight heparinoid ORG 10172 (danaparoid), and the outcome after ischemic stroke. JAMA 1998;279:1265–1272.

18   Barnett HJM, Eliasziw M, Meldrum HE: Drugs and surgery in the prevention of ischemic stroke. N Engl J Med 1995;332:238–248.

19   National Institute of Neurological Disorders and Stroke rt-PA Stroke Study Group: Tissue plasminogen activator for acute ischemic stroke. N Engl J Med 1995;333:1581–1587.

20   National Institute of Neurological Disorders and Stroke t-PA Stroke Study Group: Generalized efficacy of t-PA for acute stroke: Subgroup analysis of the NINDS t-PA stroke trial. Stroke 1997; 28:2119–2125.

21   Chiu D, Krieger D, Villar-Cordova C, Kasner SE, Morgenstern LB, Bratina PL, Yatsu FM, Grotta JC: Intravenous tissue plasminogen activator for acute ischemic stroke: Feasibility, safety, and efficacy in the first year of clinical practice. Stroke 1998;29:18–22.

22   Hacke W, Kaste M, Fieschi C, Toni D, Lesaffre E, Von Kummer R, Boysen G, Bluhmki E, Hoxter G, Mahagne M-H, Hennerici M, for the ECASS Group: Safety and efficacy of intravenous thrombolysis with a recombinant tissue plasminogen activator in the treatment of acute hemispheric stroke. JAMA 1995;274:1017–1025.

23   Hacke W: rtPA in acute ischemic stroke: European perspective. Neurology 1997;49(suppl 4):60–62.

24   Grotta J: t-PA – The best current option for most patients. N Engl J Med 1997;337:1310–1313.

25   Lyden PD: Thrombolysis: Findings and lessons of the clinical trials. J Stroke Cerebrovasc Dis 1997; 6:195–197.

26   Adams HP, Brott TG, Furlan AJ, Gomez CR, Grotta J, Helgason CM, Kwiatkowski T, Lyden PD, Marler JR, Torner J, Feinberg W, Mayberg M, Thies W: Guidelines for thrombolytic therapy for acute ischemic stroke: A statement for health care professionals from a Special Writing Group of the Stroke Council, American Heart Association. Circulation 1996;94:1167–1174.

27   Report of the Quality Standards Subcommittee of the American Academy of Neurology: Thrombolytic therapy for acute ischemic stroke-summary statement. Neurology 1996;47:835–839.

28   Caplan LR, Mohr JP, Kistler JP, Koroshetz W: Thrombolysis – Not a panacea for ischemic stroke. N Engl J Med 1997; 337:1309–1310.

29   Williams LS, Bruno A, Rouch D, Marriott DJ: Stroke patients' knowledge of stroke; influence on time to presentation. Stroke 1997;28:912–915.

30   Horner RD, Oddone EZ, Matchar DB: Theories explaining racial differences in the utilization of diagnostic and therapeutic procedures for cerebrovascular disease. Milbank Q 1995;73:443–462.

31   del Zoppo GJ, Pessin MS, Mori E, Hacke W: Thrombolytic intervention in acute thrombotic and embolic stroke. Semin Neurol 1991;11:368–384.

32   del Zoppo GJ, Randall T, Higashida RT, Furlan AJ, Pessin MS, Rowley HA, Gent M, and the PROACT investigators: PROACT: A phase II randomized trial of recombinant pro-urokinase by direct arterial delivery in acute middle cerebral artery stroke. Stroke 1998;29:4–11.

33   Caplan LR: Use of vasodilating drugs for cerebral symptomatology; in Miller R, Greenblatt D (eds): Drug Therapy Reviews. Amsterdam, Elsevier-North Holland, 1979, pp 305–317.

34   McHenry LC, West JW, Kenton EJ, Oshiro T, Jaffe ME, Cooper ES, Kawamur J, Goldberg HI: Regional cerebral blood flow and cardiovascular effects of hexobendine in stroke patients. Neurology 1972;22:217–223.

35   Cooper ES, West JW: The relation between cardiac function and cerebral blood flow in stroke patients. 1. Effect of 5% CO_2 inhalation. Stroke 1970;1:330–347.

36   Lyden PD: Neuroprotection: Before and after thrombolysis. J Stroke Cerebrovasc Dis 1997;6:198–199.

37   The RANTTAS Investigators: A randomized trial of tirilizad mesylate in patients with acute stroke (RANTTASS). Stroke 1996;27:1453–1458.

38   The SASS Investigators: Ganglioside GM_1 in acute ischemic stroke: The SASS trial. Stroke 1994; 25:1141–1148.

39   Grotta J for the US and Canadian Lubeluzole Ischemic Stroke Study Group: Lubeluzole treatment in ischemic stroke. Stroke 1997;28:2338–2346.

40   Adams HP: Trials of trials in acute ischemic stroke. Stroke 1993;24:1410–1415.

41 Dorman PJ, Sandercock PAG: Considerations in the design of clinical trials of neuroprotective therapy in acute ischemic stroke. Stroke 1996;27:1507–1515.

42 Stroke Unit Trialists' Collaboration: Collaborative systemic review of the randomized trials of organised in-patient (stroke unit) care after stroke. BMJ 1997;314:1151–1159.

43 Gordon EE, Kohn KH: Evaluation of rehabilitation methods in the hemiplegic patient. J Chron Dis 1966;19:3–16.

44 Feldman DJ, Lee PR, Unterecker J, Lloyd K, Rusk HA, Toole A: A comparison of functionally oriented medical care and formal rehabilitation in the management of patients with hemiplegia due to cerebrovascular disease. J Chron Dis 1962;15:297–310.

45 North American Symptomatic Carotid Endarterectomy Trial Collaborators: Beneficial effect of carotid endarterectomy in symptomatic patients with high-grade carotid stenosis. N Engl J Med 1991;325:445–453.

46 Mayberg MR, Wilson SE, Yatsu F, Weiss DG, Messina L, Hershey LA, Colling C, Eskridge J, Deykin D, Winn HR, for the Veterans Affairs Cooperative Studies Program 309 Trialist Group: Carotid endarterectomy and prevention of cerebral ischemia in symptomatic carotid stenosis. JAMA 1991;266:3289–3294.

47 Feinberg WM, Alpers GW, Barnett HJ, Biller J, Caplan LR, Carter LP, Hart RG, Hobson RW, Kronmal RA, Moore WS, Robertson JT, Adams HP, Mayberg M: Guidelines for the management of transient ischemic attacks. Circulation 1994;89:2950–2965.

48 Moore WS, Barnett HJM, Beebe HG, Bernstein EF, Brener BJ, Brott T, Caplan LR, Day A, Goldstone J, Hobson RW, Kempczinski RF, Matchar DB, Mayberg MR, Nicolaides AN, Norris JW, Ricotta JJ, Robrtson JT, Rutherford RB, Thomas D, Toole JF, Trout HH, Wiebers DO: Guidelines for carotid endarterectomy: A multidisciplinary consensus statement from the Ad Hoc Committee, American Heart Association. Circulation 1995;91:566–579.

49 Barnett HMJ for the NASCET Collaborators: Final results of the North American Symptomatic Carotid Endarterectomy Trial (NASCET). Stroke 1998;29:286.

50 Executive Committee for the Asymptomatic Carotid Atherosclerosis Study: Endarterectomy for asymptomatic carotid artery stenosis. JAMA 1995;273:1421–1428.

51 Biller J, Feinberg WM, Castaldo JE, Whittemore AD, Harbaugh RE, Dempsey RJ, Caplan LR, Kresowik TF, Matchar DB, Toole JF, Easton JD, Adams HP, Brass LM, Hobson RW, Brott TG, Sternau L: Guidelines for carotid endarterectomy: A statement for healthcare professionals from a special writing group of the stroke council, American Heart Association. Stroke 1998;29: 554–562.

52 Goldstein LB, McCrory DC, Landsman PB, Samsa GP, Ancukiewicz M, Oddone EZ, Matchar DB: Multicenter review of preoperative risk factors for carotid endarterectomy in patients with ipsilateral symptoms. Stroke 1994;25:1116–1121.

53 Karp HR, Flanders WD, Shipp CC, Taylor B, Martin D: Carotid endarterectomy among Medicare beneficiaries: A statewide evaluation of appropriateness and outcome. Stroke 1998;29:46–52.

54 Hsia DC, Moscoe LM, Krushat WM: Epidemiology of carotid endarterectomy among Medicare beneficiaries; 1985–1996 update. Stroke 1998;29:346–350.

55 Friday G, Lai SM, Alter M, Sobel E, LaRue l, Gil-Peralta A, McCoy RL, Levitt LP, Isack T: Stroke in the Lehigh Valley: Racial/ethnic differences. Neurology 1989;39:1165–1168.

56 Harris Y, Gorelick PB, Samuels P, Bempong I: Why African-Americans may not be participating in clinical trials. J Natl Med Assoc 1996;88:630–634.

57 Wityk RJ, Lehman D, Klag M, J Coresh, Ahn H, Litt B: Race and sex differences in the distribution of cerebral atherosclerosis. Stroke 1996;27:1974–1980.

58 Sacco RL, Kargman DE, Gu Q, Zamanillo MC: Race-ethnicity and determinants of intracranial atherosclerotic cerebral infarction: The Northern Manhattan Stroke Study. Neurology 1995;26: 14–20.

59 Maxwell GJ, Rutherford EJ, Covington D, Clancy TV, Tackett AD, Robinson N, Johnson G: Infrequency of Blacks among patients having carotid endarterectomy. Stroke 1989;20:22–26.

60 Oddone EZ, Horner RD, Diers T, Lipscomb J, McIntyre L, Cauffman C, Whittle J, Passman LJ, Kroupa L, Heany R, Matchar D: Understanding racial variation in the use of carotid endarterectomy: The role of aversion to surgery. J Natl Med Assoc 1998;90:25–33.

61   Clark WM, Barnwell SL, Nesbit G, O'Neill OR, Wynn ML, Coull BM: Safety and efficacy of percutaneous transluminal angioplasty for intracranial atherosclerotic stenosis. Stroke 1995;26: 1200–1204.
62   Duckweiler G: Interventional neuroradiologic treatments for cerebrovascular ischemia. J Stroke Cerebrovas Dis 1997;6:204–209.
63   Bettmann MA, Katzen BT, Whisnant J, Brant-Zawadzki M, Broderick JP, Furlan AJ, Hershey LA, Howard V, Kuntz R, Loftus CM, Pearce W, Roberts A, Roubin G: Carotid stenting and angioplasty: A statement for the healthcare professionals from the Councils on Cardiovascular Radiology, Stroke, Cardio-Thoracic and Vascular Surgery, Epidemiology and Prevention, and Clinical Cardiology, American Heart Association. Stroke 1998;29:336–348.
64   Antiplatelet Trialists' Collaboration: Collaborative overview of randomized trials of antiplatelet therapy in various categories of patients. BMJ 1994;308:81–106.
65   Gent M, Blakely JA, Easton JD, Hachinski VC, Panak E, Sicurella J, Blakely JA, Ellis DJ, Harbison JW, Roberts RS, Turpie AGG, and the CATS Group: The Canadian-American Ticlopidine Study (CATS) in thromboembolic stroke. Lancet 1989;i:1215–1220.
66   Deiner HC: New trials with antiplatelet drugs. Acute Stroke Manage 1997;4:12–14.
67   Caprie Steering Committee: A randomised, blinded, trial of clopidogrel versus aspirin in patients at risk of ischemic events (CAPRIE). Lancet 1996;348:1329–1239.
68   Sacco RL, Shi T, Zamanillo MC, Kargman DE: Predictors of mortality and recurrence after hospitalized cerebral infarction in an urban community: The Northern Manhattan Stroke Study. Neurology 1994;44:626–634.
69   Petty GW, Brown RD, Whisnant JP, Sicks JD, O'Fallon WM, Wiebers DO: Survival and recurrence after first cerebral infarction: A population-based study in Rochester, Minnesota, 1975–1989. Neurology 1998;50:208–216.
70   Sacco RL, Wolf PA, Kannel WB, McNamara PL: Survival and recurrence following stroke: The Framingham Study. Stroke 1982;13:290–295.
71   Alter M, Friday G, Lai SM, O'Connell J, Sobel E: Hypertension and risk of stroke recurrence. Stroke 1994;25:1605–1610.
72   Hypertension-Stroke Cooperative Study Group: Effect of antihypertensive treatment on stroke recurrence. JAMA 1974;229:409–418.

Gary H. Friday, MD, Astra USA, Inc.,
50 Otis Street, Westborough, MA 01581 (USA)

Gillum RF, Gorelick PB, Cooper ES (eds): Stroke in Blacks. Basel, Karger, 1999, pp 156–166

Rapid Identification and Treatment of Stroke in African-Americans

John R. Marler

Division of Stroke, Trauma and Neurodegenerative Disorders,
National Institute of Neurological Disorders and Stroke,
National Institutes of Health, Bethesda, Md., USA

Stroke is the sudden onset of a focal neurological deficit. The onset can occur quite rapidly and is frequently associated with a dramatic change in motor or cognitive function. The causes of stroke vary. Eighty percent of strokes are said to be caused by ischemia due to the occlusion of a brain artery by a blood clot. The other 20% of strokes are caused by brain hemorrhage, either intracerebral or subarachnoid. Whether there are significant differences in the incidence of these major stroke types for African-Americans has not been clearly established [1]. There are no proven treatments for acute intracerebral hemorrhage. There are generally accepted acute treatments for subarachnoid hemorrhage when they are caused by ruptured intracranial aneurysm. Until recently there was no proven effective treatment for acute ischemic stroke. The publication in 1995 of the results of the NINDS TPA Stroke Study which consisted of two sequential clinical trials showed that thrombolytic therapy with intravenous recombinant tissue type plasminogen activator was an effective treatment for ischemic stroke [2]. In these trials, thrombolytic therapy was administered to all patients very early within 3 h of ischemic stroke onset and in one half of the patients within 90 min of stroke onset. For this reason there is now renewed interest in rapid and acute treatment for stroke because of the potential utility of thrombolytic therapy in 80% of stroke patients. This chapter will discuss acute stroke treatment in general and, where applicable, point out specific areas that are relevant to the treatment of African-Americans.

Availability of tissue plasminogen activator for the acute treatment of ischemic stroke requires rapid identification and treatment in order to achieve maximum efficacy. Undeniably, prevention of stroke is preferable as a therapeutic goal. However, there will always be failure and the significant, serious consequences of untreated stroke warrant the extra effort required to appropriately identify ischemic stroke patients and to provide rapid treatment. In the process many strokes caused by intracerebral and subarachnoid hemorrhage will be identified early and receive appropriate care sooner, with possible improved outcome and better diagnostic accuracy. This chapter will summarize the benefits of rapid identification and treatment of patients with ischemic stroke. It will describe in general the goals of successful programs that provide rapid identification and treatment and point the way to specific methods that have been successful in the past.

Perspectives of Tissue Plasminogen Activator

Recombinant tissue-type plasminogen activator has been approved by the FDA for treatment of stroke since June of 1996. The approval was based on the two clinical trials which were published in one paper in December 1995 [2]. Both of these trials confirmed that there was a significant 12% absolute increase in the number of patients who had recovery that was either complete or left a minimal disability at 3 months. Secondary analysis of the results of these trials showed that there was not only an effect at 3 months but that there also was a major benefit even apparent in the first 24 h after treatment [3]. In addition, the survival curve of the patients showed that tissue plasminogen activator was not associated with increased mortality. When different prospectively defined risk factors for stroke were analyzed, none was found predictive of a better response to therapy [4]. This included any racial differences. Subsequent secondary analyses have also demonstrated that when considering posthospitalization cost of rehabilitation in nursing home care, the drug provided a significant cost savings [5].

The reported risk of tissue plasminogen activator in the treatment of acute ischemic stroke is primarily intracranial hemorrhage. In both trials of the NINDS TPA Stroke Study, intracranial hemorrhage occurred in approximately 6% of the patients compared to less than 1% in the placebo group. While there can be no doubt that treatment with thrombolytic therapy is associated with this increase in hemorrhage, the reader should keep in mind that there were many unreported adverse effects of the placebo treatment. For example, death by transtentorial herniation due to infarction in ischemic injury was not reported in the same manner because it was not directly caused by or could be directly attributed to tissue plasminogen activator. The fact that there was no difference in survival and there were more deaths in the placebo group in both trials, indicates that when considering the risk of tissue plasminogen activator in the treatment of acute ischemic stroke, the treating physician should not overlook the adverse effects of failing to use the treatments, such as cerebral edema. The overall risk to any group of stroke patients that are treated is the major concern. While intracranial hemorrhage is an extremely serious complication, the benefits of the treatment are immediately clear when examined in light of the overall outcome at 3 months. Recent reports have confirmed that the actual (community) use of tissue plasminogen activator in the treatment of acute stroke, as approved by the FDA, is similar to the experience demonstrated in the clinical trials [6].

There is a difference between predicting outcome from stroke based on the patient characteristics at baseline and predicting response to therapy based on the same characteristics of the patient at baseline. This concept is particularly important when considering the relative risk and benefit for a group of patients with a particular set of baseline characteristics. African-Americans are more likely to have a fatal outcome from stroke than White Americans [1]. This is true for both Black men and Black women and may indicate more frequent presentation with more severe deficits predictive of the poor outcome. However, this poorer outcome does not indicate that Black patients are less likely to have an improvement in outcome as a result of treatment with thrombolytic therapy. One surprising result of the NINDS TPA Stroke Trial was that patients who at baseline were categorized as having small-vessel occlusive disease showed a greater response to therapy than other stroke subtypes. This greater response to therapy was evident even though the outcome for patients with small-vessel occlusive disease was much better in the placebo group as well. Specifically, in both trials at 3 months, approximately 50% of the placebo-treated patients categorized at baseline as having strokes due to small-vessel occlusion had a Barthel Index with favorable outcome. This was a higher percent of favorable outcome than any of the treated groups in the large-vessel and cardioembolic stroke subtype category (see table 1).

Furthermore, the patients with small-vessel occlusive disease that were treated with total plasminogen activator had a 75% rate of favorable outcome, a much higher rate than seen in the treated group with large-vessel occlusive and cardioembolic disease. Since stroke subtype closely correlated with the severity of stroke at baseline, this says that stroke severity predicts outcome. However, the point being made here is that it does not predict the ability of the patient to respond to therapy and show an even better outcome than would be predicted from the baseline severity of the stroke. For this reason, it would be erroneous to conclude that because evidence suggests that the outcome from stroke in Blacks is worse than in Whites, one can predict that the response to therapy would be worse in Blacks than in Whites.

Table 1. Outcome at 3 months according to the classification of the stroke subtype at baseline [2]

Treatment group stroke subtype[1]	Total plasminogen activator		Placebo	
	patients n	% with favorable outcome[2]	patients n	% with favorable outcome[2]
Small-vessel occlusive	51		30	
Barthel Index		75		50
Modified Rankin Scale		63		40
Glasgow Outcome Scale		63		43
NIH Stroke Scale		47		33
Large-vessel occlusive	117		135	
Barthel Index		49		36
Modified Rankin Scale		40		22
Glasgow Outcome Scale		45		28
NIH Stroke Scale		33		18
Cardioembolic	136		137	
Barthel Index		46		37
Modified Rankin Scale		38		28
Glasgow Outcome Scale		39		31
NIH Stroke Scale		29		20

[1] Eighteen patients (2.9%) with other stroke subtypes were excluded from the analysis.
[2] Scores of 95 or 100 on the Barthel Index, <1 on the NIHSS and modified Rankin Scale, and 1 on the Glasgow Outcome Scale were considered to indicate a favorable outcome.

Thrombolytic therapy has been used most extensively in the treatment of myocardial infarction. Taylor et al. [7] have reported on the role of race and ethnicity in survival after myocardial infarction using data from the TIMI-II Phase 2 Trial. This trial randomized patients to receive one of two invasive procedures following treatment with tissue plasminogen activator within 4 h of onset of chest pain. Of the 2,885 patients, 174 were Black, the remainder were either White or Hispanic. The reported mortality in Black patients at 1 year after myocardial infarction was somewhat greater than in other groups. However, this difference was not as prominent when other baseline characteristics including age, sex, smoking, history of heart disease, hypertension, or diabetes were accounted for. The adjusted relative risk of dying at 1 year for Black patients compared with White patients was estimated at 1.1 with a 99%

confidence interval ranging from 0.6 to 2.2. The adjusted risk for reinfarction and the combined endpoints of death, reinfarction or readmission were similar for Whites and Blacks. An interesting observation was that Black myocardial infarction patients had higher baseline fibrinogen levels than White or Hispanic patients. When they were treated with tissue plasminogen activator, Black patients also demonstrated a greater reduction of the fibrinogen levels in response to treatment when compared to other patients in the TIMI-II Trial. This increase in thrombolytic activity was not accompanied by an increase in bleeding complications. The authors offered several possible explanations for the success of the TIMI-II protocol in producing equally good results in Black and White patients which included (1) selection of patients with a good prognosis; (2) equal efficacy of thrombolytic therapy of Black patients, and (3) ready access to intensive care. Patients with elevated blood pressure or a history of uncontrolled hypertension were excluded from the trial. This means that any patient with a systolic pressure > 180 mm Hg or a diastolic presure > 110 mm Hg were not included in the trial. This may have excluded a higher percentage of Black patients than White or Hispanic because of the prevalence of uncontrolled hypertension and high blood pressure in Black patients. There is a suggestion that thrombolytic therapy may have slightly different pharmacological effects in Black patients which may have helped explain the fact that no differences were found in the patency rate at 18–48 h after recombinant total plasminogen activator infusion in what otherwise would be considered a higher risk group for reocclusion or resistance to thrombolysis. The author reports that numerous studies have shown significant barriers to early intervention among African-Americans. Because of the design of the TIMI-II Trial, all patients who were enrolled received equally aggressive and complete treatment. This may be a partial explanation of the equivalent outcome observed in Black and White patients. In addition, by selecting patients treated within 4 h of symptom onset, the trial may have selected for patients who presented promptly and had already demonstrated equal access to state-of-the-art care. The removal of access barriers could be attributed to similarity of the 1-year mortality figures for all racial and ethnic groups in the TIMI-II study. It should be noted though that the number of African-Americans enrolled in this trial, 174, was 9% of the entire study population. For example, the NINDS TPA Stroke Trial, which included a total of 624 patients in the study, randomized approximately the same number of Black patients as did the TIMI-II study with 2,885 patients.

In the Gusto 1 Trial, 40,903 patients were randomized to one of four thrombolytic and anticoagulant treatment regimens [8]. 1,155 (2%) of the 40,930 patients had African ancestry. Of these, 197, or 17%, had moderate or severe hemorrhagic bleeding complications and 12 of the patients had severe bleeding complications. While the rate of moderate or severe bleeding complication was significantly higher in those patients with African ancestry, the rate of severe bleeding complication alone was approximately equal to the complication rate reported for the study population as a whole. The conclusion of Berkowitz et al. [8] was that there is a higher likelihood of bleeding in patients of African descent when treated with thrombolytic therapy. The authors speculate that this may be related to the higher thrombolytic activity previously reported in the TIMI-II Trial. Berkowitz et al. do not discuss relative benefit from the treatment so it could not be concluded that thrombolytic therapy is not beneficial for African-Americans simply because of a higher complication rate for moderate bleeding events.

In the NINDS TPA Stroke Trial, although race was considered a potential predictor of hemorrhagic complications and a potential predictor of outcome and response to therapy, race was not an evident cofactor in either response to therapy or in hemorrhagic complications [4, 9]. The NINDS TPA Stroke Trial had 170 patients out of a total of 624 patients (or 30%). While the overall trial is not as large as either the TIMT-II Trial or the Gusto 1 experience, there were approximately as many patients in the NINDS Stroke Trial as in the larger TIMI-II study for myocardial infarction. Therefore, the failure of race to appear as a predictor of either response to therapy or hemorrhagic complication in the NINDS trials suggests that Black Americans are as likely to benefit from treatment with thrombolytic therapy for stroke as do White Americans.

Early Treatment of Stroke: What Needs to Be in Place

The two NINDS trials published in December 1995 were the sole basis for approval of the use of total plasminogen activator for the treatment of acute ischemic stroke in the USA. Other trials using total plasminogen activator or streptokinase for thrombolytic treatment have not shown a positive benefit. While explanations for this failure to show a positive effect in other trials for thrombolytic therapy include considerations of the dose and the particular thrombolytic agent used, the primary difference is probably the time from the onset of symptoms to the initiation of treatment with the thrombolytic agent. Over half the patients in the NINDS TPA Stroke Trials began treatment within 90 min of the onset of symptoms and all patients in the trials began treatment within 180 min. Therefore, when the FDA approved total plasminogen activator for use in the treatment of stroke, its use was limited to the time period of 0–180 min after the clearly established onset of symptoms. This very early treatment time is a difficult challenge for the medical system but it is certainly not impossible. The TIMI-II Trial of myocardial infarction randomized over 2,000 patients in 18 months within 4 h of onset of symptoms. While 3 h is certainly a shorter time period than this, and even shorter times from onset of symptoms to treatment would be desirable, it certainly has been demonstrated that it is possible to treat a large number of patients within this time frame.

The methods required to encourage and promote the rapid diagnosis and treatment of acute ischemic stroke depends greatly on the resources available in each community. In general, when careful records and interviewing of all potential patients are initiated in the emergency room, it often turns out that there are more patients who present within 60–90 min of the onset of their symptoms than are generally known to the physicians who normally are called to treat acute stroke. The first place to begin developing a treatment effort to intervene in the course of acute stroke is in the identification of patients who already present to the emergency room (i.e., without efforts at public education). The second step is to prepare and educate a team within the hospital to respond when stroke patients do arrive early enough to be eligible for treatment with thrombolytic therapy. The third step that is logical in most situations is the education of the emergency medical transport system that received 911 calls and must move stroke patients as rapidly as possible to the appropriate emergency department where they can be treated by an established stroke team.

As the emergency medical system is developed, then efforts may begin to make the public more aware of stroke symptoms and the importance of calling 911 when a stroke is suspected. Even after all of the elements are in place (including the training of emergency department staff and developing a team or responders for acute ischemic stroke, education and training of the emergency medical system, and informing the public), there will still be many patients who arrive at the emergency department too late for treatment with thrombolytic therapy. At this point the system needs to be re-evaluated from the first point of contact with a patient all the way through to the initiation of thrombolytic therapy within the emergency department. Walk-through exercises, in which the patient arrival at an emergency department is simulated and any possible delays or bottlenecks in emergency department procedures are identified and corrected, will shorten the time from arrival at the emergency department to initiation of thrombolytic therapy, a commonly underestimated cause of delay in the treatment of acute ischemic stroke [10]. In centers with less experience in using thrombolytic therapy, the tendency to delay treatment to the last possible minute should be avoided at all cost since the likelihood is that there will be fewer patients with a beneficial response and the possibility of serious hemorrhagic complications may begin to outweigh the potential benefit of the therapy. Caution and hesitancy that causes unnecessary delay may actually do more harm to the patient in this situation.

Education of the public is a critical element of any effort to increase the number of patients who may be eligible for treatment with thrombolytic therapy or to increase the speed of diagnosis and treatment of acute stroke. Regardless of the type of stroke, it is important for patients to get to the emergency room quickly so that rapid diagnosis can determine which potential treatment and diagnostic path is required to maximize the opportunity for recovery. The public has a great deal to gain, both for their own benefit should they have a stroke, and for others should they see a stroke occur in another person. The education of the public requires the cooperation of many different organizations and skilled professionals who have an understanding of communication with the public.

Education of special subsets of the population such as African-Americans will have to be tailored to the communities in which they live. Most successful educational efforts will be headed by those who have experience with public education in general, rather than specific stroke expertise. Stroke experts often serve as resources in the content of messages for the public, but the actual delivery of the messages is often improved if public information specialists are involved in the process. In addition, especially in African-American communities, there may be different pathways for informing the public and certainly different organizations that may be more effective in these special communities.

The first efforts to develop public education and the systems needed to treat stroke rapidly should probably be directed at looking at the resources available in the community and the organizations which might have contact with patients at risk of stroke. One very useful piece of information is that more information is now included in the American Heart Association courses for cardiopulmonary resuscitation and the BLS and the ALS – the basic life support and the advanced life support courses – which are offered to emergency medical specialists [11–13]. Several national organizations such as the American Heart Association and the National Stroke Association have developed resource materials for different populations including African-Americans. In addition, other public information materials are listed on the Brain Attack Coalition Web Site [14].

The organization that recruits patients will be most successful if it has continuity and delivers a common message through different media and at different points of contact through organizations and the media. The medical professionals, involved in developing acute stroke treatment, plan to realize that in general the history of the treatment of myocardial infarction and the development of special centers for the treatment of acute trauma have demonstrated that efforts are more successful if one particular medical specialty does attempt to maintain control of each and every patient's diagnosis and treatment. Multidisciplinary teams that can be rapidly mobilized and with diverse skills are required for the complex process of treating acute stroke rapidly. In one hospital a neurologist may not be available immediately but can be called in as a consultant after 20–30 min while the rest of the process for the acute work-up of the stroke patient goes on. In academic hospitals, neurology fellows with special interest in stroke or neurology residents or internal medicine residents may be available at all times to participate in the treatment of acute stroke.

While informing the public about the availability of acute stroke treatment and providing information on the actions to take when a stroke occurs does require a great deal of modification to suit the situation in each local community, there are national efforts underway to provide the materials and to provide a background for local community efforts. To that end, the Brain Attack Coalition is a national organization that seeks to provide an opportunity for the communication between all of the different patient advocacy and medical specialty organizations that are interested in improving the speed with which stroke is diagnosed and treated. Members of the Brain Attack Coalition include the National Stroke Association, the American Heart Association, the American Academy of Neurology, the Stroke Belt Consortium, the American Association of Neurological Surgeons, the American College of Emergency Physicians, the American Association of Neuroscience Nurses, the American Society of Neuroradiology, and the National Institute of Neurological Disorders and Stroke. This organization is working for a national message to define the symptoms of stroke so that there can be consistency between the publications of all of its different members. The Brain Attack Coalition is also seeking to maintain an acute stroke toolbox for health care professionals developing systems to enable the rapid diagnosis and treatment of acute stroke. This is an Internet resource that is currently available [14]. In addition, at the regular meetings of the Brain Attack Coalition, each of the member organizations discusses the plans that they have for efforts at professional public education. While no organization devoted solely to African-Americans is part of the steering group of the Brain Attack Coalition, each of the organizations within it does seek to provide special materials and develop plans for improving communication about stroke with the African-American public.

Whatever the cause of acute stroke, it is important for the individual who has a stroke to receive as rapid as possible diagnosis and treatment. To date there is no evidence to suggest that the African-American patient would not have as much to benefit from acute stroke treatment as others. In addition, improving access to acute stroke care will provide increased quality of life and hopefully improve overall access to care for African-American patients.

In December of 1996 a major national symposium was held which developed a plan for improving the speed of diagnosis and treatment of acute stroke. This national symposium included the participation of over 50 different national organizations devoted to the rapid delivery of medical care and the treatment of stroke. From this national symposium a series of recommendations were developed [15]. In brief, the recommendations were that response systems, including optimum time frames, must be established, maintained and monitored in all emergency departments. The goals should be to: (a) perform an initial patient evaluation within 10 min of arrival in the emergency department; (b) notify the stroke team within 15 min of arrival; (c) initiate a CT scan within 25 min of arrival; (d) interpret the CT scan within 45 min of arrival; (e) insure door-to-drug or door-to-needle time of 60 min from arrival for those patients eligible to receive thrombolytic therapy, and (f) transfer the patient to an inpatient setting within 3 h of arrival.

For most stroke patients regardless of the cause of their stroke, it will not be until the CT scan is done and read at approximately 45 min after they arrive at a hospital emergency department before the cause of their stroke will be determined. In the meantime, the time from onset to the estimated time of treatment can be determined. If the stroke is not hemorrhagic and eligibility criteria for treatment have been met, then thrombolytic therapy can be given. If the patient is not eligible for thrombolytic therapy, then depending on the type of stroke and the condition of the patient, other supportive care is given.

The symposium recommendations included the concept of a chain of recovery beginning with the identification, either by the patient or an onlooker, of a possible stroke in progress and ending with a rehabilitation plan to be established in every community of the country. It was also the recommendation of the symposium that new educational initiatives must be developed and implemented for all medical personnel in the chain of recovery, including 911 dispatchers, EMS technicians, and air medical transport personnel. This will require the creation of task forces to develop model educational initiatives and standardized data sets to help insure effective research and outcome analysis.

It is important to realize that although there is treatment available for acute stroke patients, the number of these treatments will likely increase as more patients arrive early in emergency rooms and can be available to participate in clinical trials to develop new treatments. Hopefully, African-Americans will realize that as a group they are at higher risk of having a stroke and will willingly participate in clinical research aimed at the development of new therapies to reduce the serious disability that so often results from stroke.

References

1   Gillum RF: Stroke in Blacks. Stroke 1988;19:1-9.
2   The National Institute of Neurological Disorders and Stroke rt-PA Stroke Study Group. Tissue plasminogen activator for acute ischemic stroke. N Engl J Med 1995;333:1581–1587.
3   Haley ED Jr, Lewandowski C, Tilley BC, NINDS rt-PA Stroke Study Group: Myths regarding the NINDS rt-PA stroke trial: Setting the record straight. Ann Emerg Med 1997;30:676–682.
4   The National Institute of Neurological Disorders and Stroke rt-PA Stroke Study Group. Generalized efficacy of t-PA for acute stroke: Subgroup analysis of the NINDS t-PA stroke trial. Stroke 1997; 28:2119–2125.
5   Fogan SC, Morgenstern LB, Petitta A, Ward RE, Tilley BC, Marler JR, Levine SR, Broderick JP, Kwiatkowski TG, Frankel M, Brott TG, Walker MD: Cost-effectiveness of tissue plasminogen activator for acute ischemic stroke. NINDS rt-PA Stroke Study Group. Neurology 1998;50:883–890.
6   Chiu D, Krieger D, Villar-Cordova C, Kasner SE, Morgenstern LB, Bratina PL, Yatsu FM, Grotta JC: Intravenous tissue plasminogen activator for acute ischemic stroke: Feasibility, safety, and efficacy in the first year of clinical practice. Stroke 1998;29:18–22.
7   Taylor HA, Chaitman BR, Rogers WJ, Kern MJ, Terrin ML, Aguirre FV, Sopko G, McMahon R, Ross RN, Bovill EC: Race and prognosis after myocardial infarction. Results of the thrombolysis in myocardial infarction (TIMI) phase II trial. Circulation 1993;88:1484–1494.
8   Berkowitz SD, Granger CB, Pieper KS, Lee KL, Gore JM, Simoons M, Armstrong PW, Topol EJ, Califf RM: Incidence and predictors of bleeding after contemporary thrombolytic therapy for myocardial infarction. The Global Utilization of Streptokinase and Tissue Plasminogen Activator for Occluded Coronary Arteries (GUSTO) I Investigators. Circulation 1997;95:2508–2516.
9   The NINDS t-PA Stroke Study Group: Intracerebral hemorrhage after intravenous t-PA therapy for ischemic stroke. Stroke 1997;28:2109–2118.
10 Tilley BC, Lyden PD, Brott TG, Lu M, Levine SR, Welch KM: Total quality improvement method for reduction of delays between emergency department admission and treatment of acute ischemic stroke. The National Institute of Neurological Disorders and Stroke rt-PA Stroke Study Group. Arch Neurol 1997;54:1466–1474.
11 Cummins RO: Advanced Cardiac Life Support. Dallas, American Heart Association, 1997.
12 Chandra NC, Hazinski MF: Basic Life Support for Healthcare Providers. Dallas, American Heart Association, 1997.
13 Basic Life Support Heartsaver Guide: A Student Handbook for Cardiopulmonary Resuscitation and First Aid for Choking. Dallas, American Heart Association, 1993/1997.
14 Brain Attack Coalition: Acute Stroke Toolbox. URL = www.stroke-site.org
15 Marler JR, Jones PW, Emr M: Proceedings of a National Symposium on Rapid Identification and Treatment of Acute Stroke. Bethesda, The National Institute of Neurological Disorders and Stroke, 1997.

John R. Marler, MD, Division of Stroke, Trauma and Neurodegenerative Disorders,
National Institute of Neurological Disorders and Stroke, National Institutes of Health,
Federal Building, Room 8A-08, 7550 Wisconsin Avenue, Bethesda, MD 20817 (USA)

Gillum RF, Gorelick PB, Cooper ES (eds): Stroke in Blacks. Basel, Karger, 1999, pp 167–179

....

Antiplatelet and Anticoagulant Therapy in Stroke Prevention in African-Americans

Michael J. Schneck[a], *Seemant Chaturvedi*[b], *Daryl Thompson*[c], *Philip B. Gorelick*[a]

[a] Center for Stroke Research, Rush University, Chicago, Ill.,
[b] Department of Neurology, Wayne State University, Detroit, Mich.,
[c] Souers Stroke Institute, St. Louis University, St. Louis, Mo., USA

The use of antiplatelet agents and warfarin are important for stroke prevention [1–3]. This is especially true for recurrent stroke prevention in patients with transient ischemic attack (TIA) or ischemic stroke. The choice of drug depends on a number of considerations. The primary issue relates to the stroke mechanism. However, there are other contributory factors. These include adverse drug effects, patient compliance, access to follow-up care, and drug costs. At least in regard to cost, aspirin has the clear advantage. African-Americans have been underrepresented in clinical trials and there is limited data about stroke prevention in this group. The following sections describe the general use of aspirin, other antiplatelet agents, and warfarin in stroke prophylaxis with inclusion of available data on their use in African-Americans.

Aspirin

Aspirin's active ingredient is synthesized from a compound whose uses can be traced back 2,000 years. The compound, salicin, is a glycoside which is converted to salicylic acid in the body and is found naturally in the white willow tree whose bark could be chewed to relieve pain and fever. In the 1800s, European chemists extracted salicin from the willow and, in 1897, Felix

Hoffmann, in search of a pain-relieving medication for his father's rheumatism, discovered acetylsalicylic acid as a stable form of salicin.

Aspirin's mechanism of action remained a mystery until 1971 when John Vane (who won a Nobel Prize for this research) discovered that the anti-inflammatory properties of aspirin result from inhibition of prostaglandin synthesis [4–6]. Aspirin's antiaggregation effects on platelets occur by blockade of cyclooxygenase activity which reduces synthesis of thromboxane A_2. Aspirin induces a long-lasting functional defect in platelets, clinically detectable as prolongation of bleeding times. This appears to be primarily related to the permanent inactivation by aspirin of prostaglandin G/H synthase. Type 1 of this synthase is selectively acetylated by aspirin at a single serine residue causing the irreversible loss of cyclooxygenase activity. The result is decreased conversion of arachidonate to prostaglandin G_2 and ultimately of prostaglandin H_2 and thromboxane A_2, which are synthesized from prostaglandin G_2. The second isoenzyme of prostaglandin G/H synthase, which shares about 62% of its amino acids with the type 1 enzyme, is expressed only after cell activation in response to growth factors and mediators of inflammation.

The clinical pharmacology of platelet cyclooxygenase inhibition has been investigated through measurements of serum thromboxane B_2 and urinary metabolites. Single doses of 5–100 mg of aspirin result in dose-dependent inhibition of platelet cyclooxygenase activity, with 100 mg almost completely suppressing biosynthesis of thromboxane A_2 in both normal subjects and patients with atherosclerotic vascular disease. This effect is rapid and unrelated to aspirin's bioavailability. Because platelets lack the metabolic machinery necessary to synthesize new protein, defects induced by aspirin cannot be repaired during the 8- to 10-day platelet life-span. Therefore, when aspirin is discontinued, cyclooxygenase activity recovers slowly, as a function of platelet turnover. This explains the apparent paradox of a drug with a 20-min half-life having antiplatelet efficacy when administered once daily.

While the anti-inflammatory uses of aspirin inspired its initial popularity, it is aspirin's role in the prevention of vascular disease that has become of prime importance. Today, aspirin is regarded as one of the safest, most important and cost-effective therapies in the fight against cardiovascular disease. In the United States alone, estimates are that up to 10,000 additional lives could be saved annually by broader use of aspirin in persons at risk of heart attack and stroke. If aspirin were routinely used after a TIA or minor stroke, thousands of the nations 500,000 annual strokes could be prevented.

Aspirin therapy confers benefits in the acute phase of myocardial infarction (MI) and should be administered routinely to virtually all patients with evolving MI as was demonstrated in the Second International Study of Infarct

Survival (ISIS-2) [4, 7, 8]. Despite clear benefits in this setting, aspirin as a treatment for acute MI remains underused. In two recent studies, close to one third of persons, following an acute MI did not receive aspirin [4, 9, 10].

The 1994 Antiplatelet Trialists' Collaboration (ATC) meta-analysis of more than 54,000 high-risk patients with prior evidence of vascular disease showed that aspirin reduced the risk of subsequent vascular events (nonfatal MI, nonfatal stroke, vascular death) by approximately 25% [7]. These trials included patients with prior MI, stroke, TIA, unstable angina, revascularization surgery, angioplasty, atrial fibrillation (AF), valvular disease, and peripheral vascular disease. This benefit was significant for middle-aged patients, older patients, men, women, hypertensives, normotensives, diabetics, or nondiabetic patients. In absolute terms, this benefit translated to a decrease of 40 events per 1,000 patients with prior MI, stroke, or TIAs treated for 2–3 years. The specific impact of antiplatelet therapy on African-American stroke patients was not determined. However, in the Atherosclerosis Risk in Communities (ARIC) Study, aspirin use was more prevalent in Whites than in Blacks (30 vs. 11%) [11]. In Whites, there was greater aspirin use among men than women, but there was no difference in aspirin use between the sexes for African-Americans.

The most common regimen in secondary stroke prevention trials was 'medium-dose' aspirin (75–325 mg/day), and in the ATC analyses there was no evidence that either higher doses of aspirin or any other antiplatelet regimen was more effective than daily aspirin in this dose range [7]. In stroke and TIA trials, higher doses (650–1,300 mg/day) have been used, and in trials of post-MI patients, lower doses (75–325 mg/day) appeared equally beneficial in reducing stroke risks. Dyken et al. [13] and others [12, 14] have suggested that higher doses are better for stroke prevention but this remains controversial.

Persons on daily aspirin therapy have an increased risk of gastrointestinal complications. The variables that influence the overall incidence of gastrointestinal side effects during chronic aspirin therapy may include the dose and interval, treatment duration, the type of formulation (plain vs. enteric-coated), and the method of ascertainment of outcomes [4, 7, 12–14]. Therefore, it is not surprising that results of different studies vary widely. Among trials in which the daily dose of aspirin was 900–1,300 mg, the incidence of stomach pain, heartburn, and nausea was 40–60% higher among patients who received aspirin than placebo (24–44 vs. 15–32%) [4, 12, 14]. The incidence of upper gastrointestinal symptoms in patients with cerebrovascular disease who were treated with 300 mg of aspirin daily for an average follow-up of 4 years was lower than in previous trials (31% in those given aspirin and 26% in those given placebo). The proportion of strokes attributed to hemorrhagic causes was higher in primary-prevention studies of aspirin than in those involving high-risk patients. Given the relatively small number of hemorrhagic events (0.3% incidence), comparisons among different aspirin regimens is limited. However, a dose-response effect for extracranial hemorrhagic events has been found in placebo-controlled aspirin trials (the United Kingdom trial which compared the efficacy of 300 mg of aspirin with that of 1,200 mg, and the Dutch trial which compared the efficacy of 30 mg of aspirin with that of 283 mg) [4, 7, 13, 15–17]. Doses lower than 100 mg daily may be associated with bleeding complications, however [4].

Ticlopidine

Ticlopidine hydrochloride is a thienopyridine derivative which, in ex vivo studies, inhibits platelet aggregation in response to ADP, thrombin, collagen, serotonin, arachidonic acid, epinephrine and platelet-activating factor [18, 19]. Ticlopidine appears to act at the final common pathway for the ADP-induced modification of the GPIIb/IIIa glycoprotein platelet membrane receptor to form the fibrinogen binding site in platelet activation. The relative inhibitory effects of ticlopidine may decrease with higher plasma fibrinogen levels [20]. Ticlopidine has been referred to as a broad-spectrum inhibitor as it acts by several interdependent pathways and its effect on platelet function is irreversible.

Ticlopidine is metabolized in the liver and approximately 60% of an oral dose is excreted in the urine. Oral absorption is greater than 80%, and administration after meals results in a 20% increase in the AUC. In healthy volunteers over age 50, substantial ADP-induced platelet inhibition is detected within 4 days and maximum inhibition is achieved after 8–11 days. After discontinuation of ticlopidine, bleeding time and platelet function tests usually return to normal within 2 weeks. The recommended dose is 250 mg twice daily but in some patients, who are experiencing side effects, a dose of 250 mg once daily may be tried. Diarrhea (20.4%), dyspepsia (12.6%), rash (11.9%) and nausea (11.1%) are the most common side effects, as reported in the Ticlopidine Aspirin Stroke Study (TASS) [21]. The most serious adverse event is severe neutropenia ($<450/mm^3$) which occurs in about 0.9% of ticlopidine users. Neutropenia generally occurs in the first 3 months of treatment and typically reverses with discontinuation of ticlopidine. Complete CBCs are required every 2 weeks in the first 3 months of ticlopidine administration to monitor for neutropenia and thrombocytopenia; blood counts should then be obtained annually, thereafter. When compared to aspirin, there are less upper gastrointestinal side effects with ticlopidine. African-Americans may be less likely to develop side effects.

Ticlopidine has not been extensively studied in the primary prevention of cardiovascular diseases. In patients with peripheral artery disease, ticlopidine shows promise of reducing major cardiovascular disease endpoints such as MI and death [22]. Similarly, ticlopidine shows promise of reducing vascular complications in patients with unstable angina [23]. Ticlopidine has been most recently used in conjunction with coronary stents to reduce the incidence of cardiac events and vascular complications [24], and to improve long-term patency of grafts [25].

As an agent for prevention of recurrent events, ticlopidine was approved in the United States to reduce the risk of thrombotic stroke (fatal or nonfatal) in patients with stroke precursors (TIA) or completed stroke. The Canadian American Ticlopidine Study (CATS), a randomized, double-blind, placebo-controlled trial of ticlopidine 250 mg twice daily versus placebo in patients with completed stroke (n = 1,072), showed a 23.3% (p = 0.020) relative risk reduction in intention-to-treat analysis in favor of ticlopidine for the primary outcome endpoint cluster of stroke, MI or vascular death during a 24-month mean follow-up period [26]. TASS, a randomized, blinded, multicenter comparison of ticlopidine (500 mg daily) versus aspirin (1,300 mg daily) in patients with TIA or minor stroke (n = 3,069), showed a 12% risk reduction (p = 0.048) for the primary outcome cluster of nonfatal stroke or death from any cause over 3 years [21]. Subsequent posthoc analyses of the TASS data suggest certain patient subgroups might benefit from ticlopidine over aspirin. These subgroups include non-Whites, women, those with vertebrobasilar symptoms or symptoms while on aspirin or anticoagulant therapy, and patients with diffuse atherosclerotic disease rather than high-grade carotid stenosis [27, 28]. These post hoc findings should be viewed with caution unless confirmed by studies with appropriately powered statistical analyses [27, 28].

The African-American Antiplatelet Stroke Prevention Study (AAASPS) is a randomized, double-blind, National Institutes of Health sponsored trial to compare ticlopidine (500 mg daily) versus aspirin (650 mg daily) in African-Americans with mild or moderate noncardioembolic ischemic stroke. It is the first study targeted exclusively for stroke prevention in African-Americans. The window of entry is 90 days, and the primary outcome endpoint cluster is recurrent stroke, MI or vascular death [29]. Ticlopidine was chosen as an intervention for AAASPS because analyses of non-Whites in the TASS suggested that this agent might be substantially more effective than aspirin and have a better safety profile for non-Whites [27]. It is believed that non-White patients may have more cardiovascular risk factors and more severe occlusive cerebrovascular disease and thus may have greater benefit in terms of stroke risk reduction with a broader spectrum antiplatelet agent. The AAASPS is being conducted at over 40 sites throughout the United States. As of April

23, 1998, approximately 745 patients had been recruited with a goal of 1,800 patients.

Until generic forms of ticlopidine are available, it is likely that such therapy will be more expensive than aspirin, especially when the mandatory CBCs are considered. Ticlopidine is estimated to be cost-effective for secondary stroke prevention in high-risk patients but may not be cost-effective in those with less severe cardiovascular risk profiles [30]. African-Americans are at high risk for stroke and may be ideal candidates for this agent.

Clopidogrel

Clopidogrel is a new thienopyridine agent that is related to ticlopidine and blocks platelet activation by a similar mechanism [31]. Clopidogrel has been recently approved for stroke prevention by the Federal Drug Administration. A dose of 75 mg is thought to be equivalent to 250 mg of ticlopidine twice daily. In the Clopidogrel versus Aspirin in Patients at Risk of Ischemic Events (CAPRIE) study, 19,185 patients with recent ischemic stroke, MI or symptomatic peripheral arterial disease were randomized to receive either clopidogrel (75 mg daily) or uncoated aspirin (325 mg daily). Patients were followed for a mean of 1.9 years. The primary outcome cluster of ischemic stroke, MI or vascular death showed a relative risk reduction of 8.7% in favor of clopidogrel. The safety profile of clopidogrel was at least as good as aspirin. Diarrhea (0.23%), rash (0.26%) and neutropenia (0.10%) occurred infrequently.

Clopidogrel is slightly more effective than aspirin in reducing atherosclerotic events in patients with recent histories of stroke, MI or peripheral vascular disease and is safer than ticlopidine. Whether it is more effective than ticlopidine has not been determined. Of note, the dose of aspirin used in the CAPRIE trial (325 mg) was lower than in the TASS trial (1,300 mg). Whether clopidogrel's efficacy over aspirin would have been lessened if compared with higher aspirin doses is unknown. Furthermore, the CAPRIE study was not powered statistically to conclusively assess outcome events in the over 6,300 ischemic stroke patients who entered the study. Thus, it remains uncertain, for the subgroup of patients with stroke, if clopidogrel significantly reduces pertinent outcome events.

Dipyridamole

Dipyridamole is an antiplatelet agent that acts by direct stimulation of prostacyclin synthesis, potentiation of prostacyclin-induced platelet inhibition, increased platelet cyclic AMP levels and blockade of adenosine uptake. However, at therapeutic doses, dipyridamole does not block in vitro platelet aggregation or increase in vivo bleeding times [32]. Dipyridamole's efficacy in stroke prevention (in African-Americans or all stroke patients) is controversial. Prior studies failed to demonstrate that aspirin and dipyridamole were better than aspirin alone in the seconday prevention of stroke or TIA [33, 34]. A recent European trial comparing aspirin 25 mg twice daily, a high-dose modified-release form of dipyridamole (200 mg bid), and the combination of these two agents, in comparison with placebo, reported that aspirin and dipyridamole were equally effective (13 and 15% reduction of stroke or death, respectively) but combination therapy had a risk reduction of 24% [35]. It should be noted that the doses of aspirin were lower and the dose of dipyridamole was higher than is typically used in North America. Also, the dipyridamole preparation differed as it was a sustained-release form. In addition, the combination therapy results of ESPS2 were not dramatically different from results seen previously with aspirin therapy in other trials [7, 35].

Warfarin

Warfarin is the most widely used oral anticoagulant for stroke prevention. Warfarin acts via inhibition of vitamin-K-dependent clotting factors II, VII, IX and X. The pharmacology of warfarin is complex and is reviewed elsewhere [36]. The most salient pharmacological properties include: a delay in onset of anticoagulation after the initial oral warfarin doses as there is a time lag until all clotting factors are depleted; a propensity for drug interactions with other agents hepatically metabolized; an effect of patients' dietary vitamin K intake on anticoagulation effect, and the variability in patient response to warfarin requiring careful dose titration to achieve stable anticoagulation (narrow therapeutic index). Warfarin monitoring has been facilitated by development of the International Normalized Ratio (INR), which has reduced some of the variability in interlaboratory measurements of the prothrombin time. The recommended INR while on warfarin therapy is typically between 2.0 and 3.0, though a higher INR may be indicated in some circumstances.

The utility of warfarin for stroke prevention in African-Americans depends on the particular stroke subtype. Specific data about warfarin in African-Americans is limited. However, certain stroke subtypes have been presumed to be more common in African-Americans [1, 3, 37, 38]. Large-vessel atherosclerotic disease is typified by carotid and vertebrobasilar occlusive disease. For extracranial carotid stenosis, antiplatelet therapy is usually prescribed unless there is high-grade stenosis for which a patient may be a candidate for carotid endarterectomy. Some authors have suggested that low-intensity anticoagulation would be superior to aspirin in patients with carotid artery narrowing [39]. This hypothesis has never been tested by a randomized clinical trial. In the ongoing Warfarin Aspirin Recurrent Stroke Study (WARSS), patients with a variety of stroke subtypes are being randomly assigned to either low-intensity warfarin (INR 1.4–2.8) or aspirin 325 mg daily [40]. WARSS has recruited over 2,000 patients and approximately 30% of the study participants are African-American [R. Sacco, pers. commun.]. Included in WARSS are individuals with extracranial carotid stenosis. Therefore, it is possible that WARSS may demonstrate whether patients with extracranial carotid disease are better protected by warfarin or aspirin. At present, however, antiplatelet therapy is preferred.

Currently, patients with vertebrobasilar strokes may represent a large-vessel stroke subtype treated with anticoagulants. The use of warfarin for these patients is largely based on early studies which have not been replicated by modern clinical trials [41]. Thus, posterior circulation large-vessel atherosclerosis is another unsettled area for antithrombotic management. In terms of intracranial large-vessel stenosis, it has been estimated that 6–29% of cerebral ischemic events in African-Americans are due to intracranial vascular disease [37, 38]. The Warfarin Aspirin Stroke in Intracranial Disease (WASID) study was a retrospective, nonrandomized review of a multi-institutional cohort of patients with intracranial stenosis in either the carotid or vertebrobasilar system [42]. The overall rate of recurrent ischemic events was lower in the warfarin-treated group compared to patients who received aspirin. Specifically, the stroke rate was 10.4/100 patient-years for patients receiving aspirin and 3.6/100 patient-years for patients prescribed warfarin. This study included approximately 30% African-Americans. This data is intriguing and the WASID group is planning to carry out a prospective randomized trial comparing warfarin and aspirin to confirm this observation.

Cardioembolic ischemic stroke is the subtype for which warfarin has traditionally been most often used. One of the leading conditions which predisposes the patient to cardioembolism is nonvalvular atrial fibrillation (NVAF). NVAF is likely to represent an increasingly common cause of stroke in coming decades as the population ages since the prevalence of NVAF increases with age with an estimated prevalence of 5% in individuals over age 70 [43]. Several studies have shown that warfarin is very effective for primary and secondary prevention of stroke in patients with NVAF. The percentage of African-American patients in many of these studies was small, however. For example, it was approximately 4% in the Stroke Prevention in Atrial Fibrillation (SPAF) study [A. Leonard, pers. commun.]. There are no clear differences in the prevalence of NVAF among African-Americans and other groups in the United States and there is no reason to believe that warfarin would be less effective in African-Americans. In aggregate, the AF studies showed a 68% risk reduction in the incidence of ischemic stroke with warfarin therapy [44]. Therefore, unless there are specific contraindications, warfarin is the agent of choice for long-term stroke prevention in those patients with AF and a TIA or stroke or those AF patients without a history of stroke but with cardiovascular disease risk factors.

Due to a high prevalence of hypertension and diabetes mellitus, African-Americans are believed to have an elevated risk of small-vessel occlusive disease, predisposing to so-called lacunar infarction. In some studies, small-vessel strokes accounted for approximately 30% of cerebrovascular ischemic events in African-American patients [37]. The optimal antithrombotic strategy for patients with small-vessel disease is uncertain. The WARSS trial includes patients with lacunar infarction due to presumed small-vessel disease. At its conclusion, this study will provide additional information as to the role of warfarin and aspirin in patients with this stroke subtype. At present, risk factor modification and antiplatelet agents are conventionally recommended for lacunar stroke patients.

Despite the advances in diagnostic technologies, the etiology of many ischemic strokes remain undetermined or 'cryptogenic'. Ideal agents for stroke prevention in these patients are unknown. 42–54% of patients with cryptogenic stroke will have 'minor' sources of cardioembolism such as a patent foramen ovale (PFO) [45, 46]. Medical and surgical options are available for the patient with a PFO-related stroke. The medical agent of choice is unresolved but is currently being investigated. In an analysis of recurrent strokes in the SPAF study, it was found that warfarin was slightly more effective than aspirin in the prevention of cryptogenic stroke [47].

The major potential complication of warfarin therapy is bleeding. In clinical trials of AF, the rate of major hemorrhage with warfarin was 2% per year and the incidence of intracranial hemorrhage was also low at 1%. Warfarin must be monitored judiciously and patients must be selected carefully for treatment. Relative contraindications include a history of dementia, alcoholism, unsteady gait, and previous intracranial hemorrhage. The fact that warfarin use may be associated with serious complications is shown in a recent clinical trial for stroke prevention in Europe which was halted prematurely due to high rates of hemorrhagic events in the warfarin-treated group [48]. This may have been due to the target level of anticoagulation (INR 3.0–4.5).

Combination Therapies

Dose-adjusted warfarin combined with aspirin has not been studied in either AF studies or in secondary stroke prevention. The Coumadin Aspirin Reinfarction Study (CARS) and the Stroke Prevention in Atrial Fibrillation III (SPAF-III) trial failed to show any advantage for fixed-dose warfarin and aspirin as combination therapies [49, 50]. The CARS trial compared 160 mg aspirin monotherapy with 80 mg of aspirin and 1 or 3 mg of warfarin in MI patients for endpoints of stroke, MI, or vascular death and found no added benefit for combination therapy [49]. The SPAF-III compared a similar fixed-dose regimen in AF patients with dose-adjusted warfarin monotherapy [50]. Patients on the latter regimen had better outcomes. There is, however, data to support the use of combination therapy using low-dose aspirin and dose-adjusted warfarin for vascular prophylaxis in patients with prosthetic valves or unstable angina [51].

Ticlopidine and aspirin may potentiate each other when used in combination [52]. Both agents have an antithrombotic effect through different mechanisms. Data in support of combination therapy derives from coronary stenting trials [24, 52, 53]. This approach has also been adopted in stenting for extracranial carotid stenosis [54, 55]. Whether this combination is beneficial in secondary stroke prevention is unclear. Its use is limited by fears of increased bleeding complications and it is typically reserved for patients with atherothrombotic stroke (small or large vessel) who have otherwise failed monotherapy.

Conclusion

Clinical information about stroke risk profiles and stroke subtypes helps us to choose the appropriate antithrombotic agent for stroke prevention. Antiplatelet agents are used for lacunar infarcts, cryptogenic stroke and nonsurgical large-vessel disease in African-Americans. Anticoagulation with warfarin is used in patients with cardioembolism and possibly intracranial stenosis.

References

1   Gaines K, Burke G: Ethnic differences in stroke: Black-White differences in the United States population. SECORDS investigators. Southeastern Consortium on Racial Differences in Stroke. Neuroepidemiology 1995;14:209–239.
2   Modan B, Wagener DK: Some epidemiological aspects of stroke: Mortality/morbidity trends, age, sex, race, socioeconomic status. Stroke 1992;23:1230–1236.
3   Gorelick PB, Harris Y: Stroke among African-Americans. Chicago Med 1993;96:28–30.

4   Patrono C: Aspirin as an antiplatelet drug. N Engl J Med 1994;330:1287–1294.

5   Roth GJ, Calverley DC: Aspirin, platelets and thrombosis: Theory and practice. Blood 1994;83: 885–898.

6   Patrono C, Ciabattoni G, Patrignani P, Pugliese F, Filabozzi P, Catella F, Davi G, Forni L: Clinical pharmacology of platelet cyclooxygenase inhibition. Circulation 1985;72:1177–1184.

7   Antiplatelet Trialists' Collaboration: Collaborative overview of randomized trials of antiplatelet therapy. I. Prevention of death, myocardial infarction, and stroke by prolonged antiplatelet therapy in various categories of patients. BMJ 1994;308:81–106.

8   The Steering Committee of the Physicians' Health Study Research Group: Final report on the aspirin component of the ongoing Physicians' Health Study. N Engl J Med 1989;321:129–135.

9   McLaughlin TJ, Soumerai SB, Willison DJ, Gurwitz JH, Borbas C, Guadagnoli E, McLaughlin B, Morris N, Cheng SC, Hauptman PJ, Antman E, Casey L, Asinger R, Gobel F: Adherence to national guidelines for drug treatment of suspected acute myocardial infarction: Evidence for undertreatment in women and the elderly. Arch Intern Med 1996;156:799–805.

10   Sakethou BB, Conte FJ, Noris M, Tilkemeier P, Miller G, Forman DE, Cannistra L, Leavitt J, Sharma SC, Garber C, Parisi AF: Emergency department use of aspirin in patients with possible acute myocardial infarction. Ann Intern Med 1997;127:126–129.

11   Shahar E, Folsom AR, Romm FJ, Bisgard KM, Metcalf PA, Crum L, McGovern PG, Hutchinson RG, Heiss G: Patterns of aspirin use in middle-aged adults: The Atherosclerosis Risk in Communities (ARIC) Study. Am Heart J 1996;131:915–922.

12   Patrono C, Roth CJ: Aspirin in ischemic cerebrovascular disease: How strong is the case for a different dosing regimen? Stroke 1996;27:756–760.

13   Dyken ML, Barnett HJM, Easton JD, Fields WS, Fuster V, Hachinski V, Norris JW, Sherman DG: Low-dose aspirin and stroke: 'It ain't necessarily so.' Stroke 1992;23:1395–1399.

14   Hennerici MG: Aspirin dosage: A never-ending story? Cerebrovasc Dis 1995;5:308–309.

15   UK-TIA Study Group: The United Kingdom Transient Ischemic Attack (UK-TIA) aspirin trial: Final results. J Neurol Neurosurg Psychiatry 1991;54:1044–1054.

16   SALT Collaborative Group: Swedish Aspirin Low-Dose Trial (SALT) of 75 mg aspirin as secondary prophylaxis after cerebrovascular ischemic events. Lancet 1991;338:1345–1349.

17   Dutch TIA Trial Study Group: A comparison of two doses of aspirin (30 mg vs 283 mg a day) in patients after a transient ischemic attack or minor ischemic stroke. N Engl J Med 1991;325: 1261–1266.

18   Teitelbaum P: Pharmacodynamics and pharmacokinetics of ticlopidine; in Hass WK, Easton JD (eds): Ticlopidine, Platelets and Vascular Disease. New York, Springer, 1993, pp 27–40.

19   Murray JC, Kelly MA, Gorelick PB: Ticlopidine: A new antiplatelet agent for the secondary prevention of stroke. Clin Neuropharmacol 1994;17:23–31.

20   Toghi H, Takahashi H, Kashiwaya M, Watanabe K: Effect of the plasma fibrinogen concentration on the inhibition of platelet aggregation after ticlopidine compared with aspirin. Stroke 1994;25: 2017–2021.

21   Hass WK, Easton JD, Adams HP Jr, Pryse-Phillips W, Molony BA, Anderson S, Kamm B: A randomized trial comparing ticlopidine hydrochloride with aspirin for the prevention of stroke in high-risk patients. N Engl J Med 1989;321:501–507.

22   Janzon L: Clinical trials of ticlopidine in patients with intermittent claudication; in Hass WK, Easton JD (eds): Ticlopidine, Platelets and Vascular Disease. New York, Springer, 1993, pp 75–84.

23   Balsano F, Violi F: Clinical trials of ticlopidine in patients with coronary artery disease; in Hass WK, Easton JD (eds): Ticlopidine, Plataelets and Vascular Disease. New York, Springer, 1993, pp 85–98.

24   Schomig A, Neumann F-J, Kastrati A, Schuhlen H, Blasini R, Hadamitzky M, Walter H, Zitzmann-Roth EM, Richardt G, Alt E, Schmitt C, Ulm K: A randomized comparison of antiplatelet and anticoagulant therapy after the placement of coronary-artery stents. N Engl J Med 1996;334: 1084–1089.

25   Becquemin J-P for the Etude de la Ticlopidine après Pontage Fémoro-Poplité and the Association Universitaire de Recherche en Chirurgie: Effect of ticlopidine on the long-term patency of saphenous-view bypass grafts in the legs. N Engl J Med 1997;337:1726–1731.

26   Gent M, Easton JD, Hachinski VC, Harbison JW, Panak E, Roberts RS, Sicurella J, Turpie AG: The Canadian-American Ticlopidine Study (CATS) in thromboembolic stroke. Lancet 1989; i:1215–1220.

27   Weisberg LA for the Ticlopidine Aspirin Stroke Study Group: The efficacy and safety of ticlopidine and aspirin in non-Whites: Analysis of a patient subgroup from the Ticlopidine Aspirin Stroke Study. Neurology 1993;43:27–31.

28   Grotta JC, Norris JW, Kamm B and the TASS Baseline and Angiographic Data Subgroup: Prevention of stroke with ticlopidine: Who benefits most? Neurology 1992;42:111–115.

29   Gorelick PB and the AAASPS Investigators: African-American Antiplatelet Stroke Prevention Study (AAASPS). Stroke 1997;28:234(abstr 11).

30   Oster G, Huse DM, Lacey MJ, Epstein AM: Cost-effectiveness of ticlopidine in preventing stroke in high-risk patients. Stroke 1994;25:1149–1156.

31   CAPRIE Steering Committee: A randomized, blinded, trial of clopidogrel versus aspirin in patients at risk of ischemic events (CAPRIE). Lancet 1996;348:1329–1339.

32   Schafer AI: Antiplatelet therapy. Am J Med 1996;101:199–209.

33   Bousser MG, Eschwege E, Haguenau M: 'AICLA' controlled trial of aspirin and dipyridamole in the secondary prevention of athero-thrombotic cerebral ischemia. Stroke 1983;14:5–14.

34   American-Canadian Cooperative Study Group: Persantine-aspirin trial in cerebral ischemia. II. Endpoint results. Stroke 1985;16:406–415.

35   Diener HC, Cunha L, Forbes C, Sivenius J, Smets P, Lowenthal A: European Stroke Prevention Study 2. Dipyridamole and acetylsalicylic acid in the secondary prevention of stroke. J Neurol Sci 1996;143:1–13.

36   Hirsh J, Dalen JE, Deykin D, Poller L, Bussey H: Oral anticoagulants. Chest 1995;108:231S–246S.

37   Sacco RL, Kargman DE, Gu Q, Zamanillo MC: Race-ethnicity and determinants of intracranial atherosclerotic cerebral infarction. The Northern Manhattan Stroke Study. Stroke 1995;26:14–20.

38   Weisberg LA: Clinical characteristics of transient ischemic attacks in Black patients. Neurology 1991;41:1410–1414.

39   Kistler JP, Buonanno FS, Gress DR: Carotid endarterectomy-specific therapy based on pathophysiology. N Engl J Med 1991;325:505–507.

40   The WARSS, APASS, PICSS, HAS, and GENESIS Study Groups: The feasibility of a collaborative double-blind study using an anticoagulant. Cerebrovasc Dis 1997;7:100–112.

41   Whisnant JP, Cartilidge NE, Elveback LR: Carotid and vertebral-basilar transient ischemic attacks: Effects of anticoagulants, hypertension, and cardiac disorders on survival and stroke occurrence. A population study. Ann Neurol 1978;3:107–115.

42   Chimowitz MI, Kokkinos J, Strong J, Brown MB, Levine SR, Silliman S, Pessin MS, Weichel E, Sila CA, Furlan AJ, Kargman DE, Sacco RL, Wityk RJ, Ford G, Fayad PB for the Warfarin-Aspirin Symptomatic Intracranial Disease Study Group: The Warfarin-Aspirin Symptomatic Intracranial Disease Study. Neurology 1995;45:1488–1493.

43   Koefoed BG, Gullov AL, Petersen P: Prevention of thromboembolic events in atrial fibrillation. Thromb Haemost 1997;78:377–381.

44   Atrial Fibrillation Investigators: Risk factors for stroke and efficacy of antithrombotic therapy in atrial fibrillation. Analysis of pooled data from five randomized controlled trials. Arch Intern Med 1994;154:1449–1457.

45   Lechat P, Mas JL, Lascault G, Loron P, Theard M, Klimczac M, Drobinski G, Thomas D, Grosgogeat Y: Prevalence of patent foramen ovale in patients with stroke. N Engl J Med 1988;318: 1148–1152.

46   Di Tullio M, Sacco RL, Gopal A, Mohr JP, Homma S: Patent foramen ovale as a risk factor for cryptogenic stroke. Ann Intern Med 1992;117:461–465.

47   Miller VT, Pearce LA, Feinberg WM, Rothrock JF, Anderson DC, Hart RG: Differential effect of aspirin versus warfarin on clinical stroke types in patients with atrial fibrillation. Neurology 1996; 46:238–240.

48   The Stroke Prevention in Reversible Ischemia Trial (SPIRIT) Study Group: A randomized trial of anticoagulants versus aspirin after cerebral ischemia of presumed arterial origin. Ann Neurol 1997; 42:857–865.

49   Coumadin Aspirin Reinfarction (CARS) investigators: Randomized double-blind trial of fixed low-dose warfarin with aspirin after myocardial infarction. Lancet 1997;350:389–398.

50   Anonymous: Adjusted-dose warfarin versus low-intensity fixed-dose warfarin plus aspirin for high-risk patients with atrial fibrillation: Stroke Prevention in Atrial Fibrillation III randomized clinical trial. Lancet 1996;348:633–638.

51   Altman R, Rouvier J, Gurfinkel E: Oral anticoagulation treatment with and without aspirin. Thromb Haemost 1995;74:506–510.

52   Gregorini L, Marco J: Ticlopidine and aspirin interactions. Heart 1997;77:11–12.

53   Goods CM, al-Shaibi KF, Liu MW, Yadav JS, Mathur A, Jain SP, Dean LS, Iyer SS, Parks JM, Roubin GS: Comparison of aspirin alone versus aspirin plus ticlopidine after coronary stenting. Am J Cardiol 1996;78:1042–1044.

54   Yadav JS, Roubin GS, Iyer S, Vitek J, King P, Jordan WD, Fisher WS: Elective stenting of the extracranial carotid arteries. Circulation 1997;95:376–381.

55   Alberts MJ, McCann R, Smith TP, Stack R, Roubin G, Schneck MJ, Haumschild D, Iyer S: A randomized trial of carotid stenting versus endarterectomy in patients with symptomatic carotid stenosis: Study design. J Neurovasc Dis 1997;2:228–234.

Michael Schneck, 1725 West Harrison Street, Suite 755, Chicago, IL 60612 (USA)

Gillum RF, Gorelick PB, Cooper ES (eds): Stroke in Blacks. Basel, Karger, 1999, pp 180–187

....

Hypertension and Other Medical Complications of Acute Stroke in African-Americans

Edgar J. Kenton, III[a], *Edward S. Cooper*[b], *Frank S. James*[c]

[a] Division of Neurology, Lankenau Hospital, Wynnewood, Pa.;
[b] Department of Medicine, University of Pennsylvania, and
[c] Division of Cardiology, Germantown Hospital, Philadelphia, Pa., USA

Stroke is a devastating disease which frequently immobilizes the patient and sets the stage for many medical complications. Furthermore, the patients are usually elderly with hypertension and possibly other cardiovascular risk factors. Thus, they are especially prone to have heart and other vascular complications in the acute stage of illness as well as during recuperation. This chapter will review the identification, management and prevention of the most important medical complications, including hypertension, in the acute stroke patient.

Overview

The recognition and management of medical complications in the acutely ill stroke patient are continuous processes from stroke onset to rehabilitation. An alert and diverse health care team is required which possesses special expertise in the assessment and treatment of seriously ill patients with acute central nervous system disease. The neurological aspects of this subject have been covered on pp. 142–155. When the patient is seen initially at the scene of the acute brain attack, immediate recognition of stroke is helpful in order to alert and prepare the hospital for rapid assessment and management of this severe illness upon hospital arrival of the patient, preferably by ambulance. The patient's vital signs must be determined promptly. An unobstructed airway should be provided to prevent hypoxia and measures should be taken to avoid

Table 1. Complications of acute stroke in 120 patients

Complication	n	%
Urinary tract infections	24	20.0
Electrolyte	21	17.5
Pneumonia	20	16.7
Cardiac arrhythmia	13	10.8
Congestive heart failure	9	7.5
Brainstem herniation	7	5.8
Decubiti	6	5.0
Gastrointestinal hemorrhage	5	4.2
Seizures	4	3.3
Labile hypertension	3	2.5

aspiration and to secure the irrational patient to prevent injury from a fall. When adequacy of ventilation and oxygenation is questionable, oxygen inhalation therapy should be initiated and blood gasses measured. Even cardiopulmonary resuscitation might be required on occasions, although life-threatening cardiac arrhythmias, shock and cardiac arrest are much less common than in heart attack patients. For example, acute stroke is rarely the cause of sudden death except in patients with massive brainstem or subarachnoid hemorrhage or in those patients with complicating myocardial infarction or pulmonary embolism. The primary initial goal should be to keep the patients alive and supported during the early minutes of medical care and to transport them to the hospital as rapidly as possible where emergency assessment can be performed to determine the course of treatment.

Upon arrival at the hospital emergency room, prompt neurological and rapid medical evaluation is of primary importance (see pp. 142–155), along with further stabilization of the patient's general condition, if indicated. Those patients who might benefit from tPA therapy should be identified within 3 h of stroke onset. Therefore, in order to conserve time, systemic arterial blood pressure (BP) control, airway maintenance, vital signs monitoring, aspiration avoidance, seizure control and other supportive measures must be accomplished in synchrony with expeditious neurological evaluation including urgent CT brain scan. Following the emergency medical and neurological management, the patient is hospitalized either in a special stroke unit or in a hospital area where the patient's neurological and general medical status can be closely observed. It is during this period that most of the medical complications are seen and addressed. Table 1 indicates the complication rates seen in acute stroke patients, thus highlighting the medical management issues.

Hypertension

Acute stroke in African-Americans is clearly influenced by the presence of hypertension which is of considerable importance in the prevention and management of medical complications of acute stroke. Hypertension is a significant risk factor for stroke, presents a major cause of hemorrhagic, lacunar and multi-infarct stroke, prolongs hospitalization, is associated with increased cardiac disturbances and contributes to excess morbidity and mortality [1–9]. The judicious regulation of BP in the acute stroke patient is therefore of great interest but there are practically no serious studies available on this subject to guide the clinician. Thus, our discussion will be based principally on personal experience.

Accurate BP measurement and monitoring are essential to initiate treatment in the acute stroke patient. Cautious BP reduction is appropriate in hypertensive crisis with intracranial hemorrhage, ruptured cerebral aneurysm or hypertensive encephalopathy, as well as in patients with ischemic brain infarction and excessively high systolic BP levels. If hypertension is treated during the acute stage of illness, the goal is to maintain sufficient perfusion to prevent further brain ischemia. Often the BP will fall spontaneously towards normal after a few days of hospitalization. Generally, elevations of BP should not be treated acutely in ischemic cerebral infarction patients unless the systolic BP exceeds 220 mm Hg, the diastolic BP is 120 mm Hg, the mean BP remains above 130–160 mm Hg, or there is major organ failure that necessitates antihypertensive treatment. The goal is usually is to reduce BP about 15% over 24 h. More aggressive measures are used if concomitant complications exist, such as an acute myocardial infarction, pulmonary edema, and aortic dissection, as well as cerebral aneurysm hemorrhage and early in the course of cerebral hemorrhage. While there is no unanimity about which antihypertensive agent should be used in acute stroke, ACE inhibitors or labetalol are preferred because they are most favorable in regard to intracranial pressure and disturbances of autoregulation. Often, less potent oral antihypertensive agents may be chosen for routine BP lowering as they are less risky, particularly in the elderly, and can be easily continued after discharge [10]. Stroke patients, especially the elderly, frequently have impaired systemic baroreceptor responses, as well as faulty cerebral autoregulation and great care must be exercised while lowering BP [11]. In such patients, if excessive antihypertensive medication is administered, BP might fall toward shock levels because of inadequate systemic compensatory reflexes. In addition, cerebral perfusion may be further impaired because of poor cerebral autoregulatory responses. A similar instability of cerebral perfusion may develop if BP is lowered too vigorously in patients with extracranial occlusive cerebral vascular disease. These and other factors should be thoroughly considered before lowering BP in the acute stroke patient [12–16].

Acute ischemic stroke patients should not receive tPA until their systolic BP is below 180 mm Hg and diastolic below 110 mm Hg. Following the infusion of tPA in eligible ischemic stroke patients, the BP should be monitored continuously for 6 h, then every hour from the 8th hour through 24th hour, then routine monitoring. The lack of careful BP control is thought to increase the danger of intracerebral hemorrhage in patients who receive thrombolytic therapy [17–20].

Acute stroke patients who present with normal or low BP are also challenging at times. On occasions, such patients will experience significant reversal of their deteriorating neurological status following therapeutic elevation of BP, especially when BP on admission is low. Generally speaking, in order to assure adequate cerebral perfusion in these patients, BP should be maintained at 120–150 mm Hg systolic and 60–90 mm Hg diastolic or higher, if possible.

Cardiac Dysfunction

Cardiac arrhythmias, myocardial infarction and congestive heart failure are the major heart abnormalities encountered in the acute stroke patient. Cardiac arrhythmias are the most common of the heart disturbances and require continuous electrocardiographic monitoring for accurate diagnosis and also possible treatment, especially when circulatory compromise is threatened. The cardiac arrhythmias may result from intrinsic heart disease as well as from central nervous system reflex responses brought on by the brain disruption and damage [21]. The detailed management of cardiac arrhythmias is beyond the scope of this chapter. Briefly, serious ventricular dysrrhythmias require immediate intervention and cardiac consultation should be sought. Atrial fibrillation is particularly common and worrisome because of its propensity to produce thromboembolic complications and, at times, circulatory compromise. The management of atrial fibrillation in the stroke patient is discussed on pp. 129–141, but fundamentally the decision has to be made regarding the use of anticoagulant therapy and/or cardioversion. If atrial fibrillation is the cause of the ischemic stroke requiring hospitalization, then a delay of several days to a week or more is given, depending upon the size of the embolic infarct, to prevent conversion to cerebral hemorrhage.

If acute myocardial infarction is present concomitantly with stroke, such patients are usually referred to the coronary care unit (CCU), especially if the myocardial infarction is a complicated one. In the CCU, serious cardiac arrhythmias, shock, myocardial or valvular rupture, heart failure and other severe heart emergencies can be more effectively managed. If old or recent myocardial infarction with or without ventricular aneurysm is accompanied by mural thrombosis, then anticoagulant therapy to prevent recurrent stroke is usually required. Congestive heart failure (CHF) and acute stroke are a particularly troubling combination because of the generally fragile course and poor prognosis. CHF management requires the usual careful monitoring of vital signs and state of oxygenation. In addition, diuretics, ACE inhibitors and possibly digitalis along with fluid and sodium restriction may be indicated. CHF is an increasingly pervasive problem in the American population because of the growing reservoir of coronary and hypertensive heart disease victims who have not succumbed to acute attacks, as in the past. CHF is now the number 1 cause of repeated costly hospitalization of Medicare patients. The simultaneous occurrence of stroke and CHF will become more common as our population ages and the pool of high-risk patients increases.

Pulmonary Embolism and Venous Thrombosis

Because stroke patients may be immobilized for many days or weeks, they are particularly prone to develop venous thrombosis and possibly pulmonary embolism which may occur in approximately 10% of autopsied stroke patients. Stroke patients also commonly have generalized vascular disease, obesity, and CHF, which are added risk factors for venous thrombosis. To prevent venous thrombosis, the patient should be ambulated as soon as possible using early bedside introduction of physical therapy. Patients without cerebral hemorrhage should be started on low-dose heparin (5,000 units subcutaneously twice daily). Patients in whom acute pulmonary embolism is suspected should receive an appropriate combination of the following studies depending upon the height of suspicion: chest x-ray, arterial blood gasses, electrocardiography, noninvasive studies of the venous circulation of the lower extremities, venography, nuclear lung and perfusion scan and pulmonary angiography.

Routine therapy with the use of anticoagulants might be appropriate for patients who do not have brain hemorrhage. Venous umbrella may be necessary in other cases to prevent recurrent embolism in patients who are refractory to anticoagulant therapy or who have contraindications to anticoagulation.

Infections

Urinary tract infections, pneumonia and infected decubitus ulcers are the common bacterial complications in stroke patients and are not infrequently the cause of late death. Urinary tract infections are common because of the frequent use of an indwelling catheter which acts as a foreign body and because stroke often alters the functioning of the urinary bladder and its external sphincter. Urinary retention, poor emptying of bladder and infection may result. Whenever possible, indwelling catheters should be avoided and intermittent straight catheters substituted for bladder evacuation, or a condom catheter used. Bladder training, urological studies, encouragement of frequent voiding and urinary pharmacotherapy are often attempted.

Pneumonia is commonly related to swallowing difficulties and aspiration [22] and decubitis ulcers to inadequate skin care and delayed ambulation. The prevention and management of these problems are discussed in the rehabilitation section on pp. 198–209.

Metabolic Abnormalities

Hypo- and hyperglycemia, hyponatremia, hypernatremia with dehydration, depressed or elevated serum potassium levels, renal failure with azotemia and acidosis as well as other electrolyte disturbances are seen in the acutely ill stroke patient and must be addressed. Whether hyperglycemia is particularly harmful to stroke patients remains controversial but diabetes is generally closely controlled, avoiding hypoglycemia as much as possible.

Intravenous fluids are administered in the acutely ill stroke patients who have limited oral intake, to ensure adequate hydration as well as sufficient caloric intake and medication access. This is especially relevant in patients with swallowing difficulty. Extended malnutrition may become a problem in the stroke patient and may be easily overlooked, especially in elderly patients. Careful attention should be given to food intake, including vitamins and minerals. Nasogastric intubation or long-term gastric and jejunostomy feeding tubes may be placed in patients with refractory swallowing function which cannot be corrected through the guidance of the rehabilitation staff.

Seizures and Depression

These complications are fairly frequent in the acute stroke patients, seizures up to 10% and depression 30% [23–25]. Recurrent seizures must be treated with anticonvulsants to avoid aspiration, injury and status epilepticus. Depression may be overlooked by the generalist and neurologist and, if refractory, may require antidepressant therapy and psychiatric consultation. The patient's entire support system must be involved to achieve optimal success in management. How depression affects rehabilitation of the stroke patients is discussed on pp. 198–209.

Conclusion

In the setting of acute stroke in African-Americans, prevention and the careful management of medical complications will significantly reduce the morbidity and mortality of stroke. The principal medical complications are hypertension, cardiac dysfunction, pulmonary embolism and venous thromboses, infections, metabolic abnormalities, depression and seizures. The increasing economic and social burden of stroke in the Black community can be reduced. An awareness and knowledge of the medical complications of acute stroke including hypertension is essential. There is a need for further research regarding the medical management of the acute stroke patient, particulary regarding the optimal regulation of BP.

Acknowledgments

The authors thank Geraldine Davis Kenton for preparation of the manuscript.

References

1   Whispant JP: Effectiveness versus efficacy of treatment of hypertension for stroke prevention. Neurology 1996;46:301–307.
2   Burt VL, Whelton P, Roccella EJ, Brown C, Cutler JA, Higgins M, Horan MJ, Labarthe D: Prevalence of hypertension in the US adult population: Results from the Third National Health and Nutrition Examination Survey, 1988–1991. Hypertension 1995;23:305–313.
3   Broderick J, Brott T, Kothari R, Miller R, et al: The Greater Cincinnati/Northern Kentucky Stroke Study. Preliminary first-ever and total incidence rates of stroke among Blacks. Stroke 1998;29: 415–421.
4   Centers for Disease Control: Cerebraovascular disease mortality and medicare hospitalization – United States 1980–1990. MMWR 1992;41:477–480.
5   Special Report from the National Institute of Neurological Disorders and Stroke: Classification of cerebrovascular diseases. III. Stroke 1990;21:637–676.
6   Cerebral Embolism Task Force: Cardiogenic brain embolism. Arch Neurol 1989;46:727–743.
7   Mohr JP, Caplan LR, Melski JW, et al: The Harvard Cooperative Stroke Registry: A prospective registry. Neurology 1978;28:754–762.
8   Roman GC: Senile dementia of the Binswanger type. A vascular form of dementia in the elderly. JAMA 1987;258:1782–1788.
9   Kenton EJ, Gorelick PB, Cooper ES: Stroke in elderly African-Americans. Am J Geriatr Cardiol 1997;6:39–49.
10 Cooper ES, West JW: The study and management of stroke. Urban Health 1979;8:48–51.
11 Cooper ES: Cerebrovascular disease in Blacks; in Hall WD, Saunders E, Shulman N (eds): Hypertension in Blacks. Chicago, Yearbook Medical Publishers, 1985, pp 83–105.

12   Burris JF: Beyond controlling blood pressure in the Black patient: Metabolic considerations. J Natl Med Assoc 1995;87:359–362.
13   Oprail S: Antihypertensive therapy and atherosclerosis in coronary heart disease. Cardiovasc Risk Factors 1996;6:222–232.
14   American Society of Hypertension: Recommendations for routine blood pressure measurement by direct cuff sphygmomanometry. Am J Hypertens 1992;5:207–209.
15   Guidelines for Measurement of Patients with Acute Ischemic Stroke: A statement for health care professionals from a special writing group of the Stroke Council, American Heart Association. Stroke 1994;25:1901–1914.
16   Kenton EJ: Diagnosis and treatment of concomitant hypertension and stroke. J Natl Med Assoc 1996;88:364–368.
17   The National Institute of Neurological Disorders and Stroke rt-PA Study Group. Tissue plasminogen activator for acute ischemic stroke. N Engl J Med 1995;333:1581–1587.
18   Guidelines for Thrombolytic Therapy for Acute Stroke: A supplement to the guidelines for the management of patients with acute ischemic stroke. Stroke 1996;27:1711–1718.
19   Consensus Conference on Anti-Thrombotic Therapy. Chest 1991;102:426S–433S.
20   Oparil S: Clinical crossroads. A 42-year-old man with hypertension. JAMA 1997;278:1015–1021.
21   Cooper ES, West JW: Cardiac arrhythmias, cerebral function and stroke. Current concepts cerebrovascular disease. Stroke 1970;5:53–58.
22   Mulley GP: Pneumonia, stroke and laterality. Lancet 1981;i:1051–1060.
23   Feabel JH, Springer CJ: Depression and failure to resume social activities after stroke. Arch Phys Med 1982;63:276–277.
24   Szetcla B: Mood change following left hemisphere brain injury. Ann Neurol 1981;9:477–453.
25   Cooper ES: Clinical cerebrovascular disease in hypertensive Blacks. J Clin Hypertens 1987;3:795–845.

Edgar J. Kenton, III, MD, Division of Neurology, Lankenau Hospital, Wynnewood, PA 19096 (USA)

Gillum RF, Gorelick PB, Cooper ES (eds): Stroke in Blacks. Basel, Karger, 1999, pp 188–197

....
Late Sequelae of Cerebrovascular Disease in African-Americans: Vascular Dementia

Philip B. Gorelick[a], *Patrick Griffith*[b]

[a] Department of Neurological Sciences, Center for Stroke Research and Section of Cerebrovascular Disease and Neurologic Critical Care, Rush Medical College, Chicago, Ill., and
[b] Department of Medicine, Section of Neurology, Morehouse Medical School, Atlanta, Ga., USA

Vascular causes of cognitive impairment are common and may be preventable [1]. In some parts of the world where stroke rates are high, vascular dementia (VaD) may be more common than Alzheimer's disease (AD) [2]. Since African-Americans are at high risk of stroke [3], it is logical to conclude that they may be at high risk for VaD [1, 2]. Thus, African-Americans are an important group to study with regards to vascular causes of cognitive impairment. Since 1987 we have been carrying out case-control and longitudinal studies of African-Americans with stroke who do or do not have dementia associated with stroke, to identify risk factors for VaD and to refine our understanding of cognitive decline among African-Americans. In this chapter we review the findings of our epidemiological studies of VaD among African-Americans and provide an overview of the epidemiology, classification, prognosis, clinical features and treatment of VaD.

Epidemiology

Mortality
VaD patients generally have higher mortality rates when compared to AD patients or controls. In a racially-mixed study group in New York, mortality rates were 19.8/100 person-years for those with dementia after stroke

compared to 6.9/100 person-years for those with stroke but no dementia [4]. Similarly, in a racially-mixed group in Chicago the life quotient (estimated survival divided by expected survival) was 0.78 for AD and 0.57 for VaD [5].

Incidence and Prevalence

VaD rises exponentially with age and is thought to be more common than even AD in some parts of the world such as Asia where there are high stroke rates [6]. Although there is a paucity of information about the frequency of VaD among African-Americans, it is suspected that VaD rates will be high in this group as stroke rates are high [7]. In a multiethnic cohort of municipal retirees in Houston, the age-adjusted prevalence of dementia was highest for Black men when compared to White or Hispanic men, whereas the cumulative incidence was slightly higher for Hispanic men [8]. In these retirees, VaD was more common than AD.

As African-Americans are a rapidly expanding segment of our elderly population and the elderly are at high risk of stroke and AD, an important question is raised: Do African-Americans suffer a double burden of dementia? That is, a high rate of both AD and VaD [9]. We are attempting to answer this important question in a clinicopathologic study of our African-American patients who have these two common types of dementia [7].

Risk of Dementia after Stroke

Cognitive impairment is common after stroke. In a racially-mixed group of hospitalized stroke patients in New York, after 52 months the cumulative proportion with dementia and stroke was about 33% whereas for community controls the cumulative proportion with dementia was about 10% [10]. The incidence of dementia was estimated to be 8.4/100 person-years in the stroke group and 1.3/100 person-years in the control group. It is well known that cognitive function may improve after stroke. This may be most evident with left hemisphere infarction and more severe hemispheral syndromes [11]. Diabetes mellitus, on the other hand, may be associated with failure to exhibit improvement.

Risk Factors

Risk factors for VaD may be considered putative at this time as there is a lack of consistency and a general paucity of studies [1]. It is logical to conclude that risk factors for stroke will also be risk factors for VaD. With additional rigorous epidemiologic study, we believe that consistency regarding risk factors for VaD will emerge. At the present time, possible risk factors for VaD may be classified as demographic, atherogenic, genetic and stroke-related [1].

Putative Risk Factors for VaD in African-Americans

Our epidemiologic studies in Chicago have focused on potential risk factors for dementia following stroke in hospital-based referral patients [7, 12–15]. Those patients with dementia and stroke have been compared to controls with stroke but no dementia or AD patients. In one study of stroke patients with and without dementia [12], we found that advanced age, lower educational attainment, history of myocardial infarction and recent cigarette use were positively associated with dementia. Furthermore, systolic blood pressure level was inversely associated with dementia risk. In a comparison study designed to assess cranial computed tomography (CCT) predictors of dementia in stroke patients, we concluded that left cortical infarction might be the best CCT predictor of dementia associated with stroke [13].

When we extended our study to include a comparison group of African-American AD patients, distinct patient profiles emerged: African-American VaD patients had a higher frequency of cardiovascular disease risk factors, focal neurologic findings and medication use whereas African-American AD patients were more likely to have a family history of AD, Parkinson's disease and dementia, and a history of head injury with loss of consciousness [7]. These risk factor profiles were consistent with those reported in other studies of VaD and AD from different patient populations and a comparable time period. The companion CCT and magnetic resonance imaging (MRI) study showed the following trends for our African-American patients [14]: (1) on CCT, the presence of white matter lesions, nonlacunar infarcts and left subcortical infarcts distinguished VaD from AD, whereas atrophy of the third ventricle and equal distribution of white matter lesions distinguished VaD from stroke without dementia (SWD), and (2) on MRI, atrophy of the temporal sulci, temporal horns, and the third ventricle, and right hemisphere infarcts distinguished AD from VaD, whereas atrophy of the third ventricle differentiated VaD from SWD. We concluded that the qualitative CCT and MRI findings among our African-American patients were similar to those reported in other studies, and atrophy, especially at the level of the third ventricle, presence of infarcts, and white matter lesions might be good predictors of dementia subtype by CCT or MRI.

White matter lesions may be an important predictor of cognitive impairment, and African-Americans may have a higher proportion of more severe white matter lesions as diagnosed by neuroimaging studies [16]. White matter lesions have been linked to age, hypertension, cigarette smoking, lacunar infarction and lower educational attainment. At least several of these factors are more prevalent in African-Americans [3].

Table 1. Putative risk factors for vascular dementia

Demographic	Stroke-related
1. Age	1. Volume, number and location of infarcts
2. Male sex	2. Cerebral atrophy
3. Race/ethnicity	3. White matter lesions (leukoaraiosis)
(Asians and possibly African-Americans)	4. Silent cerebral infarcts
4. Blue-collar work	

Genetic
1. Autosomal dominant hereditary cerebral hemorrhage with amyloidosis-Dutch type
2. Cerebral autosomal dominant arteriopathy with subcortical infarct and leukoencephalopathy (CADASIL)
3. Apolipoprotein E polymorphism

Atherogenic	Toxins
1. Hypertension	1. Pesticides and herbicides
2. Cigarette use	2. Liquid plastic or rubber
3. Myocardial infarction	
4. Atrial fibrillation	*Psychologic*
5. Diabetes mellitus	1. Stress
6. Hypercholesterolemia	
7. Hematocrit, hemostasis abnormalities, peripheral vascular disease, alcohol consumption	

Putative Risk Factors for VaD from Other Studies

Potential risk factors for VaD are depicted in table 1 and are summarized in two recent review articles [1, 17]. At the present time, age is the only factor that can be considered a well-documented risk factor for VaD until additional epidemiologic studies emerge with consistent risk factor patterns. The factors that are outlined in table 1 are from a diverse group of subcategories that include demographic factors, genetic factors, atherogenic host risk factors, stroke-related factors and toxic exposures. Besides our own data [7, 12–15], most studies have not specifically addressed risk factors for VaD in African-Americans.

Classification and Mechanism

Diagnostic Criteria

VaD has traditionally been thought of as a syndrome of cognitive impairment in conjunction with stroke that is characterized by abrupt onset, stepwise deterioration and fluctuating course [2]. More recently, the term VaD has replaced the term MID (multi-infarct dementia) since VaD, as a descriptor, is thought to be more encompassing. Furthermore, emphasis has been placed on different stages of vascular cognitive impairment and the importance of identifying the vascular mechanism underlying the cognitive impairment to enact appropriate prevention and treatment measures [18].

Modern diagnostic criteria for VaD have evolved to include clinical, neuro-radiologic and neuropathologic aspects [19, 20]. The key components of these research criteria are the presence of dementia, a temporal relation between stroke and dementia, and the presence of impairment in several cognitive domains (e.g., memory, language, attention). While these criteria remain to be validated, data from neuroimaging and neuropathologic studies of VaD will help to sharpen these criteria and allay criticisms about lack of sensitivity, specificity and uniformity of previous diagnostic criteria [2].

Classification

VaD syndromes may be classified by site of stroke or by etiology. In the former scheme, VaD is classified by location of infarct or hemorrhage in the superficial cerebral cortex, deep white matter and surrounding structures, or combined involvement of superficial and deep structures. By the etiologic scheme, the underlying mechanism of stroke is identified (e.g., cerebral embolism secondary to atrial fibrillation, cerebral hemorrhage secondary to hypertension or amyloid angiopathy, etc.). While both classification schemes offer inherent advantages to further our understanding, definition of the stroke pathophysiologic mechanism that underlies cognitive impairment offers the most practical approach to prevention and treatment of VaD.

Pathophysiologic Mechanism

For stroke-prone groups such as African-Americans, it is important to identify the pathophysiologic mechanism of stroke in an effort to prevent further vascular damage and to lessen the likelihood of subsequent vascular cognitive impairment. African-Americans, for example, are thought to be at higher risk for lacunar infarcts and intraparenchymal hemorrhage. Both of these stroke subtypes have been linked to hypertension. Thus, control of hypertension may be important to reduce the risk of vascular cognitive impairment in African-Americans. It is also believed that some African-Americans may not have nocturnal dips in blood pressure (so-called nondippers). Such sustained hypertension could predispose to more severe brain white matter lesions which have been associated with vascular cognitive impairment [16]. Finally, small, strategically located silent cerebral infarcts (SCIs) in such areas as the thalamus and deep frontal lobe have been associated with cognitive impairment and may be more likely to occur in African-Americans. SCIs have been linked to hypertension and white matter lesions (leukoaraiosis) [21]. Prevention of SCIs could be another important avenue for reduction of vascular cognitive impairment in African-Americans.

Concomitance of AD and VaD: Are African-Americans at Higher Risk for Mixed Dementia?

A recently published longitudinal study of nuns emphasized the possible importance of cerebrovascular disease in determining the presence and severity of the clinical symptoms of AD [22]. In this study, among 61 participants who met neuropathologic criteria of AD, those with brain infarcts had poorer cognitive function and a higher prevalence of dementia than those without infarcts. Furthermore, those with lacunar infarcts in deep brain areas had a high prevalence of dementia. In this study atherosclerosis of the circle of Willis was associated with lacunar and large brain infarcts. Therefore, one may conclude that a few small infarcts in strategic brain locations could produce dementia in those with abundant AD lesions.

The implications of the above findings are important for African-Americans. First, African-Americans are at high risk of stroke and as aging occurs are at high risk for AD. Second, since stroke is preventable, cognitive impairment may be averted or at least postponed if stroke can be prevented. The study of Snowdon et al. [22] provides evidence for the 'double-burden' of dementia hypothesis. Furthermore, not only have strategically placed SCIs and white matter lesions been found to contribute to dementia and possibly set the stage for mixed AD and VaD in susceptible persons, but vascular changes such as atrophic and coiling microvessels, amyloid deposits and endothelial-derived toxin may serve as additional vascular links to AD. These findings coupled with those of possible shared genetic risk for dementia associated with stroke and AD via apolipoprotein Eε4 alleles [23] suggest an important role for mixed AD and VaD in the elderly, especially those at high risk for stroke. We have advocated a comprehensive clinical-neuropathologic study to further define this possible relationship among African-Americans [9].

Clinical Features

In contradistinction to AD, which typically has a slowly progressive and insidious clinical presentation of memory loss and other cognitive dysfunction, VaD traditionally has been characterized by more abrupt or stepwise deterioration of cognitive function in conjunction with recent stroke(s). There is a relative paucity of longitudinal systematic study about the clinical presentation of VaD and accompanying manifestations. One must maintain heightened vigilance to establish a diagnosis of VaD as somatic stroke deficits and aphasias are often the focus of poststroke rehabilitation, and vascular causes of cognitive impairment are ignored or given a lower priority in the overall examination [24].

As previously noted, the diagnosis of VaD requires the presence of a dementia syndrome and substantial evidence of cerebrovascular disease as the causative factor [19, 20, 25]. Cognitive dysfunction should be temporally linked to a recent stroke(s) and generally, there is a preponderance of cardiovascular disease risk factors. Ideally, neuroimaging studies support the diagnosis by providing evidence of cerebral infarction or hemorrhage in areas of the brain that are linked to affected cognition, and neuropsychological studies are also consistent with these findings. In the aged it may be difficult to distinguish AD and VaD at times. Furthermore, in some cases there are extensive brain white matter lesions, presumed to be vascular in origin, diagnosed by CCT or MRI, and an insidious clinical course more typical of AD. In these cases it may be difficult to arrive at a clear-cut dementia subtype diagnosis, and the possibility of mixed dementia (AD plus VaD) may be entertained.

Neurologic physical examination findings will vary depending on the location and mechanism of stroke. As African-Americans are at higher risk for lacunar infarction, these small deep infarcts may be accompanied by subcortical deficits in attention and memory, hemiparesis, hemisensory loss, ataxia, and pseudobulbar manifestations (e.g. emotional incontinence, dysarthria, dysphagia, spasticity and hyperactive deep tendon reflexes). More traditional cortical deficits such as aphasia, apraxia, and visuospatial dysfunction may occur with cardiogenic embolism or large artery thromboembolic disease.

Neuropsychiatric manifestations may be common in African-Americans with VaD. Harris et al. [26] found that irritability (57%), apathy (44%), insomnia (44%), agitation (41%), impatience (37%) and emotional lability (28%) were common features in VaD patients with multiple infarcts. Of these factors, only apathy and irritability were independent predictors of VaD.

Treatment

Control of cardiovascular disease risk factors may be effective strategies in VaD [27]. Observations from small-scale clinical trials or observational studies support this belief. Blood pressure control in the systolic range of 135–150 mm Hg may be related to cognitive improvement [28]. Daily aspirin therapy [29], cessation of smoking [28] and control of blood lipids [30] are additional strategies that may improve cognitive function in patients with VaD. These promising results, however, need to be validated in large-scale studies.

Neuroprotectant therapy to potentiate salvage of neurons that may be rendered ischemic has been studied. Pentoxifylline, a hemorheologic agent, and propentofylline, an adenasine uptake/phosphodiesterase inhibitor with neuroprotective properties, may be beneficial [31, 32]. Nimodipine, a vasoactive agent and one that protects the cell from calcium influx, could also be beneficial [33] as may glutamate antagonists and vasodilators [27]. Further study of these treatments is needed to validate their possible effectiveness.

Management of caregiver stress, behavioral symptoms and psychosocial aspects may also play an important role in the care of the patient with VaD. Standard approaches for such intervention are recommended [27].

Prevention

As there is no definitive medical or surgical treatment for VaD, prevention of stroke may offer the most viable solution to reduce the ravages of VaD [27]. Heightened public awareness about the treatment and control of cardiovascular disease risk factors is paramount [34]. This looms ever important for African-Americans as elevated blood pressure level in mid to later life may be predictive of future cognitive impairment [35, 36]. Since hypertension is so prevalent in African-Americans, its control could reduce not only the propensity for stroke, but that for VaD as well.

Closing Remarks

Vascular causes of cognitive impairment may be the most important and only major preventable form of dementia in the elderly. As a group, African-Americans are at high risk of stroke and as they age, are at high risk of AD. The susceptibility to VaD for those at high risk of stroke has been emphasized in this chapter as well as the potentially important interaction between AD and strategically located brain infarcts in determining the occurrence and severity of dementia. African-American elderly are at risk for dementia and could be vulnerable to a 'double burden' of dementia as both stroke and AD may occur in this group.

The clinical and neuroimaging signs and harbingers of VaD have become better defined. Thus, the time has come to identify African-Americans at risk for vascular cognitive impairment or who have early vascular cognitive impairment to intervene in an attempt to avert cognitive sequelae. Such simple measures as control of blood pressure, blood lipids and encouragement of other healthy cardiovascular lifestyles may lead to preservation of cognition [37]. The primary prevention of stroke through modification of treatable cardiovascular risk factors and the identification of well-documented risk factors for VaD will play important roles in our thrust against vascular causes of cognitive impairment. Cognitive impairment may not be an inevitable eventuality in the elderly.

Acknowledgment

Supported in part by National Institutes of Health contract numbers R01 NS33430-03 (P.B.G.) and R01 AG10102-07 (P.B.G.), and the MR Bauer Foundation (P.B.G.).

References

1   Gorelick PB: Status of risk factors for dementia associated with stroke. Stroke 1997;28:459–463.
2   Gorelick PB, Roman G, Mangone CA: Vascular dementia; in Gorelick PB, Alter MA (eds): Handbook of Neuroepidemiology. New York, Dekker, 1994, pp 197–212.
3   Gorelick PB, Harris Y: Stroke: An excess burden on African-Americans. Chicago Med 1993;96:28–30.
4   Tatemichi TK, Paik M, Bagiella E, Desmond DW, Pirro M, Hanzawa LK: Dementia after stroke is a predictor of long-term survival. Stroke 1994;25:1915–1919.
5   Hier DB, Warach J, Gorelick PB, Thomas J: Predictors of survival in clinically diagnosed Alzheimer's disease and multi-infarct dementia. Arch Neurol 1989;46:1213–1216.
6   Yoshitake T, Kiyohara Y, Kato I, Ohmura T, Iwamoto H, Nakayama K, et al: Incidence and risk factors of vascular dementia and Alzheimer's disease in a defined elderly Japanese population: The Hisayama study. Neurology 1995;45:1161–1168.
7   Gorelick PB, Freels S, Harris Y, Dollear T, Billingsley M, Brown N: Epidemiology of vascular and Alzheimer's dementia among African-Americans in Chicago, IL: Baseline frequency and comparison of risk factors. Neurology 1994;44:1391–1396.
8   Perkins P, Annegers JF, Doody RS, Cooke N, Aday L, Vernon SW: Incidence and prevalence of dementia in a multiethnic cohort of municipal retirees. Neurology 1997;49:44–50.
9   Gorelick PB, Nyenhuis DL, Garron DC, Cochran E: Is vascular dementia really Alzheimer's disease or mixed dementia? Neuroepidemiology 1996;15:286–290.
10 Tatemichi TK, Paik M, Bagiella E, Desmond DW, Stern Y, Sano M, Hauser WA, Mayeux R: Risk of dementia after stroke in a hospitalized cohort: Results of a longitudinal study. Neurology 1994;44:1885–1891.
11 Desmond DW, Moroney JT, Sano M, Stern Y: Recovery of cognitive function after stroke. Stroke 1996;27:1798–1803.
12 Gorelick PB, Brody J, Cohen D, Freels S, Levy P, Dollear W, Forman H, Harris Y: Risk factors for dementia associated with multiple cerebral infarcts. A case-control analysis in predominantly African-American hospital-based patients. Arch Neurol 1993;50:714–720.
13 Gorelick PB, Chatterjee A, Patel D, Flowerdew G, Dollear W, Taber J, Harris Y: Cranial computed tomographic observations in multi-infarct dementia. A controlled study. Stroke 1992;23:804–811.
14 Charletta D, Gorelick PB, Dollear TJ, Freels S, Harris Y: CT and MRI findings among African-Americans with Alzheimer's disease, vascular dementia and stroke without dementia. Neurology 1995;45:1456–1461.
15 Gorelick PB, Freels S, Harris Y, Billingsley M: Risk factors for dementia associated with stroke in African-Americans: A case control analysis. J Ment Health Aging 1996;2:51–64.
16 Liao D, Cooper L, Cai J, Toole J, Bryan N, Burke G, Shahar E, Nieto J, Mosely T, Heiss G: The prevalence and severity of white matter lesions, their relationship with age, ethnicity, gender and cardiovascular disease risk factors: The ARIC study. Neuroepidemiology 1997;16:149–162.

17   Skoog I: Status of risk factors for vascular dementia. Neuroepidemiology 1998;17:2–9.
18   Hachinski VC: Vascular dementia: A radical redefinition; in Carlson LA, Gottfries CG, Winblad B (eds): Vascular Dementia. Etiological, Pathogenetic, Clinical and Treatment Aspects. New York, Karger, 1994, pp 130–132.
19   NINDS-AIREN International Workshop Group: Vascular dementia: Diagnostic criteria for research studies: Report of the NINDS-AIREN International Workshop. Neurology 1993;43:250–260.
20   Chui HC, Victoroff JI, Margolin D, Jagust W, Shankle R, Katzman R: Criteria for the diagnosis of ischemic vascular dementia proposed by the State of California Alzheimer's Disease Diagnostic and Treatment Centers. Neurology 1992;42:473–480.
21   Kobayashi S, Koide H, Bokura H, Yamaguchi S, Okada K, Yamagata S, Tsuchiya H: Prospective study on stroke onset in silent cerebral infarction. J Stroke Cerebrovasc Dis 1996;6(suppl 1):93–96.
22   Snowdon DA, Greiner LH, Mortimer JA, Riley KP, Greiner PA, Markesbery WR: Brain infarction and the clinical expression of Alzheimer's disease. The nun study. JAMA 1997;277:813–817.
23   Slooter AJC, Tang M-X, van Duijn CM, Stern Y, Ott A, Bell K, Breteler MMB, Van Broeckhoven C, Tatemichi TK, Tycko B, Hofman A, Mayeux R: Apolipoprotein E ε4 and the risk of dementia with stroke. A population-based investigation. JAMA 1997;277:818–821.
24   Dollear W, Gorelick PB, Harris Y, Miles T, Bozzola F: Vascular dementia: A clinical and death certificate study. Neuroepidemiology 1992;11:53–58.
25   Wetterling T, Kanitz R-D, Borgis K-J: Comparison of different diagnostic criteria for vascular dementia (ADDTC, DSM-IV, ICD-10, NINDS-AIREN). Stroke 1996;27:30–36.
26   Harris Y, Gorelick PB, Cohen D, Dollear W, Forman H, Freels S: Psychiatric symptoms in dementia associated with stroke: A case-control analysis among predominantly African-American patients. J Natl Med Assoc 1994;86:697–702.
27   Nyenhuis D, Gorelick PB: Vascular dementia: A contemporary review of epidemiology, diagnosis, prevention and treatment. J Am Geriatr Soc 1998, in press.
28   Meyer JS, Judd BW, Tawaklna T, Rogers RL, Mortel KF: Improved cognition after control of risk factors for multi-infarct dementia. JAMA 1986;256:2203–2209.
29   Meyer JS, Rogers RL, McClintic K, Mortel KF, Lofti J: Randomized clinical trial of daily aspirin therapy in multi-infarct dementia. J Am Geriatr Soc 1989;37:549–555.
30   Walzl M, Walzl B, Lechner H: Results of a two-month follow-up after a single heparin-induced extracorporeal LDL precipitation in vascular dementia. J Stroke Cerebrovasc Dis 1994;4:179–182.
31   European Pentoxifylline Multi-Infarct Dementia (EPMID) Study Group: European pentoxifylline multi-infarct dementia study. Eur Neurol 1996;36:315–321.
32   Marcusson J, Rother M, Kittner B, et al: A 12-month, randomized, placebo-controlled trial of propentofylline (HWT 285) in patients with dementia according to DSM III-R. Dement Geriatr Cogn Disord 1997;8:320–328.
33   Pantoni L, Carosi M, Amigoni S, Mascalchi M, Inzitari D: A preliminary open trial with nimodipine in patients with cognitive impairment and leukoaraiosis. Clin Neuropharmacol 1996;19:497–506.
34   Gorelick PB: Stroke prevention. Arch Neurol 1995;52:347–354.
35   Skoog I, Lernfelt B, Landahl S, Plamertz B, Andreasson L-A, Nilsson L, Persson G, Oden A, Svanborg A: 15-year longitudinal study of blood pressure and dementia. Lancet 1996;347:1141–1145.
36   Launer LJ, Masaki K, Petrovich H, Foley D, Havlik RJ: The association between midlife blood pressure levels and late-life cognitive function. The Honolulu-Asia Aging Study. JAMA 1995;274:1846–1851.
37   Gorelick PB: Stroke prevention: Windows of opportunity and failed expectations? A discussion of modifiable cardiovascular risk factors and a prevention proposal. Neuroepidemiology 1997;16:163–173.

Philip B. Gorelick, MD, MPH, Center for Stroke Research,
1645 West Jackson, Suite 400, Chicago, IL 60612 (USA)

Gillum RF, Gorelick PB, Cooper ES (eds): Stroke in Blacks. Basel, Karger, 1999, pp 198–209

....

Stroke Rehabilitation in African-American Patients

Larry B. Goldstein[a], *Helen Hoenig*[b]

[a] Division of Neurology, Department of Medicine, Duke Center for
Cerebrovascular Disease, Center for Clinical Health Policy Research,
Duke University, and Veterans Affairs Medical Center,
[b] Division of Geriatrics, Department of Medicine, Physical Medicine and
Rehabilitation Service, Veterans Affairs Medical Center, Durham, N.C., USA

The treatment of patients with cerebrovascular disease involves a continuum of care with primary prevention being the cornerstone of therapy. More effective strategies to reduce the risk of stroke through the identification and management of common risk factors in the African-American population may lead to a reduced burden of disease in the future. In addition, there have been advances in secondary prevention strategies such as the selective use of anticoagulants in patients with atrial fibrillation and the performance of carotid endarterectomy in qualified patients with extracranial carotid artery stenosis. The use of tPA can improve outcomes in carefully chosen patients with acute ischemic stroke and experimental neuroprotective agents may prove useful in limiting stroke-related brain damage. However, it is likely that these measures will never be universally effective and applicable. As a result, many patients will be left with neurological deficits due to stroke. Although experimental therapies aimed at improving recovery may become available in the future, rehabilitative services currently offer the primary means of therapy and a source of hope and encouragement for both stroke patients and their families. The goals of rehabilitative therapy are to promote functional recovery and prevent stroke-related complications.

Functional Impact of Stroke and Measurement Instruments

The functional impact of stroke may be considered at several levels [1]. The World Health Organization scheme refers to stroke-related deficits at the levels of impairment, disability and handicap to fully describe the consequences of stroke. At the level of *impairment*, stroke affects specific physiologic functions such as language, spatial perception, sensation, strength and coordination. *Disability* is the result of physiologic impairments and is reflected in specific activities (i.e. bathing, walking, dressing, etc.). *Handicap* results from impairments and disabilities and refers to loss of function at a societal level (i.e. loss of employment). Handicap can be conceptualized as the interaction between disability and the surrounding environment. It is important to recognize that improvement at the impairment level may not be mirrored by improvement in disabilities and handicaps and that diminished disability and handicap may not reflect decreased impairment. For example, limb paresis may improve after stroke, but the patient may still be unable to walk without assistance (disability) or return to work as a postman (handicap). A patient with an upper limb amputation may learn to use a prosthesis and the remaining arm to dress (improved disability) and to provide childcare (reduction of handicap). Therefore, in considering the impact of stroke and functional recovery, the level of function must be clearly understood.

A variety of different clinical instruments have been developed to measure stroke-related deficits and recovery at each of the three principle functional levels. In the United States, the National Institutes of Health Stroke Scale (NIHSS) has been validated, shown to be reliable, and is now the standard stroke impairment scale [2]. Most of the individual scale items are reliably assessed and the evaluation requires about 10 min or less to perform and may be used serially. Reliability of this scale can be improved for use in multicenter trials through the use of standardized video training [3]. The European Stroke Scale is quite similar to the NIHSS and is reliable and partially validated [4]. The Canadian Neurological Scale (CNS) is more rapidly performed, but does not capture many stroke-related impairments [5]. Scales to measure specific types of impairments such as the Fugl-Meyer Assessment (motor) and the Berg Balance Scale (balance) have also been developed and validated in stroke patients [6].

Disability is commonly measured with the Barthel Index [7]. Pivotal scores have been established that correspond to severe dependence (score < 40) and assisted independence (score > 60) [7]. Instrumental Activity of Daily Living (IADL) scales attempt to bridge the delineation between disability and handicap [8]. The Functional Independence Measure (FIM) is another valid, reliable and widely used measure of disability [9]. The FIM is used for monitoring functional improvements at the level of disability through the course of rehabilitation therapy. There is no consensus definition of IADL. These scales attempt to measure the patient's ability to live independently in the home and capture certain core activities including domestic chores, household management, outdoor activities and transportation. None of the scales have been fully validated and reliability has not been fully established.

The Rankin Scale has been used as a measure of stroke-related handicap in many interventional trials [10]. However, the Rankin Scale is a global functional health index emphasizing physical disability [11]. The scale may be reliably applied, and because it is weighted towards physical function, the results correlate closely with scores on the Barthel Index [12, 13]. The Craig Handicap Assessment and Reporting Technique (CHART) was specifically designed to assess handicap and may prove applicable to stroke patients [14].

In addition to these physically based measures, it is important to assess the patient's quality of life. Issues related to proxy responses, reliability and validity in this setting have generally not been systematically evaluated in a prospective study, although some data are now becoming available [15]. Because many of the measures are lengthy, issues related to feasibility in patients recovering from acute stroke also need to be assessed. The Sickness Impact Profile (SIP), Health Utilities Index (HUI) and EuroQol have been used in the evaluation of stroke patients [15, 16]. The physical subscore of the SIP correlates with stroke-related impairments as measured with the NIHSS and CNS, but the psychosocial subscore correlates less well [13]. Disability scores measured with the Barthel Index and handicap scores measured with the Rankin Scale explain only 33% of the variance in SIP scores [17].

Rehabilitation and Poststroke Functional Recovery

Regardless of the initial severity of the neurological deficit, most stroke survivors exhibit some degree of recovery over time [18, 19]. The most rapid period of recovery occurs over the first 30–90 days after stroke, however, some patients may continue to make gains over longer periods of time. A variety of factors may influence the ultimate rate and degree of recovery after stroke. Several complex prognostic scoring systems have been developed to predict this recovery [20]. The single most important variable is the severity of the initial neurological deficit which can be measured in several ways. Patients presenting with a depressed level of consciousness have poorer outcomes than those who are alert. For example, in one study, no patient who was alert, but 37% of those whose consciousness was initially impaired died [21]. Patients with more severe motor impairments have greater disabilities 9 months after stroke than those with less severe initial motor deficits [22].

Optimization of the rate and degree of 'spontaneous' recovery is one of the primary goals of poststroke treatment. Achieving this objective requires a 'team approach' involving a variety of specialists including physicians, nurses, physical therapists, occupational therapists, psychologists, speech pathologists, and nutritionists. Two prospective studies indicate better functional outcomes for stroke patients cared for in rehabilitation hospitals compared to nursing homes [23, 24]. Similarly, a recent meta-analysis of randomized trials of organized stroke units (including rehabilitation units) showed a reduction in mortality and improved functional outcome with organized stroke care compared to traditional care [25]. Characteristics differentiating organized care from traditional care included the presence of a coordinated, multidisciplinary rehabilitation team, staff education and training in stroke, specialization of the medical and surgical staff, and the availability of a geographically distinct ward [26].

Facilitation of motor recovery is a primary goal of stroke rehabilitation because motor function is one of the major determinants of independence in activities of daily living [22]. Conventional therapy aimed at decreasing disability after stroke traditionally relies on a variety of physical training techniques based on different philosophies including those that are designed to either provide optimal compensation for particular impairments (i.e. traditional approach [27]) or to specifically stimulate neurological recovery (i.e. neurodevelopmental technique [28], Brunnstrom approach [29], or integrated behavioral-physical therapy [30]). Although definitive evidence is lacking, regardless of the treatment methodology, stroke patients appear to benefit at least marginally from rehabilitation with physiotherapy [31].

Aphasia and dysarthria represent major potential stroke-related impairments as they can affect the most basic function that make us human, the ability to communicate. Similar to motor recovery, most aphasic stroke patients recover language ability, at least to some degree [32, 33]. As discussed below, speech pathologists have a major role in the assessment of poststroke dysphagia. In addition, speech therapy is commonly used to help improve communication in stroke patients with speech and language impairments. However, controlled data regarding the efficacy of these types of interventions are in conflict [34–36]. Regardless, formal attempts to improve language recovery and promote the use of compensatory strategies are undoubtedly of great psychological value.

Based on the rapidly expanding knowledge of the fundamental neurobiology underlying normal recovery, a variety of innovative approaches for the management of stroke patients are currently being explored. For example 'forced use' [37–39], sensory stimulation [40], biofeedback [41] and suspended gait training in nonambulatory patients [42] represent some of these novel strategies.

Recent laboratory studies suggest that certain drugs that influence the activities of specific central neurotransmitters may modulate the recovery process. These drug effects may potentially be either harmful and retard recovery or beneficial and facilitate the recovery process [43]. Determining whether the detrimental effects of drugs anticipated from laboratory studies also occurs in humans is difficult, but important since many of these medications are commonly given to patients recovering from stroke [44]. In a retrospective cohort study, the motor recoveries of stroke patients who received one or a combination of the antihypertensives clonidine and prazosin, dopamine receptor antagonists, benzodiazepines, or phenytoin (drugs that were anticipated to impair recovery based on the results of laboratory studies) were compared to the recoveries of a similar group of patients who were not given any of these medications [45]. Those that received these drugs had poorer recoveries than controls. Multivariate analysis indicated a significant effect of 'drug group' even after correcting for the contributions of other variables including the initial severity of the deficit. A similar effect was found in a separate cohort of patients with anterior circulation ischemic stroke [46]. The subjects were control patients enrolled in an acute interventional stroke trial. Nearly 40% received one or a combination of drugs hypothesized to impair recovery over the first 30 days after stroke. As with the previous study, stepwise multivariate analyses indicated that drug group had a negative effect on outcome independent of the degree of the initial motor impairment, comorbid conditions and other patient characteristics. However, because both studies involved retrospective analyses, it cannot be certain that the reason for the administration of a given drug rather than the drug itself influenced recovery. Further, the impact of specific 'detrimental' drugs, dose and timing effects could not be analyzed. Although overriding medical conditions often dictate the choice of specific medications, whenever possible, drugs suspected of having the potential to impair recovery should be avoided over the first several months after stroke.

Although only preliminary data based on small numbers of patients are available, new research suggests that other classes of drugs may enhance recovery. The most extensively studied drug with this potential is *d*-amphetamine. In one exploratory study, 8 patients with stable motor deficits were randomized to receive either a single dose of amphetamine or placebo within 10 days of carotid-distribution ischemic stroke [47]. Within 3 h of drug administration, all of the patients underwent intensive physical therapy. The following day, the patients' abilities to use their affected limbs were reassessed. Overall, the amphetamine-treated group had a significant improvement in motor performance while there was little change in the placebo-treated group. Although promising, not all of the patients had a 'dramatic' motor improvement, only very short-term motor recovery was measured, and because the patients were highly selected, the generalizability of the observations is uncertain. More recently, a placebo-controlled trial of the effects of amphetamine on motor recovery in rehabilitation patients was performed [48]. Patients treated with amphetamine had significantly greater improvements in motor scores compared to placebo-treated patients and the effect was maintained as long as 1 year after drug treatment was discontinued. While encouraging, issues related to drug dose and treatment windows need to be addressed and the results need to be replicated in a larger sample of patients. As there are limited available clinical data and there are potential side effects of amphetamines in stroke patients, at present this medication should not be used outside of a study setting.

Rehabilitation and Poststroke Complications

Medical Complications

Other major medical complications of stroke include aspiration pneumonia, deep vein thrombosis and pulmonary embolism, and urinary tract infection.

Aspiration pneumonia: Regardless of whether the stroke has affected the brainstem or cerebral hemispheres, stroke patients are at risk for aspiration pneumonia and generally not fed orally until aspiration risk is formally assessed [49–51]. Aspiration may occur in 25% of patients with hemispheric strokes and over 60% of patients with brainstem strokes [49]. Selective use of video-fluoroscopy can be helpful in identifying patients at risk for aspiration who do not have overt signs of dysphagia on clinical examination [52]. Speech pathologists can play a critical role in these evaluations. Aspiration can often be prevented through compensatory swallowing techniques and family education [53]. However, in patients with persistent aspiration risk, early gastrostomy may be superior to nasogastric tube feeding [54, 55]

Deep vein thrombosis: Immobilized stroke patients are at risk for deep vein thrombosis (DVT) which can occur in up to 75% of patients with a paralyzed leg [56]. Fatal pulmonary embolus can occur in 1–2% of those with a DVT. Antiembolism stockings are commonly prescribed, but their efficacy has not been proven. Intermittent pneumatic compression devices are a promising alternative [57]. Low-dose heparin (5,000 units administered subcutaneously twice daily) is the most commonly used medical therapy to prevent DVT. Although more costly, low-molecular-weight heparins or heparinoids may be used increasingly in the future [58].

Urinary tract infection: Urinary tract infection may occur in more than 15% of stroke patients. Early removal of indwelling bladder catheters may significantly reduce the risk. Intermittent catheterization should be considered for patients with persistent incontinence.

Fever: Laboratory data show that the amount of ischemic injury is influenced by brain temperature [59]. Even small increases in temperature may significantly increase the amount of ischemic damage [60]. Therefore, fever is treated aggressively with antipyretics while definitive therapy (i.e. antibiotics for aspiration pneumonia, urinary tract infections, etc.) is provided [61].

Depression

Clinical depression is associated with impaired recovery after stroke in humans [62]. Tricyclic antidepressants are commonly used to treat mood disorders in stroke patients. These drugs may not only have effects on the mood disorder, but through modulating the levels of central neurotransmitters, they may influence the recovery process. For example, trazodone was found to improve outcome as measured with the Barthel Index in depressed stroke patients [63]. Other clinical studies have found a beneficial effect of the serotonin reuptake blocker fluoxetine [64] and no significant effect of the norepinephrine reuptake blockers maprotiline [64] and nortriptyline [65]. However, the available data remain preliminary and larger-scale trials will be needed to determine the relative benefits of different classes of antidepressant medications.

Lethargy

Nonspecific stimulant medications including methylphenidate have been used in cognitively impaired brain-injured patients for many years to improve their capacity to participate in physical therapy. The drug has also been used in the treatment of poststroke depression in patients undergoing rehabilitative therapy [66–68]. However, only limited data are available concerning the drug's impact on neurological impairments [69]. One study did not find any effect of the drug on physical performance despite significant effects on cardiovascular function [69]. Therefore, there remains no clear evidence that the use of methylphenidate or other nonspecific stimulants improves outcome when given to patients during the course of rehabilitation.

Delivery of Rehabilitative Services

Poststroke rehabilitative services may be offered in a variety of settings. Over 70% of stroke survivors receive either postacute institutional or ambulatory rehabilitation care during the first 6 months after stroke [70]. Long-term ambulatory care and nursing home costs account for over 50% of the lifetime cost associated with stroke [70]. Overall in the United States, nearly one-third of rehabilitation services over the first 6 months after stroke are provided in institutional rehabilitation hospitals, about 25% in skilled nursing facilities, 16% in

Table 1. Unadjusted and adjusted risk ratios for the use of inpatient physical and occupation therapy between Blacks and Whites [75]

	Relative risk	95% confidence interval	p
Unadjusted	1.11	0.93–1.33	0.22
Adjusted	1.06	0.89–1.27	0.42

acute care hospitals, and 11% through home health agencies [70]. The setting of care should be influenced by a variety of factors including the patient's deficits, capacity to participate in rehabilitative therapy, and potential home support. However, there are wide variations across the United States in the use of specific rehabilitation services [70]. For example, the percentage of stroke survivors admitted to a rehabilitation hospital varies from 10% in Tampa-St. Petersburg to 31% in Houston. Use of a skilled nursing facility varies from 14% in Newark to 41% in Minneapolis-St. Paul. The percentage that receive home health services varies from 19% in Minneapolis-St. Paul to 57% in Miami. Urban-rural differences are also significant. Stroke patients living in rural areas are 25% less likely to be admitted to a rehabilitation hospital, 10% less likely to receive home health services, and 41% less likely to receive rehabilitation services from independent providers than those residing in urban areas [70]. Therefore, where a patient resides may be as important as clinical and social factors in determining what rehabilitative services the patient receives.

Use of Rehabilitation Services by Blacks

Some variation in the use of rehabilitative services in Blacks as compared to other ethnic groups might be expected based on geographically based differences in population demographics. Further, Blacks can have more severe residual motor impairments and worse functional status from stroke than Whites [71, 72]. Two reports found no racial differences in the utilization of rehabilitation services, but did not adjust the analyses for stroke severity [73, 74]. Given greater stroke severity in Blacks, Blacks might be relatively underutilizing rehabilitation services relative to Whites. A more recent study [75] adjusted for patient characteristics associated with the use of physical and occupational therapy and found no racial differences in the likelihood of use of inpatient rehabilitative services. Without adjusting for important clinical indicators, relatively more Blacks than Whites received these services (66% of Blacks vs. 56% of Whites, p < 0.01). Table 1 gives the unadjusted and adjusted risk ratios for the use of inpatient physical and occupational therapy. There were also no differences between Blacks and Whites in the time to initiation of physical and occupational therapy, or overall number of days of rehabilitation as a proportion of hospital stay. This study was limited to Medicare recipients and did not address the use of posthospitalization services. Although differences in the use of rehabilitation services by Blacks and Whites may exist based on geographic and other demographic factors, there is no evidence for systematic differences in the utilization of these services based on the currently available data.

Conclusion

Rehabilitation remains a critical part of the care of stroke patients. Two primary goals of therapy during the poststroke recovery period are to avoid and treat medical complications and improve functional recovery. New therapeutic modalities aimed at speeding poststroke recovery are being developed and the theoretical effects of drugs on the recovery process should be recognized. There are significant variations across the country in the utilization of rehabilitation services. However, there are no data suggesting a differential use of rehabilitation services between Blacks and Whites. Whether there are differences in the relative efficacy of rehabilitation interventions between Blacks and Whites remains a topic for study.

References

1   International Classification of Impairments, Disabilities and Handicaps. Geneva, World Health Organization, 1980.
2   Brott T, Adams HP Jr, Olinger CP, Marler JR, Barsan WG, Biller J, Spilker J, Holleran R, Eberle R, Hertzberg V, Rorick M, Moomaw CJ, Walker M: Measurements of acute cerebral infarction: A clinical examination scale. Stroke 1989;20:864–870.
3   Lyden P, Brott T, Tilley B, Welch KMA, Mascha EJ, Levine S, Haley EC, Grotta J, Marler J, NINDS TPA Stroke Study Group: Improved reliability of the NIH Stroke Scale using video training. Stroke 1994;25:2220–2226.
4   Hantson L, De Weerdt W, De Keyser J, Diener HC, Franke C, Palm R, Van Orshoven M, Schoonderwalt H, De Klippel N, Herroelen L, Feys H: The European Stroke Scale. Stroke 1994;25:2215–2219.
5   Cote R, Battista RN, Wolfson C, Boucher J, Adams J, Hachinski VC: The Canadian Neurological Scale: Validation and reliability assessment. Neurology 1989;39:638–643.
6   Post-Stroke Rehabilitation Guidelines Panel: Post-Stroke Rehabilitation. Rockville, Agency for Health Care Policy Research, 1995.
7   Granger CV, Dewis LS, Peters NC, Sherwood CC, Barrett JE: Stroke rehabilitation: Analysis of repeated Barthel Index measures. Arch Phys Med Rehabil 1979;60:14–17.
8   Chong DK-H: Measurement of instrumental activities of daily living in stroke. Stroke 1995;26:1119–1122.

9   Data Management Service of the Uniform Data System for Medical Rehabilitation: Guide for the Use of the Uniform Data Set for Medical Rehabilitation. Buffalo, Research Foundation – State University of New York, 1990.

10   Rankin J: Cerebral vascular accidents in patients over the age of 60. II. Prognosis. Scott Med J 1957;2:200–215.

11   De Haan R, Limburg M, Bossuyt P, Van Der Meulen J, Aaronson N: The clinical meaning of Rankin 'handicap' grades after stroke. Stroke 1995;26:2027–2030.

12   Wolfe CDA, Taub NA, Woodrow EJ, Burney PGJ: Assessment of scales of disability and handicap for stroke patients. Stroke 1991;22:1242–1244.

13   De Haan R, Horn J, Limburg M, Van Der Meulen J, Bossuyt P: A comparison of five stroke scales with measures of disability, handicap, and quality of life. Stroke 1993;24:1178–1181.

14   Whiteneck GG, Charlifue SW, Gerhart KA, Overholser JD, Richardson GN: Quantifying handicap: A new measure of long-term rehabilitation outcomes. Arch Phys Med Rehabil 1992;73:519–525.

15   Mathias SD, Bates MM, Pasta DJ, Cisternas MG, Feeny D, Patrick DL: Use of the health utilities index with stroke patients and their caregivers. Stroke 1997;28:1888–1894.

16   Bergner M, Bobbitt RA, Carter WB, Gilson BS: The Sickness Impact Profile: Development and final revision of a health status measure. Med Care 1981;19:787–805.

17   De Haan R, Limburg M: The relationship between impairment and functional health scales in the outcome of stroke. Cerebrovasc Dis 1994;4(suppl 2):19–23.

18   Duncan PW, Goldstein LB, Matchar D, Divine GW, Feussner J: Measurement of motor recovery after stroke. Outcome assessment and sample size requirements. Stroke 1992;23:1084–1089.

19   Wade DT, Wood VA, Hewer RL: Recovery after stroke – The first three months. J Neurol Neurosurg Psychiatry 1985;48:7–13.

20   Fullerton KJ, Mackenzie G, Stout RW: Prognostic indicies in stroke. Q J Med 1988;66:147–162.

21   Oxbury JM, Greenhall RCD, Grainger KMR: Predicting the outcome of stroke: Acute stage after cerebral infarction. Br Med J 1975;iii:125–127.

22   Lincoln NB, Blackburn M, Ellis S, Jackson J, Edmans JA, Nouri FM, Walrer MF, Haworth H: An investigation of factors affecting progress of patients on a stroke unit. J Neurol Neurosurg Psychiatry 1989;52:493–496.

23   Kane RL, Chen Q, Blewett LA, Sangl J: Do rehabilitative nursing homes inprove the outcomes of care? J Am Geriatr Soc 1996;44:545–554.

24   Kramer AM, Steiner JF, Schlenker RE, Eilertsen TB, Hrincevich CA, Tropea DA, Ahmad LA, Eckhoff DG: Outcomes and costs after hip fracture and stroke – A comparison of rehabilitation settings. JAMA 1997;277:396–404.

25   Ottenbacher KJ, Jannell S: The results of clinical trials in stroke rehabilitation research. Arch Neurol 1993;50:37–44.

26   Stroke Unit Trialists' Collaboration: Collaborative systematic review of the randomised trials of organised inpatient (stroke unit) care after stroke. BMJ 1997;314:1151–1159.

27   Wescott EJ: Traditional exercise regimens for the hemiplegic patient. Am J Phys Med 1967;46:1012–1023.

28   Bobath B: Adult Hemiplegia: Evaluation and Treatment. London, Heinemann Medical, 1984.

29   Brunnstrom S: Movement Therapy in Hemiplegia. A Neurophysiological Approach. New York, Harper & Row, 1970.

30   Basmajian JV, Gowland CA, Finlayson AJ, Hall AL, Swanson LR, Stratford PW, Trotter JE, Brandstater ME: Stroke treatment: Comparison of integrated behavioral-physical therapy vs traditional physical therapy programs. Arch Phys Med Rehabil 1987;68:267–272.

31   Ernst E: A review of stroke rehabilitation and physiotherapy. Stroke 1990;21:1081–1085.

32   Lomas J, Kertesz A: Patterns of spontaneous recovery in aphasic groups: A study in adult stroke patients. Brain Lang 1978;5:388–401.

33   Kertesz A, McCabe P: Recovery patterns and prognosis in aphasia. Brain 1977;100:1–18.

34   Basso A, Capitani E, Vignolo LA: Influence of rehabilitation on language skills in aphasic patients. A controlled study. Arch Neurol 1979;36:190–196.

35   Holland A, Wertz R: Measuring aphasia treatment effects: Large-group, small-group, and single-subject studies. Res Publ Assoc Res Nerv Ment Dis 1988;66:267–273.

36 Lincoln NB, McGuirk E, Mulley GP, Lendrem W, Jones AC, Mitchell JRA: The effectiveness of speech therapy for aphasic stroke patients. A randomized controlled trial. Lancet 1984;i:1187–1200.

37 Wolf SL, Lecraw DE, Barton LA, Jann BB: Forced use of hemiplegic upper extremities to reverse the effect of learned nonuse among chronic stroke and head-injured patients. Exp Neurol 1989;104: 125–132.

38 Taub E, Crago JE, Burgio LD, Groomes TE, Cook EW III, DeLuca SC, Miller NE: An operant approach to rehabilitation medicine: Overcoming learned nonuse by shaping. J Exp Anal Behav 1994;61:281–293.

39 Taub E, Miller NE, Novack TA, Cook EW III, Fleming WC, Nepomuceno CS, Connell JS, Crago JE: Technique to improve chronic motor deficit after stroke. Arch Phys Med Rehabil 1993;74:347–354.

40 Johansson K, Lindgren I, Widner H, Wiklund I, Johansson BB: Can sensory stimulation improve the functional outcome in stroke patients? Neurology 1993;43:2189–2192.

41 Wolf SL, Binder-Macleod SA: Electromyographic biofeedback applications to the hemiplegic patient. Phys Ther 1983;63:1393–1403.

42 Hesse S, Bertelt C, Jahnke MT, Schaffrin A, Baake P, Malezic M, Mauritz KH: Treadmill training with partial body weight support compared with physiotherapy in nonambulatory hemiparetic patients. Stroke 1995;26:976–981.

43 Goldstein LB, Davis JN: Restorative neurology: Drugs and recovery following stroke. Curr Concepts Cerebrovasc Dis 1990;25:1–6.

44 Goldstein LB, Davis JN: Physician prescribing patterns after ischemic stroke. Neurology 1988;38: 1806–1809.

45 Goldstein LB, Matchar DB, Morgenlander JC, Davis JN: Influence of drugs on the recovery of sensorimotor function after stroke. J Neurorehabil 1990;4:137–144.

46 Goldstein LB, Sygen in Acute Stroke Study Investigators: Common drugs may influence motor recovery after stroke. Neurology 1995;45:865–871.

47 Crisostomo EA, Duncan PW, Propst MA, Dawson DB, Davis JN: Evidence that amphetamine with physical therapy promotes recovery of motor function in stroke patients. Ann Neurol 1988;23:94–97.

48 Walker-Batson D, Smith P, Curtis S, Unwin H, Greenlee R: Amphetamine paired with physical therapy accelerates motor recovery after stroke – Further evidence. Stroke 1995;26:2254–2259.

49 Horner J, Massey EW, Riski JE, Lathrop DL, Chase KN: Aspiration following stroke: Clinical correlates and outcome. Neurology 1988;38:1359–1362.

50 DePippo KL, Holas MA, Reding MJ: Validation of the 3-oz water swallow test for aspiration following stroke. Arch Neurol 1992;49:1259–1261.

51 Smithard DG, O'Neill PA, Park C, Morris J, Wyatt R, England R, Martin DF: Complications and outcome after acute stroke – Does dysphagia matter? Stroke 1996;27:1200–1204.

52 Kidd D, Lawson J, Nesbitt R, MacMahon J: Aspiration in acute stroke: A clinical study with videofluoroscopy. Q J Med 1993;86:825–829.

53 Goldstein LB, Duncan PW, SASS Investigators: Disparity between disability and motor recovery after stroke. J Stroke Cerebrovasc Dis 1995;5:103.

54 Norton B, Homer-Ward M, Donnelly MT, Long RG, Holmes GKT: A randomised prospective comparison of percutaneous endoscopic gastrostomy and nasogastric tube feeding after acute dysphagic stroke. BMJ 1996;312:13–16.

55 Allison MC, Morris AJ, Park RHR, Mills PR: Percutaneous endoscopic gastrostomy tube feeding may improve outcome of late rehabilitation following stroke. J R Soc Med 1992;85:147–149.

56 Brown M, Glassenberg M: Mortality factors in patients with acute stroke. JAMA 1973;224:1493–1495.

57 Turpie AG, Hirsh J, Gent M, Julian D, Johnson J: Prevention of deep vein thrombosis in potential neurosurgical patients. A randomized trial comparing graduated compression stockings alone or graduated compression stockings plus intermittent pneumatic compression with control. Arch Intern Med 1989;149:679–681.

58 Turpie AG, Gent M, Cote R, Levine MN, Ginsberg JS, Powers PJ, Leclerc J, Geerts W, Jay R, Neemeh J, Klimek M, Hirsh J: A low-molecular-weight heparinoid compared with unfractionated heparin in the prevention of deep vein thrombosis in patients with acute ischemic stroke. A randomized, double-blind study. Ann Intern Med 1992;117:353–357.

59   Busto R, Dietrich WD, Globus MY-T, Ginsberg MD: The importance of brain temperature in cerebral ischemic injury. Stroke 1989;20:1113–1114.

60   Busto R, Dietrich WD, Globus MY-T, Valdes I, Scheinberg P, Ginsberg MD: Small differences in intraischemic brain temperature critically determine the extent of ischemic neuronal injury. J Cereb Blood Flow Metab 1987;7:729–738.

61   Adams HP Jr, Brott TG, Crowell RM, Furlan AJ, Gomez CR, Grotta J, Helgason CM, Marler JR, Woolson RF, Zivin JA, Feinberg W, Mayberg M: Guidelines for the management of patients with acute ischemic stroke. Stroke 1994;25:1901–1914.

62   Morris PLP, Raphael B, Robinson RG: Clinical depression is associated with impaired recovery from stroke. Med J Aust 1992;157:239–242.

63   Reding MJ, Orto LA, Winter SW, Fortuna IM, Di Ponte P, McDowell FH: Antidepressant therapy after stroke. A double-blind trial. Arch Neurol 1986;43:763–765.

64   Dam M, Tonin P, De Boni A, Pizzolato G, Casson S, Ermani M, Freo U, Piron L, Battistin L: Effects of fluoxetine and maprotiline on functional recovery in poststroke hemiplegic patients undergoing rehabilitation therapy. Stroke 1996;27:1211–1214.

65   Lipsey JR, Pearlson GD, Robinson RG, Rao K, Price TR: Nortriptyline treatment of post-stroke depression: A double-blind study. Lancet 1984;i:297–300.

66   Johnson ML, Roberts MD, Ross AR, Witten CM: Methylphenidate in stroke patients with depression. Am J Phys Med Rehabil 1992;71:239–241.

67   Lazarus LW, Moberg PJ, Langsley PR, Lingam VR: Methylphenidate and nortriptyline in the treatment of poststroke depression: A retrospective comparison. Arch Phys Med Rehabil 1994;75: 403–406.

68   Lazarus LW, Winemiller DR, Lingam VR, Neyman I, Hartman C, Abassian M, Kartan U, Groves L, Fawcett J: Efficacy and side effects of methylphenidate for poststroke depression. J Clin Psychiatry 1992;53:447–449.

69   Larsson M, Ervik M, Lundborg P, Sundh V, Svanborg A: Comparison between methylphenidate and placebo as adjuvant in care and rehabilitation of geriatric patients. Comp Gerontol 1988;2: 53–59.

70   Lee AJ, Huber J, Stason WB: Poststroke rehabilitation in older Americans. The Medicare experience. Med Care 1996;34:811–825.

71   Horner RD, Matchar DB, Divine GW, Feussner JR: Racial variations in ischemic stroke-related physical and functional impairments. Stroke 1991;22:1497–1501.

72   Sacco RL, Hauser WA, Mohr JP, Foulkes MA: One-year outcome after cerebral infarction in Whites, Blacks, and Hispanics. Stroke 1991;22:305–311.

73   McElligott JM, Dolezal J, Hamilton J: Stroke, racial variations, and effective inpatient rehabilitation in a rural setting. Arch Phys Med Rehabil 1993;74:1278.

74   Kuhlemeier KV, Steins SA: Rehabilitation after stroke: Gender and racial disparities? Arch Phys Med Rehabil 1991;72:840–841.

75   Horner RD, Hoenig H, Sloane R, Rubenstein LV, Kahn KL: Racial differences in the utilization of inpatient rehabilitation services among elderly stroke patients. Stroke 1997;28:19–25.

Larry B. Goldstein, MD, Director, Duke Center for Cerebrovascular Disease,
Head, Stroke Policy Program, Center for Clinical Health Policy Research, Box 3651,
Duke University Medical Center, Durham, NC 27710 (USA)

Gillum RF, Gorelick PB, Cooper ES (eds): Stroke in Blacks. Basel, Karger, 1999, pp 210–216

....

Practical Guidelines for Diagnosis and Management of Stroke in Blacks in the Primary Care Setting

Louis R. Caplan[a], *Edward S. Cooper*[b], *Michael A. Kelly*[c]

[a] Department of Neurology, New England Medical Center, Boston, Mass.;
[b] University of Pennsylvania School of Medicine, Philadelphia, Pa.; and
[c] Rush Medical College, Chair, Division of Neurology, Cook County Hospital, Chicago, Ill., USA

Cerebrovascular disease, like vascular disease in the rest of the body, is a chronic disorder that evolves over years and decades. Cerebrovascular disease is an especially serious health problem among Blacks. Ample data cited in early chapters of this book document that Black populations suffer more morbidity and mortality from stroke than comparable White populations. The most important and most effective action that can be taken against this destroyer of minds and body functions is clearly *prevention*.

Overview

Cerebrovascular disease and strokes in Blacks share many features with strokes in Whites, Asians, and other racial and ethnic groups but there are differences. The major differences are:

(1) Hypertension is a critically important risk factor in Blacks: (a) Poorly controlled hypertension accounts for the higher frequency of lacunar infarcts due to penetrating artery disease and hypertensive intracerebral hemorrhage in Blacks. (b) Recognition and treatment of hypertension in Blacks is often suboptimal for a host of psycho-socioeconomic reasons. (c) Chronic poorly controlled hypertension contributes to the development of chronic microvascular changes in the subcortical nuclei and white matter causing vascular dementia. Dementia accompanied by abnormal motor and sensory functions is

relatively more common in Blacks as compared to Whites. Vascular dementia may be more frequent in Blacks than Alzheimer's disease, while the opposite is true in Whites.

(2) The distribution of cerebrovascular disease varies by race: (a) Blacks, especially Black women, have a lower frequency of extracranial severe arterial occlusive disease involving the most proximal portions of the internal carotid and vertebral arteries in the neck than Whites of comparable age. (b) Blacks have a higher frequency of severe intracranial artery occlusive disease involving the anterior, middle and posterior cerebral arteries and intracranial vertebral and distal basilar arteries than Whites of comparable age.

The remainder of this chapter will elaborate further on these differences and their consequences for the diagnosis and management of cerebrovascular disease in Blacks. Special socioeconomic considerations will also be discussed.

Diagnostic Workup

Knowledge of the distribution of occlusive vascular disease in Blacks is important because different strategies of testing are required to demonstrate intracranial and extracranial disease. Screening for extracranial disease involving the cervical portion of the internal carotid and vertebral arteries is best done with Duplex ultrasound scans (combined B-mode and Doppler ultrasound) of the neck arteries. Images of the neck arteries can also be obtained noninvasively by magnetic resonance angiography (MRA). In this technique, moving blood creates an image of the arteries. The neck arteries are usually imaged using a neck coil separate from that used for cranial magnetic resonance imaging (MRI). Contrast can be given during computerized tomography (CT) examinations of the brain with films taken of the neck arteries – CT angiography (CTA). These three tests – CTA, MRA and Duplex ultrasound – are very effective screening tests for severe extracranial stenosis or occlusion of the vertebral arteries. When imaging of the proximal vertebral arteries is desired, the ordering clinician must alert the physician supervising the MRA or CTA to obtain films of the brachiocephalic arteries at the aortic arch since the disease in the vertebral arteries is lower in the neck than that in the internal carotid artery.

Although less common than Whites, some Blacks do have occlusive disease of the extracranial carotid and vertebral arteries. Clues to this are: (1) the presence of hypercholesterolemia; (2) the coexistence of coronary artery disease-related findings – angina pectoris or myocardial infarction and/or claudication of the lower extremities; (3) the presence of bruits over the carotid arteries in the neck, and (4) transient monocular visual loss.

Intracranial artery occlusive disease in the larger arteries outside of the brain but inside of the skull and in the branch arteries that penetrate into the brain are more common in Black populations than in comparable White populations. Asians also have a high prevalence of intracranial artery disease. Different testing strategies are used to image and quantify vascular disease inside the skull. MRA is an excellent screening tool for recognition of narrowing of the middle, posterior, and proximal anterior cerebral arteries. The basilar artery is especially well shown by MRA. Unfortunately, in many cranial MRA films the imaging is cut off so that the beginning portions of the intracranial vertebral arteries are not included on the films. If these arteries are of interest in the patient being studied, the ordering clinician should specifically request attention to the entire intracranial vertebral arteries. CTA is also helpful. However, CTA is best at imaging a specific artery or region of an artery that is of clinical interest. For example, in a Black woman who has repeated episodes of abnormal speech and numbness and weakness of her right arm and who has an infarct in her left basal ganglia region, the artery of interest is the left intracranial internal carotid artery and its middle cerebral artery branch. CTA focused on these arteries can be quite useful.

Transcranial Doppler (TCD) ultrasound is a relatively new noninvasive test that is very helpful in screening for intracranial occlusive disease and for monitoring intracranial disease once it is recognized. Ultrasound is a very important diagnostic tool that has a number of advantages. Machines are portable. Testing is safe and without risks. Ultrasound testing can be repeated to show changes in narrowed or blocked arteries. In some centers ultrasound equipment is available at the bedside and is used by physicians to extend the vascular physical examination much as ultrasound is now used by nurses and doctors in intensive care units to monitor peripheral vessels.

Intracranial arteries are insonated using a small probe placed at regions of the skull where there are foramina or natural soft spots. The usual windows are the orbit, foramen magnum, and temporal bone. TCD probes are placed perpendicular to arteries, for example, the middle cerebral arteries, while the technician or physician performing the test listens for the characteristic pulsatile swooshing sound that shows that the probe is in the correct position. The computer allows the person performing the TCD examination to view the Doppler spectrum at successive 5-mm depths along the insonated artery. TCD measures blood flow velocity, direction and pulsatility along insonated arteries.

Most people have had the experience of trying to wash a pavement of a patio with a garden hose. When the spigot is turned fully on and the nozzle is fully open, a broad stream of water issues from the hose. When the nozzle of the hose is turned, a stronger, more targeted water spray is generated.

Turning the nozzle reduces the size of the lumen at the end of the hose. The velocity of flow in the water jet is inversely proportional to the luminal size until a critical luminal size is reached at which time flow is reduced. If the nozzle is turned fully, then water stops flowing or dribbles out the end of the hose. Similarly, if an insonated artery is stenotic, then the blood flow velocities are increased at the site of narrowing. TCD would measure and record the localized increased velocity. If the artery is blocked by an embolus or by a thrombus that has formed locally, engrafted on a region of atherosclerotic stenosis, then no or very low signals are obtained.

In a patient with a right middle cerebral artery (MCA) territory stroke, the absence of Doppler signals over the right MCA, when left MCA signals are normal, is strongly suggestive of right MCA occlusion. Subsequent appearance of signals in the right MCA, when TCD is repeated hours or days later, shows that the obstruction has moved along or passed. Similarly, much higher blood flow velocities in the right MCA as compared with the left MCA, or higher velocities in the right vertebral artery compared to the left, indicate stenosis of these intracranial arteries. Unfortunately, in some patients, especially older women, it is not possible to obtain signals from the MCAs because of the lack of a suitable temporal window. The intracranial vertebral arteries (ICVAs) can be insonated well through the foramen magnum. Using a combination of TCD and either CTA or MRA along with a brain imaging test CT or MRI, usually allows recognition of the presence, location, and severity of brain infarction and of any important severe intracranial artery occlusive disease.

Because of the complexity of clinical workup and the issues of cost-effectiveness, good practice is to obtain a neurological consultation for all stroke and TIA (transient ischemic attack) patients. However, the need for neurological consultation is more urgent when the use of thrombolytic therapy is contemplated, if there is doubt concerning the diagnosis of stroke or TIA, when no obvious stroke risk factor is present especially in the young, when study results are ambiguous, if neurological symptoms and clinical signs do not correlate well, and for other purposes such as patient and family reassurance.

Treatment

Treatment of intracranial occlusive disease may differ in Blacks compared to Whites although this has not been formally studied. Studies of the antiplatelet agent ticlopidine suggest the possibility of greater benefit in stroke prevention in Blacks, a hypothesis currently in trial. Blacks seem to have less TIAs and seem to respond less well to warfarin anticoagulation than Whites with comparable intracranial occlusive disease. Brain ischemia in Blacks might be caused more by flow-limiting narrowing of intracranial arteries caused by hypertrophy of the medial smooth muscle and connective tissue than by embolization of white or red clots that form on irregular plaques in relation to the arterial intima. Strategies to treat flow reduction include elevation of blood volume and surgery or angioplasty to dilate the arteries. Anticoagulants are effective in preventing thrombi but do not increase blood flow.

Finally, the dangers of uncontrolled hypertension hover over the entire clinical process of stroke management and prevention, especially in Blacks. Hypertension remains by far the major risk factor for stroke in Blacks (see pp. 83–93, 118–128, 142–155, 180–187); since 85% of stroke cases are seen in the >65-year-old population, substance abuse and sickle cell anemia in the young, for example, are relatively uncommon, though tragic causes of stroke. Furthermore, the rigorous control of hypertension is mandatory in the protocol for the use of thrombolytic therapy in acute ischemic stroke. Moreover, the greatest progress in stroke prevention, both primary and secondary, can be achieved by increasing the percentage of adequately controlled hypertension rates in our population from the present levels of 25–30% to a desired level of greater than 50% and upwards. This is not to denigrate the potential added benefits to be achieved by reduction of elevated cholesterol levels and heart disease rates; avoidance of tobacco use especially in Black men and now adolescents; as well as reversal of the rising obesity and diabetes rates, particularly in the Black women.

Other Practical Considerations

Kenton [9] has reviewed many of the subtle and not so subtle obstructions to the availability and utilization of quality neurologic services for African-American patients. These are particularly notable for those of low socioeconomic status. Many of these same difficulties are experienced by indigent Black patients in Africa, the Caribbean and other areas of the world. Table 1 summarizes many of the special concerns of African-American patients and health care providers. In addition to economic factors, there are cultural barriers, communication delays, (unfamiliar) inner city mores, poor compliance, residual racism and other social issues that arise. Primary physicians especially must be aware of the above limitations. They should serve as the health advocates and advisors for stroke and stroke-prone patients. The prescribed neurological evaluation and treatment processes are often complex

Table 1. Stroke in Blacks – key factors of concern for primary care

1. Prevalence and mortality rates of stroke are increased in African-Americans
2. High uninsured rates impede prevention and care
3. Aggressive detection, management and follow-up of hypertension is critical
4. Most African-Americans depend upon non-Black physicians for health care
5. Culturally sensitive health providers should be patient advocates
6. Strengthened stroke education programs are needed
7. Poverty, misinformation, cultural barriers, decreased compliance, residual racism and decreased personalized care are all access problems
8. More stroke research should be a high priority
9. Needed are more medical providers trained from underserved populations
10. Increased office paper work, increased bureaucratic delays and increased economic retrenchment disproportionately harm Blacks

and frightening to patients. The health care providers must be culturally sensitive and use affirmative techniques to reach many African-American patients who often feel lonely and vulnerable in the increasingly highly organized and impersonal health system. A smile, kind word or brief discussion of a subject of mutual interest (sports, weather, etc.) will often relax the patient, establish rapport quickly, improve compliance, facilitate family support and even help prevent future litigation.

Conclusion

The primary practitioner is a key link in the health care system for stroke and stroke-prone Black patients. The practitioner must understand the salient importance of hypertension control in the prevention of stroke in African-Americans as well as the aggravating role of other risk factors. Blacks also may have a higher frequency of severe intracranial artery occlusive disease and lower frequency of severe extracranial arterial occlusive disease which modify to some extent the diagnostic workup and treatment.

Strengthened education programs are required for the public (and health care providers) regarding stroke risk factors and early warning signs. The underserved must benefit from the new nationwide stroke control initiatives. There is an urgent need for improved access to and utilization of quality health services, as well as for additional culturally sensitive practitioners to serve as patients' advocates.

References

1   Caplan LR: Stroke, A Clinical Approach, ed 2. Boston, Butterworth-Heinemann, 1993.
2   Caplan LR: Posterior Circulation Disease: Clinical Findings, Diagnosis and Management. Boston, Blackwell Science, 1996.
3   Gorelick PB, Leurgens S, Richardson D, Harris M, Billingsley M, AAASPS Investigators: African-American Antiplatelet Stroke Prevention Study (AAASPS): Clinical trial design. J Stroke Cerebrovasc Dis 1998.
4   Johnson BA, Heiserman JE, Drayer BP, Keller PJ: Intracranial MR angiography: Its role in the integrated approach to brain infarction. AJNR Am J Neuroradiol 1994;15:901–908.
5   Ruggieri PM, Masaryk TJ, Ross JS: Magnetic resonance angiography. Cerebrovascular applications. Stroke 1992;23:774–780.
6   Wong KS, Liang EY, Lam WW, Huang YN, Kay R: Spiral computed tomography angiography in the assessment of middle cerebral artery occlusive disease. J Neurol Neurosurg Psychiatry 1995;59: 537–539.
7   Alberico RA, Patel M, Casey S, Jacobs B, Maguire W, Decker R: Evaluation of the circle of Willis with three-dimensional CT angiography in patients with suspected intracranial aneurysms. AJNR Am J Neuroradiol 1995;16:1571–1578.
8   Wong KS, Lam WW, Liang E, Huang YN, Chan YL, Kay R: Variability of magnetic resonance angiography and computed tomography angiography in grading middle cerebral artery stenosis. Stroke 1996;27:1084–1087.
9   Kenton EJ: Access to neurological care for minorities. Arch Neurol 1991;48:480–483.

Louis R. Caplan, MD, Professor and Chair, Department of Neurology,
New England Medical Center, 750 Washington Street, Boston, MA 02111 (USA)

Gillum RF, Gorelick PB, Cooper ES (eds): Stroke in Blacks. Basel, Karger, 1999, pp 217–224

....

Future Research Directions

Toni P. Miles[a], *Gloria Bonner*[b], *Yvonne Harris*[c]

[a] University of Texas Health Science Center at San Antonio, Tex.;
[b] University of Illinois, Chicago, Ill., and
[c] Rush-Presbyterian St. Luke's Medical Center, Chicago, Ill., USA

Stroke and stroke-related morbidity are a primary public health concern for African-Americans. The high prevalence rates of risk factors for cardiovascular disease (e.g. hypertension, obesity, and low physical activity) combined with the growth of the population of persons aged 55 and older suggest that the importance of stroke-related research will increase in the future. Medical management of stroke has evolved over the past 20 years. Persons with stroke are more likely to survive the initial event and less likely to be admitted to the hospital. Those who are admitted have on average a shorter length of stay. For example, Black men aged 65–74 years had a length of stay of 19 days in 1981; by 1987 it had declined to 10.8 days [1]. There are no population-level data measuring the postdischarge or long-term functional status of these survivors.

These trends underscore the efficacy of and the need for more research to develop poststroke treatment to maximize recovery of function. Analyses involving cross-ethnic group comparison have failed to identify barriers to recovery of function that may be unique to African-Americans. To yield useful results, research questions must be framed such that population-specific concerns are identified. Identifying population-specific medical complications and treatments are important. Coverage by third-party payers (particularly Medicare and Medicaid) are based on demonstrated effectiveness. Evidence-based medicine and standards of clinical practice are increasingly derived from clinical trials. Standardized care will only work to the advantage of African-Americans if the clinical trials include sufficient numbers of participants so that safety and efficacy can be measured within the group. The only other formal mechanism for accumulating these data are reports of individual adverse events. Typically, adverse event monitoring is used to identify problems with new medications – not population-specific problems. Poststroke depression (PSD) is a complication of stroke that has received attention only in the larger clinical community [2]. In this chapter, as one of the topics for future research directions, we examine current work on PSD and its potential for being a population-specific concern as a complication of stroke.

Clinical studies in stroke prevention and treatment will require researchers to develop strategies that encourage African-Americans to enroll and remain in the trials. The factors underlying barriers to enrollment and continued participation in clinical trials are examined in this chapter. Participation in a study can be thought of as an agreement between the researchers and the subjects. Each brings a unique set of expectations to the process. To date, there have been no published reports describing the attributes of researchers who successfully recruit and retain African-Americans in their studies. Clearly, more research is needed in this area. On the other hand, there has been some work describing attributes of persons who refuse to participate in trials. In this chapter we discuss those papers and their implications for study design. A third area of discussion in this chapter will be the need for better delineation of specific risk factors for stroke among Black populations.

Depression and Stroke

Mood disorders are common after stroke and may impede physical, functional, and cognitive recovery, making early identification and treatment of potential importance. The emergence of depression appears to be a biological consequence of the stroke [2–5] and independent of the hemisphere involved [6]. The occurrence of depression after a stroke among African-Americans is a poorly documented phenomenon. If nursing home residents represent a small subset of persons with stroke and depression, then African-Americans with stroke who are newly admitted to nursing homes should be routinely evaluated and treated for depression after stroke. Among African-American nursing home residents aged 65 years and older, an estimated 65% have cognitive disabilities related to stroke [1]. In this same population of nursing home residents, an estimated 10.4% meet the relatively insensitive DSM-IV criteria for depression. Anxiety disorder may further complicate the association between stroke, PSD and the likelihood of recovery. In a study of older patients, anxiety disorder significantly interacted with depression to influence the severity and course of depression, outcome of activities of daily living, and social functioning [7]. Anxiety disorder, however, did not affect cognitive impairment, which was influenced only by major depression suggesting that the existence of anxiety disorder may play an important role in the prognosis of patients with PSD. This study and pharmacological therapy data also suggest that depression and anxiety disorder may have different mechanisms.

One barrier to detection of depression is the sensitivity of screening instruments currently in use. Findings from younger patients may not generalize to older persons, and existing studies of screening instruments in older patients may have substantial methodological limitations. The Structured Clinical Interview for the Diagnostic and Statistical Manual of Mental Disorders [8] was used as a 'gold standard' in a study of persons aged 60 years or older. Two screening scales were used for comparison: the Center for Epidemiological Studies-Depression Scale (CES-D) and the Geriatric Depression Scale (GDS) [9]. In this study, both the CES-D and the GDS had excellent properties in screening for major depression. The shorter version of the GDS was also found to be sensitive and specific for major depressive disorder. However, all scales lost accuracy when used to detect minor depression or the presence of any depressive diagnosis. Development and testing of screening instruments to detect PSD for African-Americans is an important area of future research.

Recruitment

Historically, African-Americans have had less access to and use of preventive, palliative, diagnostic, and treatment services from the medical community [10, 11]. African-Americans are underrepresented in clinical trials. The problem of underrepresentation in clinical trials has been reviewed by Svensson [12]. In trials that were published between 1984 and 1986, full racial disclosure data were available for only 35 of the 50 drug trials. Twenty-three of the 35 studies had a lower percentage of African-American participants than would be expected based on the proportion living in the communities where recruitment for the trials took place. There has been some increase in the participation of Blacks in clinical trials after 1989 (table 1). This increase may be due in part to a change in federal policy that mandates inclusion of minorities and women in federally funded research.

Recruitment and retention of study subjects are key to the success of a trial. For studies focused on Blacks, the historical alienation from the medical health care system creates a special challenge [11]. A number of barriers to participation in clinical trials have been identified, including mistrust, economic disadvantage, lack of awareness of existing trials, and social isolation [13].

Table 1. Recruitment data of clinical trials

Trial	Total number of patients recruited		% Black, n	Centers, n
TASS[1] (1989)	Ticlopidine	1,529	17 (257)	56
	Aspirin	1,540	15 (238)	
	Total	3,069	16 (495)	
CATS[2] (1989)	Ticlopidine	525	27 (142)	25
	Placebo	528	29 (153)	
	Total	1,053	28 (295) non-White	
NASCET[3] (1981)	Medical	331	4 (13)	50
70–99% stenosis	Surgical	328	2 (7)	
	Total	659	3 (20)	
NINDS rt-PA[4] (1995)	Part I	291	30 (87)	41
	Part II	333	24 (82)	
	Total	624	27 (169)	
ACAS[5] (1995)	Surgical	825	3 (25)	39
	Medical	834	2 (17)	
	Total	1,659	2 (41)	
CAPRIE[6] (1996)	Clopidogrel	3,233	9 (291)	384
Stroke Subgroup Only	Aspirin	3,198	9 (288)	
	Total	6,431	9 (579) non-White	
AAASPS[7] (4/16/98)		764	100 (764)	≤ 38

[1] Weisberg LA: The efficacy and safety of ticlopidine and aspirin in non-Whites: Analysis of a patient subgroup from the Ticlopidine Aspirin Stroke Study. Neurology 1993;43:27–31.
[2] Gent M, Easton JD, Hachinski VC, Panak E, Sicurella J, Blakely JA, Ellis DJ, Harbison JW, Roberts RS, Turple AGG, and the CATS Group: The Canadian-American Ticlopidine Study (CATS) in thromboembolic stroke. Lancet 1989;i:1215–1220.
[3] North American Symptomatic Carotid Endarterectomy Trail Collaborators: Beneficial effect of carotid endarterectomy in symptomatic patients with high-grade carotid stenosis. N Engl J Med 1991;325:445–463.
[4] The National Institute of Neurological Disorders and Stroke rt-PA Stroke Study Group: Tissue plasminogen activator for acute ischemic stroke. N Engl J Med 1995;333:1581–1587.
[5] Executive Committee for the Asymptomatic Carotid Atherosclerosis Study: Endarterectomy for asymptomatic carotid artery stenosis. JAMA 1995;273:1421–1428.
[6] CAPRIE Steering Committee: A randomised, blinded, trail of clopidogrel versus aspirin in patients at risk of ischaemic events (CAPRIE). Lancet 1996;348:1329–1339.
[7] Establishing a Community Network for Recruitment of African-Americans into a Clinical Trial: The African-American Antiplatelet Stroke Prevention Study (AAASPS) Experience. J Natl Med Assoc 1996;88:701–704.

Mistrust of the medical profession dates back to the antebellum South, where Blacks were victims of medical experimentation and demonstration practices that were often brutal and unethical [14]. The Tuskegee Syphilis Study, the most widely publicized of these studies, has been referred to as 'the longest running nontherapeutic experiment and known violation of human subjects' [15]. Although modern-day safeguards are in place to prevent this type of abuse, these may be insufficient to ease fears based on historical realities.

The challenge to researchers is to overcome these barriers to participation. This will require strategic planning that should include representation of Blacks at all levels of the trial – participants, staff and researchers. To obtain optimal participation, the targeted program should be presented as a credible initiative, designed to address a concern of personal interest to Blacks. Design and implementation of these trials work best when there is bidirectional education between researchers and the community throughout its conduct [16]. Successful recruitment and retention of Blacks in trials is dependent upon community acceptance, which may be most effectively established in the preprogram planning stages of an initiative. This concept of obtaining community approval and acceptance prior to set-up is not new, and does not apply exclusively to the African-American community.

Retention and Culture

Retention of persons for longitudinal studies presents a special challenge to researchers. Sometimes, the process necessary to collect data acceptable to the scientific community requires the use of procedures that are viewed as unacceptable to the lay community. In this section, we examine one potentially offensive procedure: request for autopsy. The ability to link pathological changes with measured behavior is a 'Holy Grail' in dementia research. Obtaining brains for autopsy study requires advance permission from participants and their families as well as notification within hours of the death. Distinguishing vascular dementia from other forms requires autopsy examination. Autopsy is a traditional method used by the clinical community to identify causal factors in illness and mortality. There has been an overall decline of autopsies conducted and examination rates are even lower among African-Americans, 8% among older Whites compared to 4% among older Blacks [17–19]. Autopsy requests by researchers can be a barrier to continued participation. Data on preferences surrounding autopsy examination among African-Americans is particularly scarce. In a study of 147 patients and family caregivers, a variety of reasons for refusal were given including fears regarding mutilation of the body and distrust of the underlying purpose of the study

[Bonner, unpubl. data]. There were 34 families that gave final permission. Among these, 13 patients died and only 5 had actually had autopsies. The families that did not follow up gave the following reasons: (1) adult children overruled the primary caregiver's decision; (2) families vacillated over the decision; (3) families were in crisis at the time of death; (4) the hospital refused to release the body without the family paying additional fees. This experience suggests that intense contact will be required to see participants and their families through the process of medical research.

Future Studies of Risk Factors and Prevention Strategies

A major future research effort for stroke prevention among Blacks should be focused on multiple facets of hypertension. Efforts should be directed on elucidating the physiologic, biologic correlates and preclinical markers. Although there is burgeoning descriptive epidemiologic literature on hypertension in this population, little is known about the mechanism of blood pressure regulation and why African-Americans are more prone, and how these nuances foster end-organ damage in cerebral vascular and other major systemic arterial beds. In addition to improving our understanding of basic physiological mechanisms for blood pressure regulation, more work needs to be done identifying interactions between factors that work in concert to heighten risk. Data from epidemiologic studies of multiple populations indicate that factors such as obesity, insulin resistance, and diet are associated with increased rates of hypertension. Additional work needs to be done to identify population-specific candidate genes associated with stroke and cardiovascular disease. There is also a need to improve public health interventions for traditional cardiovascular risk factors such as physical inactivity, diabetes mellitus and dyslipidemias. Bridging gaps in access to medical care and developing better understanding of the roles of stress and racism will also be important. Population-targeted interventions such as the African-American Antiplatelet Stroke Prevention Study (AAASPS) are important [19]. AAASPS will serve as a model for the delineation of stroke in Blacks, for recruitment and retention as well as the identification of antiplatelet medications that may be safe and effective for secondary stroke prevention.

In summary, the need for more and better data about stroke prevention and treatment among African-Americans will grow as the population at risk increases in the next century. Fundamental questions about why African-Americans have more strokes and the mechanisms whereby strokes occur must be answered. Is there more to the story than just an excess of traditional cardiovascular risk factors? Furthermore, population-level data measuring post-discharge or long-term functional status of stroke survivors is needed. PSD is a complication of stroke that requires specific attention. PSD after stroke may impede physical, functional, and cognitive recovery, making early identification and treatment of potential importance. Finally, recruitment and retention of African-Americans are key to assure successful collection of these needed data. This will require strategic planning that should include representation of Blacks at all levels of the trial – participants, staff and researchers. To obtain optimal participation, the targeted program should be presented as a credible initiative, designed to address a concern of personal interest to blacks. With these considerations in mind, we can begin to answer the important questions about stroke in Blacks that will lead to heightened prevention and improvements in diagnosis and management.

References

1   Blesch KS, Furrer SE: Health Data on Older Americans. Health of older Black Americans, chapt 9. Vital and Health Statistics, DHHS Publ No 93–1411, series 3, No 27.
2   Dam M, Tonin P, DeBoni A, Pizzolato G, Casson S, Ermani M, Freo U, Piron L, Battistin L: Effects of fluoxetine and maprotiline on functional recovery in poststroke hemiplegic patients undergoing rehabilitation therapy. Stroke 1996;27:1211–1214.
3   Reding MJ, Orto LA, Winter SW, Fortuna IM, DiPonte P, McDowell FH: Antidepressant therapy after stroke. Arch Neurol 1986;43:763–765.
4   Raffaele R, Rampello L, Vecchio I, Tornali C, Malaguarnera M: Trazodone therapy of the post-stroke depression. Arch Geront Geriatr Suppl 1996;5:217–220.
5   Andersen G, Vestergaard K, Lauritzen L: Effective treatment of poststroke depression with the selective serotonin reuptake inhibitor citalopram. Stroke 1994;25:1099–1104.
6   MacHale SM, O'Rourke SJ, Wardlaw JM, Dennis MS: Depression and its relation to lesion location after stroke. J Neurol Neurosurg Psychiatry 1998;64:371–374.
7   Shimoda K, Robinson RG: Effects of anxiety disorder on impairment and recovery from stroke. J Neuropsychiatry Clin Neurosci 1998;10:34–40.
8   King DA, Conwell Y, Caine ED: The Structured Clinical Interview for the Diagnostic and Statistical Manual of Mental Disorders, ed 3. Washington DC, American Psychiatric Association, 1990.
9   Lyness JM, Noel TK, Cox C, King DA, Conwell Y, Caine ED: Screening for depression in elderly primary care patients. A comparison of the Center for Epidemiological Studies – Depression Scale and the Geriatric Depression Scale. Arch Intern Med 1997;157:449–454.
10 Straub NR: African-Americans: Their health and the medical system. Pharos 1994;57:18–20.
11 Blendon RJ, Aiken LH, Freeman HE, Coroy CR: Access to Medical Care for Black and White Americans. JAMA 1989;261:278–282.
12 Svensson C: Representation of American Blacks in clinical trials of new drugs. JAMA 1989;261: 263–265.
13 Harris Y, Gorelick PB, Samuels P, Bempong I: Why African Americans may not be participating in clinical trails. J Natl Med Assoc 1996;88:630–634.
14 Savitt T: The use of Blacks for medical experimentation and demonstration in the old South. J South Hist 1982;28:331–348.
15 Caplan A, Edgar H, King P: Twenty years later: The legacy of the Tuskegee Syphilis Study. Hastings Cent Rep 1992;22:29–38.

16 Gorelick PB, Richardson D, Hudson E, Harris Y: Establishing a community network for recruitment of African-Americans into a clinical trail: The African-American Antiplatelet Stroke Prevention Study (AAASPS) experience. J Natl Med Assoc 1996;88:701–704.

17 Shope JT, Homes SB: Pathologist's participation in post-mortem examinations for patients with dementia. Gerontologist 1993;33:461–467.

18 Harrell LE, Callaway R, Powers R: Autopsy in dementia illness: Who participates? Alzheimer Dis Assoc Disord 1993;7:80–87.

19 Lindberg GD: Attitudes towards autopsy and organ donation in Sweden and the United States. JAMA 1994;271:317.

Toni P. Miles, MD, PhD, University of Texas Health Science Center at San Antonio,
Department of Family Practice, 7703 Floyd Curl Drive, San Antonio, TX 78284-7795 (USA)

Author Index

Subject Index

Cardiac valve disorders, stroke risk
40, 41, 135
Carotid endarterectomy
stroke prevention 149, 150, 152
utilization in Blacks vs other groups
110, 111, 147
Cerebral angiography, *see* Angiography,
cerebral
Cerebral atherosclerosis, *see* Atherosclerosis,
cerebral
Cerebral embolism, *see* Embolism, cerebral
Cerebral ischemia, incidence in Blacks vs
other groups 7, 8
Clopidogrel, stroke prevention 172
Community prevention, stroke 125, 126
Computerized tomography
acute stroke management 50, 51
angiography 211, 212
costs and Medicare reimbursement 55–57
emergency evaluation of stroke patients
142, 143, 165, 181, 211
intracerebral hemorrhage 57, 60
lacunar stroke imaging 19, 20, 23, 24
Congestive heart failure
management following acute stroke 184
stroke risk effects 135
Coumadin, *see* Warfarin therapy
Craig Handicap Assessment and Reporting
Technique, stroke rehabilitation
assessment 200

Dementia, *see* Alzheimer's disease,
Vascular dementia
Depression, *see* Poststroke depression
Diabetes
Blacks vs other groups 77, 78
lacunar stroke risk factor 21, 22
outcome differences between patient
groups 15, 77, 78
prevention in stroke reduction
120, 121, 126
promotion of stroke, mechanisms 120
Diet, stroke prevention 122, 124
Dipyridamole, stroke prevention 172, 173
Disability, definition 199
Dissecting aneurysm, stroke risk 136
Dyslipidemia, *see* Lipid profile

Embolism, cerebral
cardiac sources
aortic atheroma 42
atrial fibrillation 40
myocardial infarction 41, 42
overview 36, 37
patent foramen ovale 41, 42
valve disorders 40, 41
diagnosis
patient history 38
physical examination 38, 39
transthoracic echocardiography 39, 40
etiology in Blacks vs other groups 37, 38
incidence in Blacks vs other groups
inside United States 8, 9
outside United States 72
prevalence in ischemic stroke 36
Emergency evaluation and treatment,
stroke patients 142, 143, 156, 162, 163,
165, 180, 181
Estrogen replacement therapy, stroke
prevention 125
Exercise, stroke prevention 124

Factor V Leiden, stroke association 45
Fatty acids, diet and stroke prevention 124
Fever, management following stroke 204
Functional Independence Measure, stroke
rehabilitation assessment 199, 200
Functional magnetic resonance imaging,
stroke imaging 50, 53

Handicap, definition 199
Health care, *see* Medical care
Heart disease, *see also* specific conditions
coronary heart disease as stroke risk factor
133–135
mortality among Blacks 129, 133, 137
Heparin, poststroke therapy 144, 145
Hypertension
Blacks
clinical trial design 222
comparison between Blacks of West
African origin 75, 76, 78, 79
incidence vs other groups 2–5, 16, 210
diet in prevention 122, 124
lacunar stroke risk factor 20, 21